Am I My Genes?

Also by Robert Klitzman:

A Year-long Night: Tales of a Medical Internship
In a House of Dreams and Glass: Becoming a Psychiatrist
Being Positive: The Lives of Men and Women With HIV
The Trembling Mountain: A Personal Account of Kuru, Cannibals, and Mad Cow Disease
Mortal Secrets: Truth and Lies in the Age of AIDS (with Ronald Bayer)
When Doctors Become Patients

Am I My Genes?

*Confronting Fate and Family Secrets
in the Age of Genetic Testing*

ROBERT L. KLITZMAN, M.D.

OXFORD
UNIVERSITY PRESS

OXFORD
UNIVERSITY PRESS

Oxford University Press, Inc., publishes works that further
Oxford University's objective of excellence
in research, scholarship, and education.

Oxford   New York
Auckland   Cape Town   Dar es Salaam   Hong Kong   Karachi
Kuala Lumpur   Madrid   Melbourne   Mexico City   Nairobi
New Delhi   Shanghai   Taipei   Toronto

With offices in
Argentina   Austria   Brazil   Chile   Czech Republic   France   Greece
Guatemala   Hungary   Italy   Japan   Poland   Portugal   Singapore
South Korea   Switzerland   Thailand   Turkey   Ukraine   Vietnam

Published by Oxford University Press, Inc.
198 Madison Avenue, New York, New York 10016
www.oup.com

Oxford is a registered trademark of Oxford University Press

Library of Congress Cataloging-in-Publication Data

Klitzman, Robert.
Am I my genes? : confronting fate and family secrets in the age of genetic testing /
Robert L. Klitzman.
   p. ; cm.
ISBN 978-0-19-983716-8
1. Genetic screening—Moral and ethical aspects. 2. Privacy, Right of.
3. Medical records—Access control. I. Title.
[DNLM: 1. Genetic Privacy—ethics. 2. Genetic Testing—ethics. 3. Disclosure—ethics.
4. Family Relations. 5. Genetic Diseases, Inborn. 6. Self Disclosure. QZ 21]
RB155.65.K55 2012
362.196'04207—dc23

9 8 7 6 5 4

Printed in the United States of America on acid-free paper

ACKNOWLEDGMENTS

I am deeply indebted to the men and women I interviewed for this book—for their generosity and candor. I am very grateful, too, to the Ethical, Legal and Social Implications Program of the National Human Genome Research Institute for supporting this project (ROI-HG002431-01), and also to the Greenwall Foundation. I would like to thank Jean McEwen, Elizabeth Thomson, Joy Boyer, Francis Collins, William Stubing, and David Tanner; colleagues at Columbia University and elsewhere including Wendy Chung, Karen Marder, Deborah Thorne, Carol Moskowitz, Jennifer Williamson, Edward Eden, Lori Tartell, Rubie Senie, Victor Grann, and Carolyn Kumah for valuable assistance with recruiting participants; Anke Ehrhardt and Paul Appelbaum for their support; Lisa Chin, Melissa Conley, and Meghan Sweeney for their assistance with the manuscript; Joan Klitzman, Rick Hamlin, Melanie Thernstrom, and Patricia Volk for reading drafts of this manuscript; Peter Ohlin for his unfailing and much appreciated faith in this project; Christian Purdy, Lucy Randall, Lindsay Mellor, Susan Lee, and Smitha Raj at Oxford University Press; and Charles Bieber for his help in countless other ways.

Several sections of this material have appeared in different form in the *Journal of the American Medical Association, American Journal of Medical Genetics, Genetics in Medicine, Genetic Testing, Journal of Genetic Counseling,* and the *New York Times.*

Is the whole of life visible to us, or do we in fact know only the one hemisphere before we die?

Vincent Van Gogh

We tell ourselves stories in order to live.

Joan Didion

CONTENTS

PART I

Introduction

Chapter 1

Embarking on Genetic Journeys:

Introduction

"Am I my genes?" she asked me. In her late thirties, she had breast cancer and had just learned that she had a mutation associated with the disease. She looked out the window in my office at the gray sky. We were both silent for a moment, each pondering her question. She seemed to be asking the question to herself, more than expecting a definitive answer from me.

Still, I wasn't sure what to say. I wondered to what degree exactly genes make us who we are, and how we understand what that means.

"I always knew I shouldn't have lived on Long Island for those years," another woman with breast cancer told me a few days later.

"Why is that?" I asked.

"Because *that's* why I got the cancer."

"But you have the mutation," I reminded her.

"Yes, but it was living on Long Island with all of those high tension wires, and the stress of staying in a crappy relationship that *triggered* the illness."

"I don't believe my cancer is from God or genetics," a poor African American woman from the Bronx who also had a breast cancer mutation told me a few weeks later. "It's from the environment. They dump garbage in the water and the landfills in the Bronx that they would never dump in Manhattan."

"The biggest question I face," a young, attractive blonde woman at risk for Huntington's disease said to me a few days afterward, "is whether I should just try to have kids with my husband, or adopt, abort, or have no children." She stared down into her lap, silent and sad, unsure of how to resolve her dilemma. Again, though a physician, I was uncertain what to say.

These women's statements all surprised me but, I soon saw, were hardly unique. In interviewing people confronting several diseases for which genetic tests exist, I was continually struck by the wide range of dilemmas they faced.

Genetic information forced these individuals to embark on journeys for which they had to navigate many obstacles.

They responded to genetic information about themselves as a kind of Rorschach test—interpreting this information in a wide range of ways, based on their prior views and stories about themselves and other cultural and personal experiences.

The issues they confront differ in several key ways from those of patients with other disorders for which no good genetic tests exist. The men and women I met struggle to make sense of diseases that threaten not only themselves, as single individuals, but others in their families—deceased, living, and not yet born. They feel guilty about the possibility that their mutations could harm their yet unborn children and grandchildren.

Genetic testing (also referred to below as genetic assay, assessment, and analysis) is rapidly spreading. Every year, dozens of new genetic tests are developed and offered. Over time, the amount of testing will soar. In industrialized countries such as the United States, physicians are increasingly offering genetic assays to patients and, it seems probable, will eventually sequence the entire genome of every patient. As outlined more fully below, our DNA consists of chains of four large molecules, known as nucleosides—adenine, cytosine, thymine, and guanine (abbreviated A, C, T, G)—that serve as an "alphabet." Every person has a unique set of three billion of these "letters" that constitute the genetic program that makes us. We share 99.9% of our DNA with each other, differing from one another only by about 0.1%.

Until now, many direct-to-consumer (DTC) tests have assayed at most only one out of every 10,000 letters, and only the most common of human genetic variants. Imagine comparing *War and Peace* with the Bible by reading only one letter per page—a single "A" or "C." The reader would understand nothing of either book, and could not meaningfully differentiate them.

Still, direct-to-consumer marketing companies such as 23andme.com—started and funded by the wife of one of the founders of Google—have begun providing inexpensive online testing, relying on such single letter variations. Individuals simply swipe the inside of their mouth with a swab and mail the sample. Soon after, they receive detailed information about their purported risks of numerous diseases.

Much of the information now provided by these DTC companies has little practical value, and laboratories interpret the same results in different ways. The FDA is now investigating these companies, and pursuing the possibility of regulating them.[1] But DTC testing appears likely to continue in some form. At the same time, however, the costs of mapping a person's entire genome have been plummeting—from billions of dollars to sequence the first person's complete DNA, to $100 million, to $1 million, to $100,000, to $10,000, and will shortly be even cheaper—$1,000, and eventually even less.

Thus, we are now beginning to read the equivalent of entire books, allowing us to identify and make sense of them. Soon, we will be able to sequence each of our entire genomes, permitting previously unimaginable discoveries.

Eventually, physicians will probably order complete genome sequencing tests on all of us. The Mayo Clinic and Vanderbilt University now already collect and permanently store DNA samples of all patients who walk in the door. Many other academic medical centers are trying to arrange to do the same. Ultimately, DTC testing may well include whole genome sequencing as well.

In upcoming years and decades, the usefulness of many tests, though not all, may thus increase. We will soon have more biological information about ourselves than ever before. But are we ready for it? What will it mean? What will we do with it, and how will we understand it?

In the mere 50 years since DNA was discovered, researchers have made extraordinary advances. Genetics appears likely to enhance our comprehension and treatment of many diseases, and our understandings of important aspects of ourselves. In 1986, investigators identified the first mutation for a human disease—Huntington's disease (HD). Since then, they have found mutations associated with thousands of other disorders, including cystic fibrosis, sickle cell anemia, and breast cancer. In 2003, an entire human genome was sequenced. Currently, doctors routinely check infants and pregnant mothers for genes associated with dozens of disorders, some of which are readily remediable. Scientists are also reprogramming stem cells, which have not yet specialized to become parts of particular organs (whether liver, muscle, or brain). Researchers are working to turn these protean cells into whatever types of tissue an injured body may need (e.g., heart, pancreas, or spinal cord), hoping to develop new treatments for many disorders. In 2009, researchers found that altering merely four genes can transform a skin cell into many other types of cells in the body. In May of 2010, the scientist Craig Venter announced he had "synthesized life," using a computer and four chemicals bought off a shelf to replicate the DNA of a bacteria that then took over another cell[2].

Increasingly, in the United States and elsewhere, the field is also affecting human reproduction. Assisted reproductive technologies or ARTs, once criticized for producing "test tube babies," now account for 7% of all births in some European countries, and 1% in the United States. These numbers are soon expected to reach 10%—equal to the proportion of infertile couples. Preimplantation genetic diagnosis (PGD) enables women to select which embryos to implant into their womb, based on the presence or absence of over 5,000 different mutations. Thus, couples are now eliminating certain lethal mutations from their future descendants, and in some cases, deciding the gender of their future children. Many men and women now buy and sell eggs and sperm on the Internet to assist other couples and individuals in having children, though critics argue that such transactions "commodify" these essential and sacred components of human beings—turning them, and thus us, into mere marketplace goods.

Pharmaceutical companies seek to develop "personalized medicine"—tailoring drugs for specific individuals based on the individual's genetics. Through this field of pharmacogenomics, genes are being identified that predict responsiveness to particular medications, rather than diseases. Our individual DNA may thus help determine *which* medication for an ailment will work best for each of us. Genetics may then be used not only to assist in foreseeing and diagnosing certain diseases, but in treating them, too. Knowledge is swiftly advancing about not just genes but the mechanisms through which they make and assemble proteins and regulate themselves, launching new, larger fields of "genomics" and "proteinomics." Just as antibiotics shaped the last century, eliminating certain epidemics of infectious disease, many researchers argue that genetics is beginning to alter several aspects of the twenty-first century.

Yet while researchers are discovering that single mutations are responsible for thousands of rare diseases, far more common ailments such as diabetes, cancer, heart disease, and depression appear to result not from single isolated mutations but rather from complex interactions, not yet well-understood, between *multiple* genes and other, environmental inputs. DNA mixes and sorts, and combinations of genes and gene-environment interactions, rather than single point mutations, appear to be responsible for most common diseases. Debates thus rage about the current and future extent of genetic knowledge—whether genetics is overly hyped, and if so, to what degree. Some critics have become wary of the ability of genetics to provide much new, useful information.

Clearly, at times, much hype and "genetic reductionism" occur, but the study of DNA is also still in its infancy. Our comprehension of genetics and its potential effects is still young. Now, at the start of a new millennium, it is impossible to predict what the future, or even just the next 50, 100, or 200 years will bring. To profound and unique extents, our DNA clearly helps shape us—for example, key aspects of how we look and whether we may be predisposed to develop certain diseases. To what degree and how exactly it does so, however, remain unknown.

Countless uncertainties persist. For instance, when scientists first cracked the human genome many were astonished that it contained so few genes compared to other mammals, and that we shared 99% of this DNA with primates, and 85% with mice. How humans thus look and act so differently from other species is not wholly clear. Scientists still think that half of our

DNA is "junk," its function still murky. They do not yet fully know what information and instructions it may hide that they might soon begin to decipher. In upcoming years the functions of countless additional genetic sequences will undoubtedly be discovered.

As the effects of combinations of sequences are explored, understandings of genetics will most likely increase—most likely not to the full extent that some hope, but far more than at present. Use of genetics is becoming ever more common in clinical medicine, confronting patients and their families and physicians with tests associated with medication responses, modestly increased risks for common diseases in conjunction with other, nongenetic risk factors, and genetic modifiers and suppressors that may contribute to illness, but are not primary causes.

This burgeoning genetic knowledge will continue to pose ever-new dilemmas. It is uncertain how people do or will see or fathom such information—whether they want it, and what, if anything, they do with it. Fears, myths, and misunderstandings about genes persist among patients, policy makers, scientists, and the public at large. Many critical aspects of the roles that genetics plays in our lives, and how we in fact view these, remain uncharted.

In numerous ways, genes are counterintuitive. In *The Selfish Gene*, the British biologist Richard Dawkins asserts that all species are essentially machines that genes have developed for reproducing themselves. Yet people frequently think of themselves as having free will and a transcendent spirit—not as resulting from an egg and a sperm that formed a cell that has kept dividing to produce us. Science suggests that we consist of mere molecules (mostly of carbon, hydrogen, and oxygen) and wouldn't exist otherwise, and that DNA contains the instructions for building the underlying machine or hardware that constitutes much, if not most, of us. Clearly, environmental factors also shape key aspects of us, though which aspects and to what extent remain uncertain. But in addition to these environmental influences, many people believe that genetics still insufficiently accounts for human beings—feeling, for instance, that we also have an incorporeal soul that results from nonchemical elements of our being. Crucial questions therefore arise of how people understand and make sense of these paradoxes, conceptualize themselves in relation to their genes, and make decisions as a result.

Fears also exist that eugenics may overly shape the use of this scientific knowledge. At the extreme, some caution that use of genetic information can easily slip down the slope toward the horrors of Nazi Germany. They caution, too, about the dangers of tampering with Nature, invoking images of Aldous Huxley's *Brave New World*, Mary Shelley's *Frankenstein*, and the 1997 film *Gattaca*, which portrayed a future society that tested newborns to permanently classify them as genetic "desirables" or "undesirables.'"

Many anthropologists and postmodern critics fear genetic determinism and reductionism, arguing instead that disease is "socially constructed." Barbara Katz Rothman and other scholars have criticized overemphasis on genetics as "the cause" of many disorders[3]. "Geneticization" in a variety of social realms claims too much for the potency of DNA. News headlines regularly announce the discovery of "the fat gene," "the gay gene," or the "alcoholism gene." Yet each of these traits in fact appears to involve highly complex interactions of genes with other biological, social, and psychological factors. Patients, too, may inappropriately apply the notion that genes predict certain diseases to other, multi-causal behaviors in which genes may in fact play relatively small roles.

Still, regardless of how much genetics may be oversold, we and future generations will have to live with this ever-expanding field. Every day in the United States, countless people wrestle with whether to get tested, and many proceed to do so. We need to prepare as best we can for these challenges, and the possible meanings of genetic information for us and our descendants—to understand how people perceive the current and potential meanings and implications of this information.

Genetics also sparks other, broader social challenges related, for instance, to privacy, stigma, and discrimination. Many government officials seek to establish genetic databases for law enforcement and public health. Though the U.S. Health Insurance Portability and Accountability Act (HIPAA) of 1996 aims to protect medical privacy, apprehensions persist. The burgeoning electronic storage of personal information heightens these worries. Identity theft has occurred, and hackers have broken into secure computer systems, stealing sensitive data. In 2008, Congress passed the Genetic Information Nondiscrimination Act (GINA), and most states have enacted their own genetic privacy laws. Yet these acts vary widely, and numerous challenges remain.

Genetics can pose larger psychological and metaphysical questions, too, about fate. From oracles in Ancient Greece to crystal balls in medieval tales, and psychics today, people have yearned to predict future events. In the case of HD and various enzyme deficiencies for which mutations with relatively high penetrance have been found, DNA can potentially inform many people about aspects of their future. Genetics may provide some information about the relative likelihood of certain future diseases, though surely not to the degree that some media hype may suggest. After all, genetics is still a relatively new field, and current scientific knowledge remains limited. The future can never be wholly known, and much genetic information will be in terms of relative probabilities, rather than absolutes.

Just as the ancient Greek Oracles famously offered ambiguous messages that recipients misinterpreted, so, too, genetic information will surely present us with complex puzzles and uncertainties. The information will often no doubt involve relatively small augmentations in risk, shaped by many other, still unknown factors. Nevertheless, depending on the specific details, some people may seek these relatively small increases in the chance of a disease, even if the overall predictiveness is still not very high (e.g., learning that one has a 10% or 20% chance, rather than a 1% or 2% likelihood, of getting a particular disease). Such information could potentially help motivate preventive behavior. Yet direct-to-consumer genetic testing companies are taking advantage of wide-spread popular desires to prophesy the future, aggressively marketing these tests as fortune-tellers, alluring many people. Every day, millions of people read their horoscopes, and many are now beginning to seek genetic tests as well.

As one of my teachers, the late anthropologist Clifford Geertz, has written, to understand complex social phenomena, and avoid external observers imposing their own preconceived notions onto a situation, it is crucial to understand these phenomena from the views of individuals within them.[4]

Hence, I decided to explore in-depth *how* individuals in fact now confront and understand some of these complex, multifaceted issues in their daily lives by interviewing a wide range of individuals who have, or are at risk for, several genetic diseases, in order to obtain a "think description." I interviewed 64 individuals who faced HD, breast and ovarian cancer, or Alpha-1 antitrypsin deficiency. I decided to concentrate on these three diseases, each with different characteristics, to try to grasp in a more fully and nuanced manner several ways in which genetics can affect people, and experiences individuals are now facing.

The degree to which genetic risks affected the whole span of their lives, from birth to death, surprised me. I found how these participants each wrestled with genetics, which has vast implications for their lives and those of their families. These men and women all struggled to make sense of their predicament and its causes, to discern how genetics may influence their lives, at times against their will. In the face of scientific uncertainties, they tried to comprehend these tests and probabilities; avoid fatalism, anxiety, despair, stigma, and discrimination; and find hope and meaning, and a sense of wholeness. They confront a series of quandaries, each explored in a different chapter here—whether to test; whether to disclose their genetic risks to parents, siblings, spouses, offspring, distant relatives, friends, doctors, insurers, employers, and schools; how to view and understand themselves and their genetics; what treatments, if any, to pursue; whether to have children, adopt, screen embryos, or abort; and whether to participate in genetic communities, and if so, how. These decisions are among the most difficult many have ever faced. Forced to wander through a wilderness of shifting sands, they chart paths that many others may eventually follow. They are pioneers, encountering quandaries that many of us, too, will soon face.

These men and women try to fathom their predicament, and are often both allured and frightened by the possibility of knowing key elements of their future, wanting to avoid stigma and rejection, and maintain a sense of hope and control in their lives. Yet these goals conflict. Complex social contexts—relationships with immediate and extended families, friends, health care providers, insurance companies, coworkers, and patient communities—all shape these choices. Genetics forces people to balance competing external and internal pressures. These men and women attempt to mediate and negotiate with, or work around, these social contexts. This book illuminates how these issues affect these individuals' lives.

Genetics compel these individuals to venture on long journeys, encountering many challenges. First, genetics can potentially provide certain information about the future—though generally as inexact probabilities, not absolutes. Secondly, genetic information relates to not just one individual, but to his or her family, too. Tensions can result, however, since genetic and social bonds can differ, posing questions about responsibilities toward various family members. An individual must decide, for instance, whether to disclose a mutation to certain relatives, who may then become distraught about their own future. Thirdly, diseases for which definitive genetic tests exist tend to be rare, and thus poorly understood by most people. Fourthly, new reproductive technologies permit screening of embryos and elimination of genes from descendants, posing additional moral and psychological dilemmas. Fifthly, physicians and direct-to-consumer companies offer, but at times oversell, genetic tests. And, finally, fears linger that genetic information can prompt stigma and discrimination in insurance and employment. With increasing electronization of medical records, and a fractured, yet rapidly evolving health care system, genetic information is also becoming available in a dramatically changing landscape. Other organizations—including schools and police departments—would often also like individuals' genetic data. In part in response, many individuals choose to enter genetic communities, but then face dilemmas—for example, whether to participate in research that will aid others, but not themselves. These phenomena combine, affecting each other.

In facing these moral tensions, individuals often follow implicit "gut feelings" more than explicit ethical or logical principles per se. Superstitions and beliefs about fate prove potent—not necessarily related to established religions, but rather mirroring underlying desires for coherence in one's life over time.

The bulk of this book examines the series of experiences through which these individuals pass. Heretofore, the medical literature has generally discussed each of these domains separately, with distinct sets of studies examining testing, *or* disclosure, *or* understandings of disease, *or* reproduction. Instead, I have sought to bring these facets together to explore how they fit into the whole of people's lives. From these patients' own perspectives, I probed how these issues interact. Such an effort may seem ambitious, but, I think, is vital to advance our knowledge of these realms.

This book groups these experiences into four broad domains concerning, respectively, genes in "the family," "the mind," "the clinic," and "the wider world." As a brief overview, the first of these parts, "Genes in the family," explores, in chapter 2, how individuals learn of their genetic risk (usually from other family members), how they decide whether to get tested or not, and how they interact with providers about testing issues, and view and interpret the probabilities and uncertainties involved. Chapter 3 probes how individuals decide whether and what to communicate about genetic test results to other family members. Individuals who get tested must balance ethical mandates to disclose to kin (and perhaps encourage other family members to undergo testing) against the psychological difficulties of doing so, due to shame, fear, denial, or estrangement.

In the second part of the book, "Genes in the mind," chapter 4 examines how individuals weigh possible causes (i.e., genetics and/or environment) and larger cosmological questions of "why me?" Their understandings of causality and fate powerfully shape their decisions about testing, treatment, reproduction, and disease prevention. Chapter 5 explores how individuals make sense of their "genetic identity"—how they understand information about their genes and integrate it with their past and ongoing notions of themselves, deciding how and to what degree to see their genes as part of their identity. Chapter 6 examines myths and misunderstandings of genetics as individuals struggle to make sense of complex probabilities—how they comprehend their genetic risks, and grasp murky probabilities.

In part IV, "Genes in the clinic," chapter 7 explores how individuals confront treatment decisions. Chapter 8 probes how these individuals decide whether to have children, and if so, whether to screen embryos, undergo amniocentesis and abortion of affected fetuses, or adopt. Chapter 9 looks into experiences with insurance companies, loss of insurance and privacy, and dilemmas about whether to use insurance for testing and treatment, and how to maintain confidentiality in a world with increasingly fluid electronic medical records.

Part V, "Genes in the wider world," investigates, in chapter 10, the implications of these issues for disclosures to coworkers and bosses, friends, dates, neighbors, and schools. Patients face potential discrimination, stigma, and decisions about "going public" to varying degrees. Chapter 11 probes the structures and functions of genetic communities—both in-person and, increasingly, online—that affect how individuals process and convey information. These communities can provide benefits, but also expose members to much sicker patients, generating fear and creating questions of whether, and to what degree, to join disease organizations. Chapter 12 explores the broader implications of these experiences for public health policy, widespread clinical testing and screening, professional and public education, law enforcement, and society. The concluding chapter synthesizes many of these themes.

I have arranged these discussions to reflect broadly the sequences of social space and time through which individuals tend to encounter these issues. But these domains are closely interwoven and do not fully follow a fixed progression. Rather, understandings and decisions evolve over time. Myths about genetics affect disclosure decisions, and vice versa. People divulge their genetic risks to ever-widening circles—from immediate to extended family members, friends, physicians, and employers—but not always in this same exact order.

As we will see, several key medical, social, and psychological factors also shaped these domains, including symptoms (whether patients displayed physical evidence of a disease or not), genetic testing (whether they had been tested or not, and if so, whether they had a mutation), family history (whether family members had the disease, and if so, who), socioeconomic status, age, gender, ethnicity, religion, education, other personal experiences (e.g., past trauma), and psychological traits (appearing more or less comfortable with, or able to tolerate, ambiguity). Usually, for each person, one or more of these phenomena proved more potent than others, yet no one characteristic wholly determined an individual's views.

A major overarching theme of this book concerns the degrees to which experiences and responses concerning genetics are in fact *social*. Specifically, these men and women confront these challenges in interpersonal contexts that profoundly shape the outcomes. DNA involves not simply a single patient at a time, but rather a complex social milieu involving family members (past, present, and future), physicians, pharmaceutical and biotechnology companies, policymakers, and others.

While controversies rage between "socially-constructed" versus biological or "essentialist" approaches in understanding human beings, these men and women highlight intricate negotiations and interactions between these two broad perspectives, highlighting how social and biological factors can in fact interplay.

Of note, genetic reductionism or determinism does not easily sway these interviewees. Rather, these individuals hold much more complex and nuanced perspectives. For instance, in seeking to make sense of their genetic risks, these men and women seek, too, to avoid fatalism and despair. They desire a modicum of control, and frequently a scapegoat for their problems. Genetic determinism competes with beliefs in "being able to control your fate." In confronting the fact that genetics may lie beyond their control, they struggle with quandaries of what, if anything, they can do about it. They have to balance others' rights to this information against their own fears of stigma and rejection.

THE DISEASES AND THEIR SYMPTOMS

The three disorders I focus on here vary in several ways, including prevalence, treatability, and their predictability.

Since genetics involves several complex concepts, with which some readers may have little familiarity, Appendix A provides a brief "Genetics Testing 101," offering additional background in the field.

Huntington's Disease

The first human disease for which a mutation was discovered, HD, is a fatal autosomal dominant disorder that starts in adulthood—usually in a patient's forties or fifties. Each of a patient's children has a 50% chance of having the mutation as well. A person who possesses this mutation will eventually die of it (unless succumbing to another fatal condition first), usually at about the same age as did the affected parent. The disease causes neurological and psychiatric symptoms—including discoordination, psychosis, and loss of memory and cognition—and has no proven treatment. One of the most frightening aspects of the disease is that the patient, in losing his or her mind, seems to become a different person. The mutation actually consists of a sequence of DNA that gets repeated too many times. The severity of the illness increases with the number of abnormal repeats. The mutation is more common among people of Western European descent; worldwide, it occurs in 1 in 20,000 people.[5,6] Patients' adult offspring face quandaries of whether to be tested. After Woody Guthrie died of the mutation, his son, Arlo Guthrie, publicly decided not to undergo testing. Evolutionarily, the mutation has spread because it occurs late in a patient's life—ordinarily after one had already had children and passed it on to them.

Alpha

Alpha-1 antitrypsin deficiency (AAT or "Alpha") is the only disease for which the U.S. Equal Employment Opportunity Commission has ruled that genetic discrimination has occurred.[7,8] Resulting from defective production of the enzyme Alpha-1 antitrypsin, the disease was discovered in 1963,[9] and affects the liver and lungs. If left untreated, it can cause early death. In severe cases, organ transplant can extend life. Symptoms can occur in homozygotes (with two copies of the mutation, one from each parent) and to a lesser extent, heterozygotes (with the mutation from one parent, and a normal gene from the other parent). Early genetic testing can prompt avoidance of environmental factors that can exacerbate illness (e.g., smoking and certain pollutants), enzyme replacement therapy, organ transplants, and reproductive planning to avoid transmitting the disease to offspring.[10]

In the United States, approximately 60,000 people (1 in 5,000) are homozygotes,[11] yet only 5% have been diagnosed.[12] Worldwide, about 10,000 patients now receive treatment.[13] Of Americans who would benefit from treatment, over 80% do not receive it. Many physicians remain unaware of the illness.[14] Diagnosis itself can cause depression and anxiety.[15] The World Health Organization,[16] the American Thoracic Society,[17] and the European Respiratory Society have recommended that in Europe and North America, given the relatively high prevalence of the disease, physicians should test certain patients, including those with emphysema, chronic obstructive pulmonary disease, asthma with air flow obstruction, and unexplained liver disease, and relatives of patients with Alpha.[10] To what extent doctors follow these recommendations is unknown, however. In fact, despite the increased attention given to this disorder since its discovery, between 1968 and 2003 diagnoses by physicians did not increase, and the length of time between symptoms and diagnosis increased.[12] Patients often report insufficient genetic counseling.[14,15]

Breast Cancer

Each year in the United States, over 250,000 women are diagnosed, and over 40,000 die of breast cancer, the second leading cause of cancer death among women.[18,19] In the early 1990s, the *BRCA1* and *BRCA2* mutations were discovered, and account for 5 to 10% of all cases.[19,20] Of women, 12% in the general population, and 40–60% of those with the *BRCA 1/2* mutations will eventually develop breast cancer.[21] Treatment can include chemotherapy, radiation, and surgery. The American Cancer Society now recommends that women start screening at age 40, and that those at high risk (a greater than 20% lifetime risk) receive both a mammogram and a MRI yearly.[22] The molecular diagnostic company Myriad Genetics has marketed genetic testing for the two mutations, which cost approximately $3,000–$5,000, and are not always covered by insurance. The number of *BRCA 1/2* tests performed so far is unknown.

METHODS

To understand these issues as fully as possible, I interviewed a cross-section of individuals who did and did not have symptoms, and had and had not had genetic testing. Over time, many people had in fact occupied more than one of these categories (going from asymptomatic to symptomatic, and from untested to tested). Table 1.1 summarizes these participants.

Table 1.1. SAMPLE CHARACTERISTICS (*N*=64)

		Disease			Total*
		BRCA	HD	Alpha	(N=64) N (%)
Gender	Female	32	9	7	48 (75.0%)
	Male	0	12	4	16 (25.0%)
Age	20–29	3	3	0	6 (9.4%)
	30–39	8	12	0	20 (31.3%)
	40–49	13	3	1	17 (26.6%)
	50–59	3	3	5	11 (17.2%)
	60–69	5	0	3	8 (12.5%)
	70–79	0	0	2	2 (3.1%)
Ethnicity	White	21	18	11	50 (78.1%)
	Black	6	2	0	8 (12.5%)
	Asian	2	0	0	2 (3.1%)
	Hispanic	2	1	0	3 (4.7%)
	Other	1	0	0	1 (1.6%)
Education	High School	4	4	2	10 (15.6%)
	College	15	10	8	33 (51.6%)
	Grad School	9	7	1	17 (26.6%)
	Unknown	4	0	0	4 (6.3%)
Symptom Status	Symptomatic	20	6	11	37 (57.8%)
	Asymptomatic	12	15	0	27 (42.2%)
Tested	Yes	20	14	11	45 (70.3%)
	No	12	7	0	19 (29.7%)
Test Status*	Positive	8	10	11	29 (64.4%)
	Negative	11	4	0	15 (33.3%)
	Indeterminate	1	0	0	1 (2.2%)
Total		32	21	11	64

*Percentages are of the total of those tested (45).

This book aims to illustrate the themes that emerge as richly, but concisely as possible, and thus includes quotations from 62 of these interviewees: 46 women and 16 men. Of these, 30 (all women) confronted breast cancer, 21 faced HD, and 11 Alpha; 49 were Caucasian, 7 were African American, 3 were Hispanic, and 2 were Asian; 44 had had genetic testing, of which 29 had a mutation; 36 had symptoms, and 26 did not.

In brief, as described more fully in Appendix B, I first conducted pilot interviews, and then further developed and refined the interview guide (see Appendix C) to obtain detailed descriptions of these issues. I recruited participants through staff and advertisements in medical clinics, patient organizations, a breast cancer registry, and through word of mouth. Individuals contacted me if they were interested. I interviewed each participant in-depth for two hours concerning experiences of being at risk for a genetic disease, undergoing genetic testing, and/or learning their gene status. I conducted the interviews at participants' offices or homes or in my office—whichever was more convenient for them.

These men and women spoke not only of their own experiences, but those of siblings, parents, other family members, and friends as well. I interviewed relatively fewer patients with Alpha because their experiences were, overall, more uniform. Known patients with this disorder have essentially all undergone testing because of symptoms. With HD and breast cancer, patients included those who had tested but not had symptoms, had symptoms but no testing, and had neither symptoms nor testing. Given these additional categories, I conducted more interviews regarding these two disorders.

As we shall see, overall, between these three diseases, the similarities in themes far outweigh the differences. Hence, I have presented the themes for these diseases together. Yet "genetic disease" is not monolithic, and when differences arose, I have presented these as well. I use the term "genetic disease" to refer to these three diseases, since strong genetic components have been identified for each.

Many of the issues here do not relate primarily to the fact that the diagnosis is associated with a genetic marker, but to other aspects of these disorders as well. To completely disentangle genetics from others features of these diseases is impossible. Stresses concerning genetics occur in addition to other challenges a diagnosis presents. Nonetheless, I have tried to tease out, and focus on, these genetic realms.

I have set out to convey how these individuals see and experience the predicaments they face—how they frame concepts to make sense of these psychological, social, and moral dilemmas, and what words they use. I was continually struck by their eloquence as they conveyed their struggles, physical and metaphysical concerns, and quests for meaning. For this reason I have presented their views in their own voices, as they chart what they learned and how they changed.

I have woven together these individuals' stories, presenting here a tapestry that portrays a series of journeys. In doing so, I beg the readers' patience and indulgence: I could have instead focused on only one of these diseases, or picked merely a handful of these people to present, and just ignored the rest. But that would have limited the range of insights that could be presented about genetics as a whole. Each of these men and women underwent a somewhat different journey, and offers unique perspectives. They varied in whether they had genetic testing, symptoms, or affected family members; were single or married; and wanted children or not. Each brought their individual background and past experiences to the quandaries they now faced.

Consequently, to illuminate the wide and varied realms of life that genetics affects, and the array of issues and experiences they encountered, I have presented a group portrait. Given that genetics continues to evolve, to understand as full a range as possible of these challenges is vital. Though this approach may make it harder for readers to grasp the full details of any one person's life, at various points I also draw on particular people more than others, providing more of a sense of a person's perspectives and experiences. Their names (all pseudonyms) are listed below, (see Table 1.2) here along with brief descriptions. In addition, each interviewee also appears in the index, along with a list of the pages on which he or she is quoted, allowing readers to refer back to other quotations by that person. To protect confidentiality, I have changed a few identifying details.

A critic might aver that these interviewees' experiences, confronting mutations that are relatively predictive of particular disorders, have little, if any, relevance to the issues that future, additional types of genetic testing may pose. In upcoming decades, more widespread testing may identify genetic markers that predict responses to medications, and only modestly increased risks of disease.

Yet though genetic discoveries advance, our comprehension of their multiple ethical, legal, social, psychological, cultural, and medical implications lags woefully behind. Hence, understanding experiences in the present can best help us anticipate challenges that may emerge in the future. Moreover, though scientists will most likely find that the most common diseases do not result from a single mutation, researchers may discover that several of these markers together, at times also in conjunction with environmental factors, may prove somewhat predictive. Unfortunately, we do not yet fully know what these future kinds of genetic tests will be (e.g., how much they will predict medication responses or small increased chances of disease) or how individuals will respond to all of this information. Certainly, however, future generations will encounter growing and bewildering amounts and types of genetic data.

Table 1.2. Individuals Interview

Name	Disease Confronted	Symptomatic	Genetic Test Results	Family History
Albert	HD	No	Mutation-positive	Yes
Anna	BRCA	No	No testing	Yes
Antonia	HD	No	Mutation-negative	Yes
Arlene	BRCA	No	No testing	Yes
Barbara	Alpha	Yes	Mutation-positive	Undiagnosed
Beatrice	BRCA	Yes	Mutation-negative	Yes
Benjamin	Alpha	Yes	Mutation-positive	Undiagnosed
Betty	Alpha	Yes	Mutation-positive	Undiagnosed
Bill	HD	No	No testing	Yes
Bonnie	BRCA	No	No testing	Yes
Brian	HD	Yes	Mutation-positive	Yes
Carmen	BRCA	Yes	Mutation-positive	No
Carol	BRCA	Yes	Mutation-positive	Yes
Charles	Alpha	Yes	Mutation-positive	Undiagnosed
Chloe	HD	No	No testing	Yes
Denise	BRCA	Yes	Mutation-negative	Yes
Diane	BRCA	Yes	Mutation-negative	No
Dorothy	Alpha	Yes	Mutation-positive	Undiagnosed
Evelyn	HD	No	No testing	Yes
Francine	BRCA	No	No testing	Yes
Georgia	HD	Yes	No testing	Yes
Gilbert	Alpha	Yes	Mutation-positive	Undiagnosed
Ginger	Alpha	Yes	Mutation-positive	Undiagnosed
Harriet	BRCA	No	Indeterminate genetic variances	Yes
Hilda	BRCA	Yes	No testing	Yes
Isabelle	BRCA	Yes	Mutation-positive	No
Jan	BRCA	Yes	Mutation-negative	Yes
Jennifer	Alpha	Yes	Mutation-positive	Undiagnosed
Jim	HD	Yes	Mutation-positive	Yes
Joan	BRCA	No	Mutation-negative	Yes
John	HD	No	Mutation-negative	Yes
Joyce	BRCA	Yes	Mutation-negative	Yes
Karen	BRCA	Yes	No testing	Yes
Karl	HD	No	Mutation-negative	Yes
Kate	Alpha	Yes	Mutation-positive	Undiagnosed
Kym	BRCA	No	No testing	Yes
Laura	BRCA	No	Mutation-positive	Yes
Linda	HD	No	Mutation-negative	Yes
Mary	HD	Yes	No testing	Yes
Mildred	BRCA	Yes	Mutation-positive	Yes
Oliver	HD	Yes	Mutation-positive	Yes

Table 1.2. (CONT'D)

Name	Disease Confronted	Symptomatic	Genetic Test Results	Family history
Ori	BRCA	Yes	Mutation-negative	No
Pablo	HD	No	No testing	Yes
Patty	HD	No	No testing	Yes
Peter	Alpha	Yes	Mutation-positive	Undiagnosed
Rachel	BRCA	Yes	Mutation-positive	Yes
Rhonda	BRCA	Yes	Mutation-positive	Yes
Roberta	BRCA	Yes	No testing	Yes
Roger	HD	Yes	Mutation-positive	Yes
Ron	HD	No	Mutation-positive	Yes
Samantha	BRCA	Yes	Mutation-negative	No
Sarah	BRCA	No	Mutation-negative	Yes
Sherry	BRCA	Yes	No testing	No
Shilpa	BRCA	No	No testing	Yes
Simone	HD	No	Mutation-positive	Yes
Susie	BRCA	No	Mutation-negative	Yes
Tim	HD	No	Mutation-positive	Yes
Tina	HD	No	No testing	Yes
Vera	BRCA	Yes	Mutation-positive	No
Walter	HD	Yes	No testing	Yes
Wilma	BRCA	Yes	No testing	Yes
Yvonne	Alpha	Yes	Mutation-positive	Undiagnosed

The three disorders here are not the most common diseases, but the insights these men and women offer are thus nonetheless critical. Given that the predictiveness of genetic markers discovered in the future remains unclear, we need to prepare ourselves as best we can in the meantime, based on what we can now know.

It is impossible to gauge definitively whether a larger sample of interviewees, or one recruited from a different culture or with other sociodemographics, would generate the same themes as those here. These data are not necessarily generalizable to other groups, but are valuable in and of themselves as embodiments of fundamental human issues. Indeed, perhaps most importantly, the stories of the men and women here illuminate how people seek to understand, at the most profound levels, themselves, their lives, and their world. Qualitative research can generate key hypotheses and insights, and elucidate the experiences and views of interviewees. But no psychosocial data are generalizable to all people everywhere. Surely, individuals from other cultures will differ in certain ways. But I would suggest that the men and women here highlight crucial underlying tensions—for example, whether to test, whom to tell, what genetic risks mean, how to view fate, identity, and family bonds, and how others will see them as a result—and that these broad challenges will probably have strong underlying similarities to those that arise among other individuals confronting genetic risks in the future. These interviews are noteworthy, too, because no other book has brought together this breadth of experiences concerning the roles of different genetic markers in individuals' lives. Clearly, further research is also needed to determine how often and in what ways the issues here appear among persons facing different diseases in other cultures.

But importantly, these men and women have much to teach us, suggesting that people confronting future tests will most likely also struggle to make sense of this bewildering information. New assays will also no doubt serve as Rorschachs, with which individuals grapple to construct narratives. The themes here reflect key universal dilemmas related to who we are as human beings, and in what ways, and to what degrees biology defines us. These men and women illustrate how genetics throws into bold relief numerous ancient, timeless conundra. In fact, one of the major findings here—concerning the considerable difficulties people have making sense of these genetic risks, and the subjective ways they wrestle to frame and construct understandings— will most likely be of ever-increasing importance, since future tests of less certain predictiveness will, I suspect, be harder, rather than easier, to comprehend.

Over coming years and decades, we cannot fully foresee what science will bring, but we will, it seems, have more control over our future and certainly that of our children. Genetics will no doubt continue to challenge key aspects of how we see ourselves, but many of us will be unsure how to proceed. Countervailing pushes will continue, based on religion, wariness of science, notions of social construction, and other views and beliefs. Unintended consequences will result. Increasing genetic information is also entering into a world of widening gaps between the haves and have-nots. Corporations will seek to profit as much as they can from genetics. The wealthy will seek to use it to help themselves and their offspring. The poor will have less access to it, given that many still lack basic health care. Unfortunately, among some people, certain discoveries may fuel racist attitudes. Challenges will thus persist in how we understand, seek, use, discuss, and respond to genetic tests.

Hence, the feelings, reactions, and lived experiences of the individuals here, confronting a series of dilemmas posed by current science—even if due to relatively rare disorders—are valuable. Their tales can help us, shedding crucial light on issues that many of us—whether as patients, family members, friends, coworkers, or voters—may one day face.

PART II

Genes in the Family

CHAPTER 2

"Do I Want to Know?":

Testing Decisions

Is information power, or is ignorance bliss? These men and women often remain unsure, and look to family, friends, and health care providers for answers.

"Knowledge doesn't always give power," Susie said. "Sometimes it opens Pandora's Box and other unknowns." She works for an HIV organization, and has a strong family history of breast cancer, but no symptoms or mutation herself. She and others struggle to decide which of the above scenarios would result from genetic testing. She tries to balance complex uncertainties, and the pros and cons in assessing when information may be either helpful or too frightening.

From the moment they learn they are at risk, these individuals all have to navigate through a difficult series of decisions—initially, whether to undergo testing or not. Moral dilemmas emerge of whether to obtain genetic information for the sake of one's family, despite its potential costs to oneself.

Since the HD mutation was identified in 1986, issues concerning genetic testing among at-risk individuals have been discussed, but many critical questions remain. In the 1980s, studies suggested that most at-risk individuals would opt for testing.[1,2,3,4] But rates of testing have been much lower (e.g., 5%–20%[5,6]), raising questions of how individuals at risk for these diseases in fact make these decisions.

Researchers have probed the reasons why individuals decide to test or not, but as I will show, almost all of this research has been based on rational choice models that assume that people make logical decisions. In contrast, I was struck by several aspects of these decision-making processes that have tended to receive less and less attention—for example, how these decisions are made in complex social contexts, and involve misunderstandings.

In addition, almost all testing studies have focused on *why* at-risk individuals make decisions, rather than *how* they make and view these decisions and what their experiences are like.[7] Much of this prior research has also tended to be quantitative, not qualitative—that is, measuring phenomena, rather than describing them verbally—and presenting the voices of these men and women themselves.

In the case of HD, early data, often collected before any testing was available,[8] assessed knowledge and attitudes,[9] and found several main reasons people might test or not. Reasons for testing included obtaining certainty, future planning and helping children,[10,11,12] and knowing risk to children if one tested positive. Reasons for not testing included lack of a cure, threat to health insurance, testing costs,[13] and fears of depression or problems coping with the result.[14] For several diseases other than HD, reasons for and against genetic testing often cut across diagnoses and include perceptions of advantages versus disadvantages, related to: perceived risks, ability to cope with results, intrusive thoughts, employment status, health insurance, helping affected relatives, knowledge about genetics, confidentiality, logistics involved, depression, age, education, children, and past disease experiences.[15,16,17,18,19]

Several theoretical models have been proposed to understand these issues. For instance, three types of stories have been described about how individuals make decisions about testing: proceeding to get testing without expressing any doubts, evolving toward the decision, and experiencing a pivotal moment when they decided to test.[7] Other researchers have proposed that individuals pass through four stages—of precontemplation, contemplation, action, and maintenance.[20,21,22] Yet though a "precontemplation" stage, for example, has been suggested,[21,22] what exactly occurs then, and what factors are involved, remain unclear. Such models have also been challenged since such stages may not be discrete, and individuals may occupy several simultaneously.[23] At-risk individuals monitor themselves for signs or symptoms of illness,[22] but it is not clear how exactly they do so, and how they view and experience these processes.

A health belief model has been proposed, positing that health behavior is shaped by perceived susceptibility, disease severity, and costs and benefits of the behavior.[24,25] Models of "stress and coping" have categorized coping strategies as either "problem"- or "emotion"-focused.[26] Yet with regard to genetic testing, these two models appear limited.[27] Health information itself has been seen as meeting either cognitive or emotional needs,[28] and individuals have been grouped as either seeking ("monitoring") or avoiding ("blunting) information.[29,30] In hypothetical situations, monitoring has been associated with preferences for testing,[31] and perceived threat and unpredictability.[32] In general, individuals tend to be risk averse.[33,34]

Yet testing decisions may not be matters of "rational choice."[7] *Subjective* issues have begun to be explored,[35] but require much more examination. For instance, generally, individuals seek to "manage" stigmatized information and pass as "normal,"[36] but in the case of genetics, this phenomenon requires further elaboration.

The meanings and experiences of genetic risk and testing decisions occur within multiple intra- and interpersonal frameworks and temporal contexts,[35] and perceived responsibilities toward others may play roles in testing decisions.[37] But how exactly social factors in fact operate or shape various stages and decisions has received little attention.[21,22] For Tay-Sachs disease and Fragile X syndrome, one Israeli study found that the major reason patients were not tested was that physicians did not refer them for the test.[38] Of primary care providers in the United States, only 31%–56% have ever ordered genetic tests for patients.[39,40]

Researchers have tended to view interactions with family members dichoto-mously: as coercing or permitting at-risk individuals to undergo testing.[22] Yet in general, sociological interactions can involve a broad array of dynamic, complex pressures and inputs that individuals can accept, resist, or negotiate.[41] Questions thus remain of how and when individuals weigh these and other criteria, and with what consequences.

Individuals may decide to delay testing,[22] but *why* and *how* they make these decisions is also not known. Though other studies have examined aspects of *coping* (e.g., related to post-test distress[12,42,43,44,45] and partner relationships[46]), the possible implications for understandings of testing decisions have rarely been studied. Suggestions have been made to decrease the amount of counsel-ing for genetic diseases.[47] But better understanding of how individuals progress through the testing decision process can help future doctors, patients and their families, and others.

LEARNING THAT ONE IS AT RISK

These individuals enter the world of genetics through a series of stages—each of which affects subsequent ones. Repeatedly, familial and other social contexts shape decisions and responses. Medical and personal concerns mold these decisions as well. But social milieus play critical roles that prior research has generally ignored. These social influences often combine in complex ways with other factors, based on the strength or salience of each.

As we will see, even before confronting decisions about testing, these inter-viewees learn from others—family members or physicians—that they are at risk of a familial disease. Yet they vary widely in how and when they receive this information. As offspring of affected parents, they may be told or not, and may or may not in turn tell their own offspring. Some first learn that they are at risk when a relative is diagnosed, posing a double whammy: hearing of a threat both to a family member and to themselves. The moment of revelation can be shocking, even if the information is not altogether unexpected. These issues arise with all three diseases, but news of HD in the family proves particularly disturbing. Several participants remember the exact date.

The fact that genetic disease, by definition, occurs in families has many profound implications. Within a family, a genetic mutation can cause multiple stressors, as any one member confronts not simply his or her own risk of disease, but relatives becoming ill as well. These individuals face not only their own choices regarding testing, disclosure, privacy, stigma, and having children, but also those of parents, aunts and uncles, cousins, and siblings. Ron, for instance, a 42-year-old, said, "I know what it's like watching my brother die. It's gone on and on and on for thirteen years." His brother committed suicide rather than suffer further. Ron has not yet had any symptoms of HD, but has the mutation. His experience watching his father and brother leads Ron to continue to ride a motorcycle—to enjoy life as much as he can now, while still symptom-free.

Some learn of a mutation in the family, and hence of their own risk, only when they are contacted by long-lost relatives. Brian, a former teacher, said:

> We got a phone call from a relative I never met. She was a nurse and mentioned that HD ran in the family. My wife took the call. I never spoke to her myself. She found our name through the phone book. My father and I have the same name. I don't remember meeting any of his relatives. I left the South when I was six months old.

He underwent testing and found out he had the mutation. Knowledge about distant relatives can thus be scant; some people don't have even basic information about the number or names of their parents' siblings. But in the age of genomics, such knowledge may suddenly be vital.

RESPONSES TO LEARNING OF RISK

Risk information can come as a complete surprise. The fact that the news is bad colors responses to it. Some patients wrestle with whether to blame the messenger, or family members who pushed to get the information. Brian did not like that this relative called. He thought, abstractly, that he would be better off knowing, but remains ambivalent.

Even when individuals know that a disease is in the family, they can be shocked, since it may not have been known to be genetic. Patty, a fashion designer who has not yet had HD testing or symptoms, explained:

HD being in my family came up *subtly* because no one really realized that it was HD and was so debilitating. We knew my grandfather had something, but they thought it was Parkinson's. We had no idea it was hereditary. Then, when I found out my mom had it, the doctor's reaction upset me. I thought: "Wow. Why's everybody making a big deal out of it? Grandpa had it; he was fine."

She and many others assumed that HD is like other neurological diseases without genetic markers such as multiple sclerosis or Parkinson's. Hence, one may not realize that one is at high direct risk for it oneself. Doctors also may not give, and/or patients may not remember, genetic details.

Not surprisingly, hearing that one is simply *at risk* can be devastating. When his mother was diagnosed with HD, John, who worked for a financial company, was in graduate school, and dropped out.

I just lost it. I took a job and got booted out after a year. I became irrational . . . obsessed over whether or not I had the disease. I changed how I viewed myself: from a healthy to an unhealthy person. When my mother was diagnosed, I was 27—taking on responsibilities, getting married, having kids. The news put off moving on to a more normal life. I just regressed. I couldn't handle things, started drinking and doing drugs.

Eventually, he learned that he lacked the mutation, but the prior stress had already encumbered his life.

Similar stresses arise with Alpha, too. Scientific knowledge about many genetic markers is still relatively new and therefore scarce. Hence, a disease in a family member may not be recognized as being genetic, and information about it may be communicated poorly, if at all. Family history may not be known, due in part to prior misdiagnoses. Yvonne, who had lung transplants for Alpha and, as we shall see, wanted to move to the South to avoid possible environmental exacerbants, said, "My father's sisters and brothers *could have* had Alpha. A cousin died at 35 of emphysema. At that time, they didn't know what Alpha was." Known as a diagnosis only since 1963, Alpha was often missed. "My cousin's father was *possibly* a carrier,"she continued. "He was turned down during World War II—I think because he had asthma or something like that." But she remained unsure of the exact reason. She and others were generally the first ones in their family to be diagnosed, and often faced vast uncertainties.

For breast cancer, too, risk may be perceived only indirectly, if at all. The quality of information, even when sought, can be poor, in part since families may not want to talk about a relative's diagnosis. "My father's first cousin had some sort of cancer," Karen, a lawyer with breast cancer, explained. "I don't get a straight answer from anyone about what it really was: uterine, ovarian, endometrial." Secrets can persist in families for years, blocking knowledge and obscuring ongoing risks.

Even once a disease is known to have occurred in a family member, to know whether it is genetic or not can be hard. It is difficult to determine whether a strong family history results from a clear genetic marker. Karen continued, "The doctors said, 'Possible genetic link.' They wouldn't say yes or no." As a smart lawyer, the lack of answers frustrated her.

PRE-TEST ASSUMPTIONS AND SELF-MONITORING

Particularly for HD, once learning of their risk, many people try to gauge themselves to determine whether or not they possess the lethal gene. To elude the pain and possible stigma of obtaining a definitive mutation-positive test result, they assess themselves in various ways, generally by comparing themselves to others.

Individuals usually do not just start thinking about testing when they enter a genetic counselor's office, but have instead pondered the questions for years, even decades, making guesses about their gene status that then shaped their testing and other decisions. People who learn that they may have a mutation, but do not wish to test for it immediately, face paradoxes of how to proceed with knowledge of that risk, and how to view themselves and their future. They often draw lines in the sand—striving for certainty and lower anxiety in the present, even if it implies turmoil in the future. Overall, three patterns emerge: assuming one has the disease, assuming one does not, and avoiding thinking about it at all. Interviewees make these assumptions about their genetics in the context of social relationships—judging themselves vis-à-vis ill relatives and others. These issues arise with particular force among people confronting HD, given its lethality and lack of treatment, but emerged for the other diseases as well.

Assumptions of Being Gene Positive

Surprisingly, many assumed they would be mutation-positive. Not until Simone, a 29-year-old bookkeeper, got engaged did her mother disclose that HD was in their family. Since then, Simone said that she "always thought I would have it." Eventually she tested, and found that she indeed has the mutation, though she has not had symptoms. "It's simply been proven," she said wryly. Still, in her twenties, her attitude, trying to minimize the mutation and its impact on her life, helps her cope—to feel less surprised—reflecting desires for continued life, and relative order and calm. Her belief allows her to feel, too, that she still has a future.

Even as early as adolescence, some individuals assumed that they would eventually develop a disease, based on seeing an ill relative. The fact that at-risk individuals usually observed HD in other family members made the diagnosis somewhat less surprising, even if still anxiety-filled.

As we will see, misunderstandings and myths about genetics develop—that one will develop HD simply because of *physically* resembling an affected parent. Bill, a salesman, said,

> I figured I was going to definitely have HD because I look the most like my dad . . . If you see pictures of him as a kid and me, we looked exactly the same. When they told me it was hereditary, I thought, "Well, then, I guess I'm going to have it."

Yet Bill's brother then developed the disease, and Bill has remained asymptomatic, and has not been tested. He now cares closely for his sibling.

Desires for certainty and lessened anxiety can outweigh desires for future health, which may be more abstract. Certainty can be easier than uncertainty—even if it entails assumptions of eventually having a deadly disease. These assumptions can in fact organize one's life. Ron, the motorcyclist whose twin committed suicide, and who eventually learned that he also has the HD mutation, although he has not yet had any symptoms, said:

> If you told me that I *didn't* have HD, I'd have to go out and find a new way to live my life, reassess 20 years of decisions, every relationship I've ever had. It made sense of my life.

Many at risk of breast cancer also felt they would have the disease, though these assumptions generally caused less distress. Some always assumed that they would get breast cancer, given its high prevalence in their family. Kym, a South Asian doctor, said,

> With all the cancer in my family, I've always just sort of felt I'm going to get it. I almost became O.K. with that. My mother's had it twice; it's been in my house four times now. I'm used to it.

Kym has not yet had any symptoms or been tested for it, but accepts it as a possibility, and seeks to prepare herself, in part to elude despair.

Indeed, as will be described later, a strong family history of breast cancer may prompt assumptions of developing the disease, as a result of observing it in family members—even without explicit knowledge of the genetics involved. Rhonda, a nurse, assumed even as an adolescent that she would get breast cancer because it affected her mother and aunts. Her father's warnings to her about it, and the trauma of her mother's early death, contributed to this presentiment. "You relate to what's happened to your family," Rhonda explained. "When I was six, my mother died of it. Even as a teenager, my dad gave me articles on self-exams." She ended up having breast cancer and the mutation, and feels that her forebodings were thus accurate.

Among women confronting breast cancer, those I interviewed may seem to ponder genetic issues more than some other women facing this disease. In part, I recruited interviewees through a registry of families with breast cancer, so they often had a family history of the disease. Breast cancer patients with no family history may be less inclined to view their disease in genetic terms, yet many are still clearly concerned about whether their children, siblings, and other family members may get the disease. In addition, awareness of the genetic bases of many cases of breast, ovarian, and other forms of cancer is rapidly advancing.

Assumptions of Being Mutation-Negative

Not surprisingly, others want to be disease-free, and assume they are mutation-negative. Karl was unfortunately sexually abused by his HD-affected father, underscoring the terrible possible effects of this disease in a family. Karl felt that he himself did not have the HD mutation, because he did "not want" to have it. The possibility horrified him. He also did not notice any early possible symptoms, bolstering his belief and hope. Luckily, his assumption turned out to be correct.

Others deny the very *possibility* of being affected. For breast cancer as well as for HD, despite a family history, some never thought that they themselves would be affected. Karen, the lawyer, verged on denial, saying she never imagined she would get breast cancer.

> There's a lot of cancer in my family, but I always thought I would get *colon*, not breast cancer. It just didn't click for me. In some ways, I still haven't totally dealt with it. I talk very openly about being a breast cancer survivor—it's influenced the way I live—but it's still not *real*.

She suggests how full acceptance and acknowledgement of disease can vary, and be difficult.

Others avoid attributing physical symptoms to a possible diagnosis. They assess themselves for possible evidence, and see their continued ability to function as welcome demonstration of being mutation-free. Yet such assumptions can turn out to be wrong. Walter had worked in government, and recently developed symptoms of HD. He went on disability, though he has not been tested. He said, sadly:

> I play the flute, go on the treadmill at the gym every day, and work out with dumbbells. I said, "There's no way I would have HD." But it snuck up on me. I can still do pull-ups and chin-ups. But not like I used to . . .

Such self-monitoring can clearly vary in accuracy, costs, and benefits. Some compare themselves to others, seeking confirmation of being mutation-free. Patty, the fashion designer without HD testing or symptoms, said,

> I've been taking a body sculpting class, based on balance and dance . . . As long as I . . . can stand on one foot with the other foot extended, just like everybody else, I'm still O.K.

Others go further, and may overcompensate to prove their healthiness to themselves and others. Ron motorcycled, as mentioned earlier, and gauged himself by the fact that he was still able to do so. Though asymptomatic, he eventually learned he had the HD mutation. "The fact that I was riding motorcycles seemed to mean that the odds were slightly in my favor. It was a sign that I didn't have the disease," he said. Yet his continuation of this relatively dangerous activity suggests that he may still be denying the severity of his risk.

On the one hand, such assumptions of being mutation-negative can prompt decisions to undergo testing. If one assumes that no mutation is present, the risk of bad news is low. Susie, for instance, worked for an HIV organization, and had benign ovarian cysts and a strong family history of breast cancer, but no clear symptoms of it herself. She knew a lot about genetics, and thought she did not have a *BRCA* mutation.

> [A friend] said, "If you don't get the testing, you might want to treat yourself *as if* you're positive, just to be on the safe side." That was too intense, so I ended up seeing a doctor. I met with her once and decided to test. I had to find out if I'm positive or not. The counselor made the whole family chart, and showed my percent risk. There was a higher chance that I didn't have it. That emboldened me. It just got to a certain point where

I had to find out. Ignorance is bliss, but the amount of ignorance I had was decreasing.

Luckily, she found out she lacked the mutation.

Generally, assumptions of lacking a mutation were not seen as guaranteed substitutes for definitive tests themselves. Indeed, these assumptions can prove bitterly wrong, and hence, generate much uncertainty and angst. As Susie continued,

> I was scared. It had become such a worry on my mind, wondering: am I stupid not to know? What if we find some great new breakthrough? I thought there's a better chance that I'm going to be negative. But I started to think I could die young. That was always in the back of my mind. I was worried sick.

In the end, she felt that only a test result would alleviate her anxiety.

Given the stresses of these pre-test assumptions, a few people tried to avoid thinking about their mutation status altogether. Yet this stance was hard to maintain as external events and worries impinged on one's life.

SELF-MONITORING AND ITS LIMITATIONS

As suggested above, these self-assessments are difficult, and under- and over-diagnosis occur. Uncertainties hover even as to *what* exactly constitutes symptoms, and whether these are present. Detailed knowledge about a disease can remain low, even among those who have it. Outside observers may assess at-risk individuals as well, and offer external judgments that may be unwelcome, if not resented. As Ron, the motorcyclist, said, "I lost my temper, and one girlfriend asked me whether *that* was a sign." Yet HD can be hard to diagnose in oneself or others, in part because psychiatric symptoms such as depression and anxiety can be nonspecific. Still, people sought psychological evidence to support diagnostic assumptions.

These assessments of oneself or others can induce tremendous fear, while still shrouded in uncertainty. Chloe, a 28-year-old secretary who worked with her sister, was at risk for HD, and described this tension: "I was really irritable, and thought, 'Oh my God, I'm turning into my dad.' Little things pissed me off. That was *his* first symptom." Yet she has chosen not to be tested. Testing can reduce uncertainty, but also diminish hope.

Assumptions about whether one will get HD raise questions of fate, and can become the stuff of superstitions. "There's so much hocus-pocus around whether people who are positive sort of know it," Linda, an art teacher who eventually tested negative for HD, said. "You can't remove superstition, spiritual dabbling."

Some consulted psychics, desiring definitive knowledge of the future without risking discrimination that could result from an actual documented mutation. These consultations reflected, too, the degrees to which beliefs about metaphysics and fate can underlie views of genetic risk. Evelyn, a housewife and mother in her thirties, said that her husband did not want her tested for HD because he feared the results would upset them. Consequently, though asymptomatic:

> I went to a psychic reader. She immediately said, "You have bad news in your family." My father-in-law had just died. I thought she probably means *that*. But she said, "No, I'm not talking about the death." She said, "I'm talking about the devastating news in your family. You have a very important decision to make, and don't know which way to go, and time is running out." She said, "Could you tell me what the decision is?" "I'm planning on being tested in two months, and really want to do it." She said, "You don't carry the gene. . . . You're fine and your children are fine. I'm not talking about the *rest* of your family." A weight lifted off me. I didn't feel the strong urge to be tested. I stopped at the liquor store and bought champagne.

Whether the psychic was correct remains unknown, but Evelyn and many others looked to fortune tellers to help make diagnostic and testing decisions, illustrating the degree to which these dilemmas evoke metaphysical notions.

The unpredictability and unreliability of these soothsayers can pose difficulties. Simone, the 29-year-old bookkeeper who, only after she was getting married, was told by her mother about HD in the family, went to twelve psychics, picking the prognostications she liked, before getting tested. Simone realized the "madness" and questionability of her beliefs, but remained undeterred, seeking surety. She and many others believed that a psychic could divine their future, and thus mutation status, without having to face the stress of a definitive result.

Unfortunately, interpretations of symptoms may not be clear. Physical signs of disease can be ambiguous and nonspecific. With HD, a vicious cycle can ensue of self-monitoring, oversensitivity to symptoms, and increased anxiety that can lead to further monitoring and sensitivity to symptoms. Anxiety can be viewed as evidence of HD—exacerbating fears. As Linda, the art teacher, said about the period before she tested mutation-negative:

> The whole HD nightmare: you drop or forget something. After starting genetic counseling, I got more freaked out. I lost my concentration, got *more* clumsy — because I became more and more self-conscious.

Her eventual mutation-negative test result revealed that her prior perceptions of possible symptoms were inaccurate. Anxiety can thus arise independently of the disease's direct symptoms.

Still, this worry complicates self-judgments and, as mentioned earlier, can become self-perpetuating. Physical—not only mental—symptoms can also become part of a self-perpetuating cycle, as fears lead some individuals to exercise aggressively, to prove to themselves they are healthy, though such exercising could then cause injury.

To support assumptions of being mutation-free, individuals desperately sought rationalizations—for example, that many others also displayed possible symptoms (such as anger) unrelated to the disease. But self-monitoring can, because of fear, take over and shape one's very being. Over time, anxiety and symptoms can become overwhelming, such that testing is the only relief. "Finally, I couldn't get away from it," Linda said, "until I found out about my status."

LEARNING ABOUT, AND BEING OFFERED, GENETIC TESTS

Unfortunately, not everyone who might benefit from a genetic test is offered one, or learns that such a test exists. Rather, the opportunity to undergo genetic testing occurs in specific interpersonal contexts. For HD, at-risk adults have usually seen the disease in a parent, and hence know that testing is possible. But for other diseases, the possibility of testing may never arise, or does so less directly or forcefully. For Alpha, a rare disease, patients may only get tested when a savvy physician happens to know about, and suggest the test. Many doctors don't consider ordering an assay. As Yvonne, who eventually had lung transplants for Alpha, described:

> None of the 20 doctors [I saw] tested me for Alpha, or knew what it was. Finally, one happened to send in a simple blood test. I was always being diagnosed with asthma and bronchitis.

Indeed, when eventually diagnosed, the delay could have high costs. She continued:

> When they finally detected it, it was too late. If doctors detect it earlier, they can treat it at the beginning, and extend your life. But by the time they found out, I only had a quarter usage of my lungs.

Especially for rare diseases such as Alpha, physicians may under-test. As the disease is uncommon and its genetic basis relatively new and hence little known, physicians may have little awareness of it. She added, "I still come across doctors who don't know what it is. I say I've got Alpha, and they say, 'What is that?'"

The rareness of the disease contributes to the low recognition of it among providers. She explained, "Doctors don't know about it, therefore it's missed."

Diagnosed Alpha patients argue strongly that certain types of specialists, in particular, should be aware of the disorder, but sadly often are not. As a result, as Yvonne said, "A lot of patients . . . know more about this than the doctors," which can create strains in receiving treatment and interacting with providers.

Alternatively, doctors may know of a rare genetic disease, but not think of it in diagnosing a patient—in part because they have not seen it before. Hence, some patients may learn about their disease only through the experiences of relatives—even offspring. Jennifer, a schoolteacher, was diagnosed with Alpha only after a physician tested her son.

> I had been sick for a while, not responding to antibiotics. Then my son came home for Christmas and had pneumonia, which he's been prone to since a young child. He was on an antibiotic. But I sent him down to my doctor and made my son promise to have tests done when he got back to his own home. He did. I asked him a couple of months later. He said, "Well, yeah, as a matter of fact, I have something with a missing enzyme, and they said it's not a concern right now." A month or so later my family doctor asked me if he had had testing done. I said, "Yeah, they told him he had some kind of missing enzyme," and the light bulb went on for my doctor. He said, "Alpha Antitrypsin. My God, I'll bet that's what you have."

Yet a doctor may not tell a patient to disclose the diagnosis to at-risk family members. She added,

> My son's doctor did not say, "You should tell your parents to get themselves checked out." It was a gift from the gods that the scenario played out the way it did. If I hadn't asked, I wouldn't have found out.

Providers' limited knowledge of a diagnosis—especially a relatively unusual one—can also lead them to dispense inaccurate information about testing and the disease. Without much understanding, physicians may give patients incorrect prognoses and advice. At times, only the patient's persistence prompts eventual assessment and testing. Doctors may not catch the diagnosis, and may later send the patient to specialists. Yet such secondary or tertiary referrals may serve to keep knowledge or experience about Alpha low among primary care providers, furthering a vicious cycle.

Patients may feel frustrated by referrals that require further travel and logistical difficulties, not understanding the need for the referral, and realizing only in retrospect that such consultation may be best. Patients may see only the final outcome as justifying the effort. For rare diseases, reliance on specialists may enhance care, but lessen the motivation of general practitioners (GPs) to acquire added experience.

For breast cancer, too, provider confusion and poor communication linger. Providers do not always discuss the potential of genetic testing to women at risk of breast cancer. Despite a strong family history, some women report that no one had ever mentioned the possibility of such testing to them. Providers may under-test, and not raise the issue when they perhaps should, reflecting low knowledge about genetics among doctors generally.

Yet patients may wrongly assume that tests, if not offered, are neither needed nor potentially helpful. Bonnie, a 24-year-old saleswoman who, at the age of twelve, saw her mother with breast cancer, now feels that young women at risk receive too little attention. She described a friend who did not test because doctors did not mention this possibility. This friend concluded that because she wasn't told about testing, she did not need it. Yet such assumptions can clearly be incorrect. Bonnie felt that physicians may miss the diagnosis, since they may believe that some women are simply "too young" to have breast cancer.

> When my friend said, "I feel a lump in my breast," the doctor said, "You're only 30. Don't worry about it." She finally went to another doctor, and found out it was cancer. She could have died. If she didn't push, her doctor could have just said, "Oh, it will go away. It's a gland." A lot of doctors think that way.

In the end, patients, not doctors, may end up initiating discussions about testing.

At the other extreme, some doctors may test too frequently, actively encouraging it for clinical or research reasons. Vera, a marketing executive with breast cancer and no family history, was asked to test because she was Asian.

> A doctor called me and said she was spearheading the genetic testing in the area, and they were having difficulty getting Asians. They offered it—that's the only reason I did it. I thought: What the hell? It's only blood.

She would not have sought testing on her own because no one in her family had been diagnosed with the disease. Yet surprisingly, she turned out to have the mutation.

Many physicians are unsure how to proceed, because of deficits in their knowledge and experience concerning genetic testing. They may not always get separate informed consent, or offer any or adequate genetic counseling, and may test patients without sufficiently considering the potential complexities involved. Indeed, studies have shown that physicians often have serious deficits in knowledge in this area.[48,49,50,51]

Doctors may have not only deficits in knowledge about genetics, but deficient training in the nondirective approaches that genetic counseling requires—in which practitioners do not make recommendations, but encourage the patient to consider all the pros and cons, and choose what he or she thinks is best. Genetic counseling thus necessitates a different kind of training than the directive stance medical school instills. Unfortunately, the United States and other countries have shortages of genetic counselors, as a result of which physicians may often need to take on this role. Kym, the South Asian physician with a strong family history of breast cancer, said,

> We're all supposed to be impartial, but with genetics, emotions and biases can come into it—beliefs about terminations of pregnancies, and who has the right to get pregnant. But there's either no genetic counselor, or a three-month waiting list. Most doctors are not offering or doing counseling.

Moreover, doctors may be insensitive to patients' difficulties considering and undergoing genetic tests. Physicians may see these tests as merely routine, not much different from other laboratory assays, expecting that, as with many other evaluative diagnostic tests, at-risk patients would of course undergo testing. Laura, a graphic designer with a breast cancer mutation but no symptoms, said,

> Doctors forget that there's a whole lot of emotional baggage that comes along with testing. It's really a huge decision. It's not the same as: you have an ear infection or not. This affects your identity. But when I started going to doctors, the first question I would get was always, "Did you get tested?" It's a knee-jerk reaction. It makes it easier for them.

WHY TEST?

The reasons for testing varied somewhat with each of these diseases. For Alpha, physicians more than patients usually initiated testing, and no strong disadvantages appeared. People facing risks of HD and breast cancer confront a range of intra-personal and social reasons to test or not. On the one hand, many decided to pursue testing because they felt the information would be beneficial—that information is power, valuable in and of itself—the more, the better. Yet that attitude in itself usually evolved from other past events. In deciding to test for HD, Karl, who had been sexually abused by his HD-affected father and consequently ran away as a teenager, drew on his broad life experiences. "The more I know about a situation, the better off I am," he surmised. The fact that he found he lacked the mutation contributed to this belief.

The perceived definitiveness of these tests also allure many. Despite having a normal neurological exam and no symptoms, some sought genetic testing to provide a firm answer. Karl continued,

> The *neurological* exam would tell me how affected I was, *if* I were getting sick. But I wanted *objective understanding* of what was happening, so I wouldn't be completely on my own, in the middle of the ocean, trying to figure out what's going on with my brain.

The test's objectivity and definitiveness appeared more appealing than knowledge that one was simply "at risk." Karl also didn't know to what degree to hold his father (vs. the disease) accountable for the abuse, exacerbating this desire for definitude.

As described more fully below, for breast cancer, too, mutation-positive tests prompt individuals to monitor themselves for symptoms more vigilantly. For breast cancer, such a result was felt to be important to know even for patients who had already been diagnosed, since the likelihood of disease recurrence then increases.

As we shall see, many feel that testing will allow them to do something about the increased risk. For Alpha, effective treatment with Prolastin can then be started. But this belief motivates decisions to test for breast cancer as well, for which the only treatment for asymptomatic people is prophylactic surgery.

Many see information as beneficial because it allows for possible future action, even if such a course is not yet clear. Roberta, an African American former nursing student, had breast cancer, and contemplated testing. "The kind of person I am, I'd rather know, because you can't do something about something you don't know about." The fact that she worked in health care, and had seen countless medical interventions on patients, contributed to this attitude.

The possibility of undergoing prophylactic surgery can also prompt testing. Beatrice, a Latina math teacher, had breast cancer, and was finished with childbearing. She underwent testing in part since she decided that if she had the mutation, she would have her ovaries removed. "I didn't need my ovaries anymore," she said. "They could take them out. I have two kids, and was about to enter menopause." As a math teacher comfortable with numerical assessments, she was very matter-of-fact about the risks she faced.

Testing can occur due to belief in its possible advantages for prevention—even when these may be unclear or illusory. For breast cancer, preventative health behaviors such as self-examinations and mammographies may help, though the value of the early use of these has recently been contested.[52] Evidence of the illness in a family member, even without genetic testing, could also potentially, in and of itself, impel such proactive assessments. Arguably, women should monitor themselves carefully anyway. But for many, a mutation-positive test substantially strengthens vigilance. A genetic test for breast is not definitive—other, still unidentified mutations besides *BRCA 1/2* no doubt exist, and women may or may not develop cancer, regardless of whether they are found to have a mutation. But many women feel that a genetic test offers advantages in leading to enhanced prevention. A genetic test may not be fully predictive, but still seems to offer a modicum of definitiveness.

Some assume that in general, knowledge is power—without in this particular instance fully understanding why or how. In fact, with genetic testing, more knowledge can be confusing and uncertain in meaning, and hence may not always provide such clear and unequivocal benefits. Carmen, a 49-year-old Latina former clerical aide, had breast and thyroid cancer, and a *BRCA* mutation. She suggested to her nieces and nephews in their twenties that they get tested for the mutation as well:

So they won't go through what my sister and I are going through with cancer. The doctor would be able to do the right tests. Don't wait! Test just in case! And follow up. If you don't know, the doctor won't really follow up. If you know, you will be more careful.

Yet these relatives disagreed.

An immediate family member's diagnosis of cancer can in itself, at least for awhile, motivate additional prevention efforts. But knowledge of one's own mutation appears to motivate one far more powerfully. Individuals who do not think they are directly at risk may more readily ignore the potential dangers. People may simply disregard threats that they judge to be of low probability—whether that assessment is accurate or not. As Shilpa, a Hindu medical student, born in India, with a family history of breast cancer, said: "If people are not directly affected by it, they are not going to really think about it." She has not had symptoms, and thus not been tested.

Hence, for many, a positive genetic test proves far more powerful than knowledge that they are simply at risk. Family history alone could potentially increase awareness as well, but generally does not do so to the same degree as knowledge of actually possessing a mutation.

The presence of mutation in a patient often leads doctors to follow up more vigorously as well. Isabelle, a social worker who found she had a breast cancer mutation, described how it further motivated her providers.

> If you know you have the gene, it's more of an incentive, more *real*. Since the doctors know I have the gene, they're really on top of it. I am sure they are that way with any woman with breast cancer—but for me there was *no question* about doing an MRI. They don't do that for everyone.

One could argue that a positive genetic *BRCA* test should not increase a doctor's preventive efforts, but it appeared to do so, suggesting again the powerful psychological and symbolic meanings of these tests.

Indeed, some patients test so that their physicians *will* monitor and follow them more closely. Questions then arise of how much of an increased probability of disease prompts what degree of increased quantity or quality of monitoring by providers and patients.

Since other medical tests that doctors offer have clinical utility, many patients believe that new genetic tests must do so as well. But, as mentioned earlier, the increasing marketing of new genetic tests, without clearly demonstrated clinical usefulness, takes advantage of these beliefs. Therapeutic misconception has been described in research—whereby many individuals in a research study, in which they may or may not be given an effectual treatment (e.g., a placebo), tend to believe, even if informed otherwise, that the researchers will certainly give them an effective treatment.[53] In the case of genetic testing, a similar phenomenon may exist of "diagnostic misconception."

For HD as well, individuals often feel that testing will allow them to act differently in some way. But such prevention is in fact not yet possible. Nonetheless, if the result is mutation-positive, one can potentially plan one's life accordingly. Testing tells one whether one has a limited amount of time to live, in order to set and attain appropriate goals. Pablo, a single Latino in his early thirties without symptoms or testing for HD, said:

> I want to know, to be aware of how much time I have left, before I get any symptoms. I have certain goals: I'm an artist. I want to know how much time I have left before trouble begins, to accomplish my ends.

He has not yet decided to undergo testing, but sees benefits to doing so. Testing can help in arranging for future financial needs, and reprioritizing time and resources.

Testing to Reduce Worry

For HD and breast cancer, many individuals test to lower anxiety. The uncertainties of being "at risk" can shadow and haunt one's life. Antonia worked in neuroscience, and was asymptomatic for HD, but tested because "it's always hanging over you, in the back of your mind that you could have this." The possibility of relief due to absence of a mutation can thus outweigh the risk of stress because of learning one has a mutation, tipping the scales toward testing. Luckily, she learned that she lacked the mutation.

Testing was sought, too, to eliminate the anxieties surrounding ongoing self-assessments and examinations, which themselves induce stress. Yet this motivation may prove strongest among those who believe they lack the mutation. Testing can also result from wishes to reduce anxieties about possible symptoms—for example, to ascertain that momentary forgetfulness is normal, rather than due to HD. Yet, as mentioned, with HD these issues can become very complicated, since anxiety can itself be a symptom of the disease. Evelyn, the housewife without any clear HD symptoms, has not yet undergone testing but is leaning toward doing so, and in the interim, like several others, consulted a psychic.

> I forget everything. My kids are in a million different activities, and I'm constantly running here and there. That's probably why I forget everything. But in the back of my mind, I'm always thinking, "What if . . ." I want to know one way or the other.

Unfortunately, testing for this reason runs the risk of yielding unwelcome news. Hence, individuals have to struggle to gauge the *exact amount* of anxiety they can tolerate. As Patty, asymptomatic and untested for HD, monitoring herself in a body sculpting class, said: "If I obsessed and thought about it *too* much, and it overtook my life, I would be tested. But, at this point, it doesn't." This relative amount of worry can range widely between people. Individuals differed in their capacities both to tolerate such anxiety, and to *predict* how much angst they could manage in the future. These characteristics can vary by personality and temperament. Some drew on their sense of how anxious they were. Yet anxiety could result either *directly* as an HD symptom or *indirectly* as an emotional response.

The Type Who Does Better Knowing

Many individuals think that people should test if they are the type of person who does better knowing, but gauging whether one fits into this category is not always easy. Some feel they are this type, which gives them a sense of control. As Rhonda, the nurse who at age six saw her mother die of breast cancer, and later developed the disease as well, said:

> *I'm a need-to-know person.* It's personality. Knowing me, the way I am, I wanted to know, to feel empowered, in control—though obviously there's not much you can do. But feeling a little more: maybe I *can* do something about it.

This trait contributed to her decision to become a nurse, and was in turn strengthened by her career. She found she had the mutation, and has worked hard to accept it.

For HD, too, individuals discussed this notion of a "type" who want to know. Tim, a young lawyer, tested for HD, though asymptomatic. "With someone like *me*, it makes sense to get tested," he said. "If something is knowable, I would want to know, rather than be uncertain." In part, as an ambitious and successful young attorney, he has tended to do well planning and achieving long-term goals.

Other psychological characteristics, such as assertiveness, can motivate testing, too. Some think that people who are knowledge seekers should get tested. Simone, the 29-year-old bookkeeper, tested for HD because "if people are as aggressive as I am, they definitely need to get tested." This description evokes theories concerning "monitors" versus "blunters" among people confronting medical information, but suggests that the desire for knowledge is part of larger desires and personality types.

But how exactly individuals do or should define, gauge, and predict this trait, and know in advance if they possess it—especially with regard to genetic information—remains unclear. Many have difficulty sufficiently self-assessing the presence or absence of this characteristic—how well they would handle sensitive information in the future. Linda, the art teacher who found she lacked the HD mutation, said:

> People boiled it down to: are you the type of person who does better knowing information, or not? I was very much on the fence. So, my six to eight months with the genetic counselor became about where I actually am. Finally, I was over on the other side. But it took forever. . . . I always assumed I was a person who did better *not* knowing, but that was not the case.

A sharp divide seems to separate these two camps, but deciding whether oneself or others fit this type or not was complicated, and ultimately, highly subjective.

Interest and Education in Science

Education and professional experiences shape these testing decisions as well. Several of these men and women worked in health care, and appeared more likely than others to want to know. They were familiar and experienced with handling such medical information. Several others who had a long-standing interest in and substantial amount of medical knowledge also tended to want to know. Some may simply be more medically oriented than others. Roberta, the former nursing student, distinguished herself from her mother who was "anti-doctor": "Unlike my mother, I've always been a doctor bug: Let's see what's going on."

Testing can also occur because of another family member's diagnosis, or discovery of a mutation—for example, because a sibling or parent is found to have the mutation, or dies of the disease. The presence of a mutation in a family member, not family history of disease alone, might impel testing. Sarah, a computer programmer with a family history of breast cancer, said,

> Before my sister underwent genetic testing, I had seen TV shows about genetic tests, but was lazy. Nothing kicked my butt to do it, until my sister was positive. My mother was sick, but who knows if that was from genetics or not. It's easier to make rationalizations, if you don't have somebody else's positive tests.

Luckily, Sarah lacked the mutation, and has not had any symptoms. For her, the genetic assay provided the information she wanted.

People balanced these tensions in the context of medical and economic factors as well. Testing appeared easier in the apparent absence of symptoms.

Consequently, a seeming lack of symptoms can encourage testing, but did not always guarantee that a mutation was in fact absent. Simone, the young bookkeeper, felt asymptomatic for HD, but found she had the mutation. "If you don't have symptoms, it's easier to test, because you have a chance of being gene negative," she said. "That's a huge bonus." Unfortunately, her gamble turned out to be wrong, but she still supported the logical basis of her decision—in part because, as described below, she had undergone intensive genetic counseling, carefully weighing each of these possible scenarios.

The costs of genetic assays play roles here, too. Insurance occasionally covered testing but, as we will see later, often did not do so, and discrimination could result. A few people had their insurance company pay because it was willing to, and they thought that the odds of future discrimination were low. Still, uncertainties loomed. Rachel worked in publishing and had breast cancer. Much of her family had died in the Holocaust, which left her without much knowledge of her family's medical history, and she was concerned about the possibility of future discrimination. She engaged in a complicated calculus, weighing the odds of discrimination against the lab costs (approximately $3,500). In the end, she opted to test, largely because her insurance would cover the fee.

> I didn't know what it would mean for getting other coverage in the future. The insurance company wouldn't know the results, but the truth is: if they found out I got the test, and I then started having surgeries, they could put two and two together. At the time, I wasn't really thinking about that. I just really didn't want to pay for it myself. I thought: I pay for this insurance, and don't want testing to be a financial burden.

But even when insurance would cover testing, not everyone wanted the results on their medical record. Individuals whose insurance covered the charges thus faced dilemmas of whether to submit an insurance claim for the laboratory bill. Many avoided using their insurance for this purpose.

As suggested earlier, though lack of insurance coverage could impede testing, women who already had breast cancer would presumably not face additional discrimination because of the assay, facilitating testing.

Individuals with insurance had to weigh whether to use it against perceived benefits of testing. The presence of insurance coverage was often a necessary— but not sufficient—reason to undergo genetic analysis. Beatrice, the math teacher with breast cancer, said, "$3,000 was a barrier, but I tested because at some point, my daughter or son would need that information." She had to put a price on the value of the information to herself and her family, and made an economic decision, factoring in the value to their health.

Others tested only because to do so was free through an investigative study, which at times in fact motivated them to participate in research that they probably would not otherwise have entered—raising ethical questions that we will explore later.

WHY NOT TEST?

In opposition to these reasons to undergo testing, several counterarguments arose. Some of these cons cut across diseases, while others were more unique to one condition.

A key factor was whether treatment was available. For HD, for which no effective therapy exists, many people felt that testing would confer little if any benefit. If the result were positive, they could do little about it medically. Mary, a housewife who already had early symptoms, concluded that "there's no point in finding out."

Yet for breast cancer as well, these interviewees differ as to whether the advantages of testing outweigh the disadvantages. Kym, the South Asian doctor with a strong family history of breast cancer but no symptoms, felt that learning one has a breast cancer mutation without the availability of treatment (other than prophylactic removal of her breasts and ovaries), would be "a mental jail." Others eschew testing because they do not *like* the potential treatment options—particularly, having to consider prophylactic surgery.

Many feel that a mutation-positive result will upset them, and they thus seek to avoid the news. A genetic analysis, they fear, would confirm their worst suspicions, and they would have trouble coping. They do not want to have to deal with diagnosis or its ramifications, and thus do not test. Patty, asymptomatic and untested for HD, said about her risk, "I push it under the rug. I am a very optimistic person, almost to the extreme. So, that's how I deal with things: very much in *denial*."

For breast cancer, too, anxieties about the possible result could block testing. Carol, who had cancer and a mutation and decided to have her breasts and ovaries removed prophylactically, observed that "a lot of women don't want to be tested because of fear. That's foolish." Having opted for very aggressive treatment, she disparaged the alternative: avoidance.

Others fear that an assay could harm more than benefit them because they would become fatalistic. Bonnie, the 24-year-old who, at age 12, was terrified to see her mother's breast cancer, is asymptomatic and opposes testing:

> The information would hurt more than help me. When a test says, "Yes, you're going to have cancer," you risk feeling, "Why should I bother living? I'm going to have cancer anyway." It would feel like a death sentence. There's no point to condemning yourself, your life.

The assay would indicate whether she had an increased likelihood—though by no means a 100% chance—of getting the disease. Yet her memories of her mother's illness made her fear the worst.

Younger people at risk for HD or breast cancer, in particular, may avoid testing because of their age. They have not yet made their major personal and professional life decisions, and fear that knowledge that they possessed a mutation would too powerfully mold their choices. In part, this foreknowledge generates stress because it is not clear how to respond. Bonnie expressed these existential quandaries, continuing:

> It's like someone says to you, "I see in your future: you're going to die on a train." Does that mean never leave the house? The test tells you the cancer genes are there. It doesn't mean they're going to be active. Why live with that fear in your life thinking: "I have cancer, I'm going to die"?

Those who already had breast cancer and then considered genetic testing may not pursue it because of fears that a positive result will depress them with the possibility of future recurrence. Karen, the lawyer with breast cancer who had not undergone testing, wasn't sure if she "could deal with a positive result. I spend a lot of energy convincing myself: I'm three years out from my cancer. It's time to start living."

Explicitly and/or implicitly, many fear the potency of this knowledge itself. She added,

> I hate palm readings and tarot cards, because I'm *too susceptible* to what they may say—too afraid that if they tell me something, I'll make it true, or unconsciously make decisions to fit the predictions.

Knowledge of one's fate can thus become imbued with metaphysical and magical properties. She fears that the test will somehow become a self-fulfilling prophecy, and that the information will acquire more power in her life. The potential danger would become less theoretical and more real. Consequently, some do not test because they want to think as little as possible about their risk. Kym, the South Asian physician at risk for breast cancer, opposed testing because it would then grant the disease potency over her.

> I don't want to give it that much attention. I'd rather just not know. I don't want to start focusing on it, or giving it that much power, where I'd feel like I have to start doing preventive testing and procedures.

Her mother had both renal and breast cancer. Kym is terrified of both.

Resistance to these assays stems, too, from concerns that the results may not be completely accurate (even though they overwhelmingly are for these diseases) in detecting the presence or absence of a mutation. Therefore, these doubts about accuracy may represent or verge on rationalizations, but still be strong. Bill, the salesman who thought he would get HD because he looked like his dad, and who has not had symptoms or testing, said, "I've read that the test is not 100% accurate. The last thing I want is to find out, 'You have it,' and then not have it. Or they say, 'You don't have it,' and then I do." Thus he avoids testing, though he continues to fear he has the disease.

With HD, though not mentioned in prior literature, direct symptoms of the disease can themselves affect testing decisions. Denial may represent either psychological resistance to the possibility of testing, or direct psychiatric symptoms of the disorder that can impair personality and judgment. Cognitive signs of the disease itself can hamper awareness of other symptoms. Karl, who had been sexually abused by his affected father, said,

> My brother was very resistant to testing. Maybe by the time I started discussing this with him, he was already symptomatic, which might have affected his discussion with me. He doesn't know how sick he is. He can't tell. You can't tell him, and he can't understand, because cognitively, he's impaired. He keeps saying, "I'm fine. My brain's growing back. Everything's going to be cool." But it doesn't look cool.

Not Testing Because of Pre-Test Assumptions

As suggested above, assumptions of being mutation-*negative* could further reduce perceived needs to test, because of beliefs that testing would be superfluous. Yet these underlying assumptions about the result may be erroneous. Genetic tests could eliminate room for both doubt (i.e., that one is in fact, negative), and hope (that one's fears might be unfounded). Bill, the salesman, decided not to test: "I'm 36, and have no outward signs. Doctors told me that if I haven't had any outward signs by now, most likely I don't have the disease." He also feared losing his job.

He is aware that his assumption may be wrong, but still would prefer not to know definitively. Even though he appeared to lack the mutation, the small risk of being wrong frightened him more than the comfort he would receive from being right. He thus highlights both inherent human risk averseness, and the degree to which individuals, in the end, often view and weigh definitive tests far more than mere assumptions. Conclusive knowledge proves far scarier than inference alone.

Not Testing Because of Costs

As suggested earlier, financial costs can themselves also hamper testing. Individuals who do not have or want to use insurance could potentially pay out-of-pocket, but then have to weigh this expense against the perceived advantages. "I really wanted to be tested," Patty, the fashion designer who pushes her HD risk "under a rug," said, "until I found out that it costs almost $1,000 dollars. I don't want to know *that* bad." She and others have to weigh exactly how much they want to know *vs.* how much the test costs, tragically trading off one against the other.

Worries about possible discrimination, including job loss, also deter testing. These concerns often reflect anxieties about having to confront the disease directly oneself. Evelyn, the housewife who consulted a psychic, and is asymptomatic and untested for HD, said:

> My sisters are so afraid that if their company finds out, they might get fired. They don't want to be tested because of that. If I say, "Come to the clinic, it's anonymous," they still don't want to know. I'll say, "Guess what I just read . . .?" "I don't want to hear it. If it's not good news, don't even tell me." They didn't want to know anything about it.

Unemployed, and asymptomatic, Evelyn was less afraid of the possible dangers of the information.

Breast cancer and Alpha, too, generate concerns about insurance and employment discrimination. Yet given the availability of treatment for Alpha, symptoms, when they became too severe, outweigh these apprehensions. "The people who test for Alpha," Jennifer, a schoolteacher, observed, "are already very sick."

While individuals who work in health care may be more likely to seek testing, others may be more wary of discrimination, and consequently avoid testing because of their professional background or experiences. For example, if she were not a lawyer working on health discrimination, Karen would have been tested. A range of personal and professional experiences can thus spawn fears of discrimination and deter testing.

SOCIAL FACTORS

Since genetic information is about not just one individual, but his or her family as well, families can have high stakes in any member's testing decision. These members can pressure each other either to test or not. An at-risk individual may want to acquire genetic information, but not do so because of opposition from his or her family, or vice versa. Spouses, too, though ordinarily not at risk of having each other's mutations, are much affected by each other's decisions and can exert strong force. Partners may want a genetic analysis in order to get an answer and resolve uncertainty, though they will then have to cope with the stress if a mutation is found.

Testing to Help Others

Many test because they think the information can help their kin. Such testing might be seen as benefiting adult relatives in making testing, treatment, or reproductive decisions. Yet as we will see, questions arise about how and when to balance such altruism (testing for the benefit of others) versus autonomy (one's right to decide what is best for oneself). Surprisingly, with regard to genetics, issues of how to negotiate these tensions have received little if any attention. One's own views of how one should balance altruism versus autonomy and self-interest may clash with how others think one should weigh these competing principles. Quandaries then emerge of how to proceed—how to weigh one's own versus others' views.

On the one hand, several women tested for breast cancer because they felt it would help their sisters confront risks of the disease. Denise, a banker with breast cancer and a family history, said,

> I got tested because if any information can be useful for my sisters, mother, or niece, I wanted them to have it. Since I had cancer, nobody was going to discriminate against me at this point. The driving force was: maybe my sisters could have it.

Luckily, she learned she lacked the mutation. Yet uncertainties remained as to the implications for her relatives. She continued, "If I tested positive, they might have considered getting tested. Everybody breathed a sigh of relief that I was negative. But that doesn't *really mean* that they're negative." Still, her results lowered the likelihood that they had the *BRCA 1/2* mutations (i.e., that her cancer was genetic).

Samantha, a single actress in her twenties with breast cancer but no family history or mutation, went further, declaring that, "the *only* reason to test," if one already had breast cancer, is "for the sake of your family."

Nonetheless, some who have a family history of breast cancer, but no symptoms themselves, may also undergo genetic testing in order to help others. Joan, a psychiatrist, had an extensive family history of the disease, but was asymptomatic. "I think of myself as using my body *to educate my children*," she said. She tested after her daughter's diagnosis. "I wanted most to alert everybody in my family—the kids—to the possibility of genetic transmission. They have to pay attention to this. I would like my daughter to get genetic testing." Luckily, Joan found she lacked the mutation.

Ori, a 55-year-old Israeli with breast cancer but no family history, also tested to help her daughters. She felt that her daughters had not taken care of their health as well as they should. Testing can then become part of larger ongoing family tensions and dynamics.

> I thought: if this is genetic, I should know, to guard my 26- and 21-year-old daughters. They can avoid risk factors—mixing estrogen and alcohol, stressing the body with no sleep.

She felt that her daughters, more assimilated into the United States than she was, partied too much. She saw her own testing as another way to get them to alter their behavior. But she found she was mutation-negative.

Conversely, others decided *not* to undergo testing because they do not have offspring or relatives who could benefit from the information. Wilma, for example, with breast cancer and bipolar disorder, thought testing would not aid her or her family because "I only have a brother, but no sisters, and no children. If I had sisters, or girls, I think I would go for it: to protect them, so they could take the proper precaution, like tamoxifen." She does not think the information would help her in any way, and unlike some others, she is not interested in obtaining the information for its own sake. In part, she feels she already faces enough stress, having manic depression and cancer. She admitted that men can get breast cancer, but she does not feel that the prevalence is high enough to warrant her testing for her brothers' sake.

Relatedly, others tested *only* when they decided to have children. Reproductive desires could thus impact decisions to test, particularly for HD, given its lethality. Bill, the asymptomatic, untested salesman who fears developing HD because he resembles his dad, said, "if I was going to try to have children, I would find out. And if I had the gene, I would consider adopting, or using donor sperm and egg."

Conversely, others, if HD negative, would have a child as soon as possible. "If I'm tested and it's negative," Pablo, the Latino artist, said, "I'm going to get my girl pregnant as soon as I can afford it."

Yet reproductive issues are not decided unilaterally. Rather, they involve spouses, and multiple other factors, "accidents," and desires. In these contexts, genetic results can potentially tip the balance one way or the other. John, who dropped out of graduate school because of his HD risk, was asymptomatic, but tested in the end to prevent transmitting the mutation if he had it.

> When I learned there are ways to protect yourself from carrying a fetus with HD, I said: I'm going to do that. I tested so I could protect my kids from HD, and free myself from all this worry, and my wife could avoid IVF. The negatives were just: if I tested positive for the gene, it would worry me.

He alludes to the fact that individuals at risk for HD can opt for pre-implantation genetic diagnosis (PGD), in which patients undergo in vitro fertilization (IVF) and screen embryos for mutations, implanting only mutation-negative ones into the womb. But, in part as a Catholic, he opposes IVF. He also illustrates how people weigh several competing reasons. In the end, he values his perceived responsibilities to his wife and future children over his own potential distress, and decided to test. Fortunately, he found he did not have the mutation.

A few tested for even broader altruistic reasons—to help not only their family, but science more widely. Harriet, an African American schoolteacher, had indeterminate results (in part since fewer African Americans than Caucasians have tested). Still, she would encourage others to undergo genetic analysis to aid science and others in society. "Even if there is no care for you today, it can help somebody else, give them strength," she said. Still, balancing the benefits to others versus the potential harms to oneself can be difficult.

Albert, a policeman who tested for HD only when his children were thinking of becoming parents, wondered afterward if his decision was right since he found that he had the mutation, which horrified both them and him. He faced a terrible tradeoff—ignorance versus knowledge and fear—highlighting these dark, stark choices.

Yet individuals may also test for family members who do not then appreciate the act, or want the results. Rhonda, the nurse, who at age six had seen her mother die of breast cancer and now had the disease herself, tested in large part for her aunts. Yet only one of them ended up being interested in the results, and not sufficiently so to undergo testing herself. Rhonda was surprised—suggesting how even family members can have difficulty gauging each other's interest in genetic analysis.

Adult children may also fear—and avoid learning—the results. Laura, the graphic designer, said that her mother checked for *BRCA* mutations to help Laura, who then, however, did not want to know the result—due not to denial, but to fears of discrimination. "I didn't want my mom to tell me," she said. "I don't know how paranoid to be about being discriminated against in getting health care." If Laura didn't know the result, she could truthfully claim ignorance of any mutations in the family if an insurance company asked her.

Yet family members can proceed further, and in fact *push* each other to undergo genetic assays. Spouses, siblings, and parents often feel strongly that a family member should get tested, leading at times to pressure, conflict, and bad news. Testing decisions can thus get made in the context of complex family dynamics. "My wife wanted me to get tested," Brian, the former teacher who learned of his HD risk when contacted by a long lost relative, said. His wife "wanted an answer. So she pushed me. After my mother's death, I was depressed. She thought that having the test would eliminate one possibility. It turned out just the opposite."

The reasons for pushing a relative to undergo an assay varied somewhat with each disease and each person's role in the family (i.e., as a parent, sibling, or child). With breast cancer, individuals often thought that genetic information could potentially motivate certain family members to recognize their risk and monitor themselves. Parents, in particular, may push adult offspring to undergo testing. Susie, who worked for an HIV organization, had benign ovarian growths and a family history of breast cancer on her father's side. Her mother thus pressed her hard to test, without acknowledging the potential disadvantages. Susie was asymptomatic and aware of potential health discrimination and resisted testing, but eventually succumbed in part to placate her mother. Fortunately, she found she lacked the mutation.

Such pressure can be hard to oppose, though it impinges on one's own autonomy and right to make decisions for oneself. Thus, at times people balanced their own desires to avoid testing against their perceived obligations to others. They often prioritized assistance to their children over both fears of discrimination to themselves, and stresses of learning that they themselves had a mutation.

In the end, pressure from others could be the decisive factor, but also produced strains, concerning not only whether but when to test. John said that his sister-in-law pressured his brother to get tested "because she wanted to have kids." John's brother, "delayed, which she resented," causing ongoing intra-familial strife.

Families may vary in the degree of pressure they apply. Siblings may not encourage each other to test as much as they try to persuade others in the family, who might transmit the mutation, to do so. Families may also not push a member whom they see as fragile. Antonia, a neuroscientist, asymptomatic for HD, found that she lacked the mutation and then tried "to push my brother into testing" because she sensed that he had early symptoms. "But we're very different: I am very open, outgoing, confident," she said. "He is totally the opposite: very shy, stuttering, much more delicate." Yet such traits, potentially indicating the disease, may also impede decisions to test—to elude receiving bad news about which one can do nothing.

In encouraging a genetic assay, families frequently appealed on moral grounds, arguing that for a member not to test was unjust to *them*. Karl, sexually abused by his HD-affected father, thought that his untested but possibly symptomatic brother should be genetically screened. Acutely aware of the potential dangers of HD symptoms in a parent, Karl argued, "it's fine for *you* not to get tested, but it's not very fair for your wife and children." Not surprisingly, such pressure may be unwelcome.

To avoid any such coercion, some discussed these decisions with few people—at times only with their spouse. Yet these issues can then become shrouded in secrecy, and individuals may forego support that they might otherwise receive. A person may also pick and choose with whom to discuss this decision, in order to receive support for his or her own inherent preferences.

As we will see, testing decisions get made within the context of family dynamics that can shape how these issues of altruism versus autonomy are framed and approached.

Family Opposition to Testing

As suggested, family members can not only encourage testing but deter it as well, prompting conflict. A person may seek not only to push for testing, but also to prevent certain relatives from undergoing it—for the sake of either him- or herself, or others. Desires that a person does not test can range from mild preference to active blockade.

"The only thing stopping me is my husband," said Evelyn, the asymptomatic mother and housewife. As an interim action, she had thus consulted a psychic. She added:

> I want to get tested by the time my oldest son is 18. That's the magic number I have in my mind—he'll be an adult. I have two more years. I'm not pressing it now. But I *will*. My husband disagrees: We have such a good life right now, why chance that? . . . He's scared I will find out I carry the gene, and be nervous or sad. We're going to fight about this. Ultimately, I'm going to test—for the kids, and for me.

He opposes her testing in part because he wants to have another child beforehand, and wishes to avoid stress on her and their relationship. Evelyn has to weigh her perceptions of the benefits to both her and her children against her husband's perceptions of the potential harms. Some resolve this tension by agreeing not to test now, and deferring it to the future. But eventual consensus may be hard as well.

For breast cancer, too, family members often oppose an individual getting tested because it might suggest that *they themselves* have the mutation as well. Rhonda, the nurse who as a 6-year-old had seen her mother die of breast cancer, and now has the disease and the mutation, added,

> Though people in my support group who are already diagnosed are all interested in getting tested, their family members have reservations, because [they think] "if she has it, then maybe *I* do. If my sister has cancer, fine. But if she's got cancer *and* that gene, then maybe *I* have the gene, too."

Even patients who already had breast cancer may oppose a family member testing, since a mutation-positive result would mean that these patients themselves are then at risk of disease recurrence and should consider prophylactic surgery, and could also transmit the mutation to offspring. Therefore, these patients may not want to know the results if their family members undergo testing.

Patients may discourage siblings, too, from assaying genes. Karen, the lawyer with breast cancer but no testing, didn't want her sister tested because "if she's positive, *I* could be positive. I told her that if she tests, I don't want to know that, or the results." As a lawyer, Karen is also wary she might eventually have to disclose her sister's result to insurers, and then face discrimination. Perceived inadequacies in laws to prevent insurance discrimination could thus impede communication in families.

Though family members may also oppose an individual getting tested because they feel that he or she is ill-equipped psychologically or too young to handle the information, disagreements about these judgments can arise. Paternalistic feelings emerge, too, that for others, ignorance is bliss.

With HD, given the lack of treatment and the possible psychiatric symptoms, at-risk individuals may even try to stop relatives from testing. Antonia, the neuroscientist, sensing early HD symptoms in her brother, eventually concluded that he would not cope well with the result.

> I think my brother has it. That's why I don't push him anymore to get the test. Huntington's people get a look in their eyes . . . even when there's no signs or symptoms—a glazy, spaced-out look.

Desires to avoid secrets or painful disclosures to children, if the result were positive, could also prompt avoidance of testing altogether. Tim, the lawyer with the mutation but no HD symptoms, said, "My brother's decision not to test had to do with his kids . . . You don't really want to tell them, "Oh, by the way, you have a fifty-fifty chance of getting this disease."

Alternatively, patients could test but not tell younger offspring the results. Still, keeping the knowledge secret can itself create burdens and guilt.

People may also simply worry about a family member who finds out he or she has a mutation but cannot do much about it. Such relatives may then feel only anxiety or guilt. Isabelle, the social worker with breast cancer and the mutation, said:

> My mother said she thought she should also undergo testing. I had mixed feelings about it. She's healthy. What's the purpose at this point in her life? She's not going to have preventative surgery, but just be left feeling guilty because she passed it on to me.

As a social worker, Isabelle was very aware of the possible psychological difficulties that could ensue.

Roles of Health Care Workers in Testing

Clinicians can also shape these decisions one way or the other, though varying widely in their knowledge and comfort regarding genetics. Though genetic counselors are trained to be nondirective, physicians are taught both implicitly and explicitly to be more directive. Still, individual practitioners range in their approaches. Linda, the art teacher who eventually tested to eliminate the "HD nightmare" and lacked the mutation, said,

> The clinic staff thought I should get tested. Just a couple of the people did not give me the feeling that I would be *a bad person* if I didn't get tested. My GP and Ob/Gyn were like, "You should be tested. It's irresponsible if you don't." Easy for them to say.

For breast cancer, too, clinicians may encourage testing implicitly or explicitly, and their recommendations can be hard to oppose. Karen, in part as an accomplished lawyer, has thus far resisted these inputs, but is heavily affected by her providers' views: "The doctor just saying, 'I think you should be tested' is very powerful."

Physicians can push strongly for testing. Samantha, the actress, supported holistic, non-Western views of disease and treatment, but agreed to a genetic assay simply to silence her doctors. She was 27 and had breast cancer, but no family history.

> Everybody kept saying, "You really have to get this done. You would only get this disease because of a gene." I was freaking out: "No! Forget the gene." I tested to shut everybody up.

She felt conflicted in part because of her belief in complimentary and alternative medicine (CAM). "I was making my doctor mad, because my beliefs basically threatened his whole life," Samantha explained. "He always says, 'Stop the herbs and colonics. It can stir up cancer cells.'" In the end, she recognized the need for the test, given her risk for ovarian cancer, but she resented the pressure. She turned out not to have a mutation.

Physicians may be overeager to test, overvaluing a test for its own sake, and undervaluing the possible psychological and ethical costs. Some even proceeded to test children without parental permission, reflecting in part deficits in knowledge about relatively rare disorders and the ever-growing field of genetics. Betty, a designer who has to carry a portable oxygen concentrator machine in a bag wherever she goes, reported:

> My son went to new pediatricians. I told them I was Alpha. The doctors were more recently trained, and tested him for it, without telling me. The doctor was just overzealous—interested in disease. I assumed they'd first ask.

She knew that her adolescent son was too young to have symptoms, and she wanted to spare him as long as possible the stigma and ordeal of possible treatment. The doctor's overzealousness was well-intended, but unnecessary, and potentially dangerous.

Obstacles from Providers

Physicians, because of explicit or implicit attitudes or behaviors, can not only encourage and push testing but hamper and even impede it. Some doctors may be biased by being overly wary of genetic knowledge. Ron, who continued motorcycling despite his HD mutation, felt that providers "tend to terrify you to a certain extent, in hopes of scaring off anyone too sensitive." He recognizes the reason for their intense scrutiny, but finds it uncomfortable.

At other times, providers may go too far, opposing testing because of their own personal attitudes or knowledge deficits. Antonia, the neuroscientist asymptomatic for HD, said,

> My doctor told me, "Go away. Don't be silly. Why would you want to have a test? There's much more chance of you dying of a heart attack or breast cancer. You shouldn't worry about it." I didn't like that response. But I didn't do anything about it for a few years.

His response served to delay, but ultimately not prevent, her testing. Eventually, she found that she lacked the mutation, but she remains wary of GPs' involvement in genetic testing and sees a need for specialized expertise.

Providers may oppose an individual's reasons for wanting to test, and challenge his or her desires. Evelyn, asymptomatic for HD, whose husband opposed her testing, reported:

> The staff said, "You're not being tested for a reason such as wanting to start a family." I did not have a good reason. I just wanted to know. They didn't think that was a *good enough* reason.

In part as a result, she consulted the psychic.

Due to their insufficient knowledge, providers might also not suggest or order testing because they do not *know* to offer it. Genetic tests are increasing in number, and doctors in various fields are often inadequately trained, or prepared to deal with these assays. Alternatively, physicians may know enough only to raise the topic, but not to follow through with it. They may not be able to refer patients to genetic counselors, or prepare patients for the complexities involved. Susie, who worked for an HIV organization and had benign ovarian cysts and a family history of breast cancer, continued,

> My gynecologist said, "I don't know much about the testing. But I know you're at high risk. Why don't you get counseling?" She couldn't tell me much, which was off-putting. Maybe she doesn't want to talk about it for an hour because she has other patients. But it was unsettling.

Susie eventually found that she lacked the mutation. These issues are of concern since patients are confronting these issues in an increasingly fragmented health care system.

THE STRESSES OF WEIGHING PROS AND CONS

These decisions cause confusion because they require weighing relative risks and benefits, all clouded in uncertainty. These multiple competing pros and cons require balancing both intra- and interpersonal conflicts. Testing could reflect and affect deep-seated feelings about oneself—one's body and future— generating enormous internal struggle and a wide range of emotions. Linda, the art teacher and mother who tested to escape the overwhelming "HD nightmare" and discovered that she lacked the HD mutation, said,

> At the beginning of the decision process, I dreamt: I had this insect larva that was propagating madly. I couldn't stop it. My husband said: it's because you can't stop the life already started.

People tend to be risk-averse,[33] but the individuals here reveal complicating concerns—risks in both directions. These interviewees vary in where they perceive the highest risk, and what actions they must then eschew. These decisions force them to confront competing, inherently subjective perceptions of danger—for example, the burden of possible bad news versus the potential relief of a negative result; and the anxieties of not knowing versus the risks of feeling stressed if the result is positive. "If I have the HD mutation," Chloe, the 28-year-old asymptomatic secretary who worked with her sister and feared she was turning into her father, said, "it would be much more damaging than the relief of knowing I don't have it."

Risk aversion could also prompt decisions to undergo testing to avoid the chance of later being shocked if one develops symptoms without having adequately anticipated them. "Better safe than sorry," Carmen, the former clerical aide who had both thyroid and breast cancer, said. She also felt that "maybe they will find some treatment."

These calculations entail not merely the statistical odds of each risk occurring, but the emotional valence and implications of each possible outcome. Individuals might try altering each others' assessments in these calculations, but to little avail. Even family members, with the same perceived risk, differ widely in how they weigh the relative chances on each side.

Most people agreed that ultimately, each person had to face these existential dilemmas and decide for themselves. Even support groups try to maintain neutrality, urging caution in these decisions. As Linda, the art teacher who eventually found she had no mutation, commented,

> I would never advise anybody. The most respectful and true thing I can do is just acknowledge the situation they are in, and let them hash it out. Any advice *I* got was toxic.

Others would offer only general advice ("make sure you're able to handle bad news"), not definitive answers.

WHEN TO TEST

These competing pros and cons of whether to assay genes also affect *when* individuals decide to do so. Testing occurred in not only social but *temporal* contexts—amidst shifting psychological and biological processes. Other types of medical tests occur much more closely tied to periods of disease or treatment. But genetic testing can reveal a constant, permanent aspect of oneself, and can be performed at any time, before any symptoms may occur, or be delayed. Medical, psychological, interpersonal, and logistical factors therefore play key and complex roles here. How do people approach these competing timelines? Surprisingly, these issues have received almost no attention.

On the one hand, some seek to test immediately, or very soon after learning of their risk. Yet clinicians and others generally dissuaded such haste—especially for HD, given its 100% penetrance. In retrospect, most eager patients came to see their prior haste as rash.

In the end, most decided to postpone HD testing, but to varying extents. Waiting times could be medically based—delaying until symptoms become clear. Some individuals ended up observing early symptoms or suggestions of disease for several years before seeking genetic analysis. Often the final straw was when symptoms progressed to the point where key functions were impaired, such as driving a car. Roger, a single 33-year-old man, initially resisted testing and possible symptoms of HD:

> But two years ago, my balance and driving started getting much worse. One day, the car veered off the road. At that point, I wanted to get tested. I was at peace with what was going on.

For breast cancer, too, assays often occurred only after particular medical events—either one's own or those of family members. Susie, who worked for an HIV organization, tested after developing benign ovarian growths—a "tipping point": "These cysts tipped the balance. At that point I had to know: it's real. It could happen. I've had many relatives die of cancer, but was getting more anxious." Still, she delayed for several more months.

Embarking on such a momentous decision can require first gathering more social support, and carefully considering all the alternatives—which can take time. She added,

> I needed a reality check from rational people I trusted, who love me, to say, "Testing isn't ridiculous, you're not obsessed." I have a very supportive partner. But it took a little while to get there.

She sees herself as generally not procrastinating once she makes a decision—though arriving at *this* decision took time.

Some resolved these conflicts by bargaining or negotiating with themselves or others that they would test at a certain point in the future. For instance, several people who confronted HD vowed that they would check for the mutation before having any children. In the meantime, they deferred from making a decision. For breast cancer, too, several people decided they would test in the future, prior to having offspring.

Others, who already had children, thought they would check for mutations before becoming grandparents. But to prearrange such timing could prove difficult, since it involved the prospective parents' actions. "I wanted my children to have all the information available before they had children," Albert, the policeman who ended up having the HD mutation, said. "But one had a baby quicker than I thought." Adult offspring may become pregnant without forewarning.

Others waited until they had more resources—funds for the assay or insurance (to avoid later having a "pre-existing condition" that could impede insurance). At times, genetic counselors explicitly advised patients to delay for this reason. Karen, the lawyer, said about breast cancer,

> Since my diagnosis, I have tried to buy additional disability, life, and long-term care insurance, but have been told I have to wait five years out from my cancer. So, if I were smart, I would probably buy all of that insurance and *then* get tested.

She and others fear discrimination, and are wary of the protection that legislation might provide—in part since laws can change.

Alternatively, others waited because of psychosocial reasons, such as until arriving at particular personal or professional junctures—getting married, having children, or being at a "stable point," defined in various ways. Oliver, in his twenties, decided to continue to pursue a PhD despite learning he had the HD mutation. His sister decided to delay until she was more secure—"to be at a more stable moment in her life: when she had support." Yet understandably, some simply end up continually deferring.

Some undergo an assay only when having to face major career decisions. The uncertainty of not knowing how to move forward professionally could outweigh fears of having the mutation. "I had known about it for a decade," Antonia, the neuroscientist, said about her risk for HD, while lacking any symptoms.

> It came to a point where not knowing was as bad as having it. You convince yourself you have it, so you might as well find out . . . It was the uncertainty of not knowing: should I go on to do a PhD, or have kids early and get a house and a mortgage—career or family? . . . If I had HD, I would have a family. It turns out, I didn't have the gene, so I did my PhD.

If she had had the mutation, she would have chosen a different career. "I would have changed paths totally, and made money, to have financial security," she said. "I wouldn't have had the luxury of just pursuing what I wanted to do." Fortunately, she turned out to be mutation-free.

Testing may be delayed, too, until reaching certain milestones such as a particular age. "I was turning 40," Ron, the motorcyclist, said. He hadn't perceived any clear symptoms of HD, but he "didn't want to be 65 and find I didn't have it." Unfortunately, he learned he possessed the mutation. Still, he continued to motorcycle to live life to the fullest.

Other family members' medical events can also prompt testing. A relative's death can powerfully shape decisions of whether and when to proceed. Such a death can have both direct and indirect effects—jolting an individual with harsh reality, and perhaps reorienting the person from caregiver to potential patient.

The counseling process itself is designed to compel individuals to fully consider all of these options—which can take time. Yet tensions could result if individuals want to move ahead more swiftly. "I was fighting with staff," Evelyn, the asymptomatic mother, whose husband opposed her testing, said about her desire to proceed. "They said, 'We'd really like you to wait six months.' 'How dare you tell me I have to wait?'" This imposed delay contributed to her decision to consult a psychic.

As one strategy for navigating amidst these conflicting currents, suggestions arose for at-risk individuals to begin the counseling process and consider genetic analysis earlier, and reassess with the passage of time. Karl, who had been sexually-abused, and then ran away from home, said, "I'd tell others not to get tested, but to participate in the testing procedure and see what happens." He valued "doing something" to resolve problems. Time itself could help.

THE TESTING PROCESS ITSELF

Once deciding to test, many people encountered challenges as part of the counseling and testing process itself. Experiences vary widely in ways that could influence subsequent events. Institutions that provide genetic assays range from specialized centers with strong social service supports, to GPs' offices. Clinics differed widely in their experiences and abilities with diagnosing and testing. Some had handled few, if any, prior cases. Pablo, the Latino artist, untested and asymptomatic for HD, reported:

> My sister is in a private hospital. The doctor said they were 90% positive it was HD, but wanted to test. I said, "Has the hospital ever dealt with HD?" They said no. "Has the doctor personally ever dealt with HD?" No . . . "Has anybody in the team ever dealt with HD?" No. This pissed me off.

Differences emerge related to how and to what degree physicians, as opposed to genetic counselors and other clinicians, were involved. A few individuals felt that physicians tended to favor testing, while nonphysician health care providers (e.g., genetic counselors) were more wary—perhaps as a result of differences in professional training. Linda, the art teacher who was mutation-negative for HD, said,

> Medical people tend to have a definite opinion one way or another, and are not afraid to let you know. Maybe that's why social workers tend to swing so far to the other side . . . to be a little bit more respectful about how hard

it must be; and acknowledge that they have no idea what you're going through.

Physician training emphasizes more directiveness, and doctors often have less time to address patients' psychological difficulties.

Variations in Quantity and Quality of Counseling

These individuals also provide many insights about the counseling process itself that are important as the amounts and types of genetic testing expand. Counseling experience varied from good to bad—from relatively more to less helpful or traumatic. From the very initial contacts—even the first phone call—patients evaluated their counselors, which affected eventual decisions of whether to test. "On the phone, the genetic counselor sounded very reasonable," Beatrice, the math teacher with breast cancer, said. Beatrice ultimately tested because, if positive, she wanted to have her ovaries removed: "I went to meet her. Within five minutes, I knew I wanted to do it."

Trust plays an important role in these decisions, yet is strongly shaped by perceptions. Diane, a Spanish language teacher, underwent surgery for a lumpectomy and woke up to find that the surgeon had instead performed a mastectomy because he thought it was indicated. Later, a doctor suggested genetic analysis.

> At first, I was not convinced. But I liked this doctor—her approach. Some kind of a trust established right there. *That* made me consider it. I didn't reject it outright, which I usually do from doctors.

Despite her prior wariness, she underwent the assay, and learned she lacked the mutation.

Yet occasionally, counseling was minimal, leading to negative experiences. Karl learned that he lacked the HD mutation, but was nonetheless dismayed by the process. "This doctor wrote the prescription for the test," he said. "That was it . . . No counseling, no nothing, just that. That was a mistake."

The process can be highly traumatic because of what it represents—the possibility of disease and even death. Not surprisingly, anxieties persisted throughout these processes, even after individuals decided to have blood drawn. Fears can hover not only before and during the counseling, but even after individuals decide to proceed. "It's a sword of Damocles hanging over you," Karl continued. "Especially the period between giving them the blood and receiving the results."

At other times, more counseling occurred, but still fell short—providing insufficient follow-up or support over time. Albert, the policeman who checked for the mutation to help his children and found he had it, reported:

> The doctor said, "If you need to come back, talk to us" . . . I called . . . but they were moving the office. I tried to reach out, but couldn't get anyone . . . They never got back to me.

These worries can culminate in picking up the results. Counselors themselves also responded to these fears by, for instance, agreeing not to know the result before revealing it to the patient. As Linda, the art teacher who found out she lacked the mutation, said:

> I was most scared about the walk from the waiting room to where they were going to tell me . . . How the hell do you walk from one place to the other with a person who knows? So the counselor actually set up this elaborate plan where she was not going to know, and was going to pick me up and walk me from the waiting room to the room where I found out. So I wouldn't have to walk with someone who knew when I didn't know.

She highlights the multiple complex stages involved in this process.

For breast cancer as well, anxieties and uncertainties continue, particularly during the waiting period. Women here, too, wonder whether the counselor yet knows.

Providers, regardless of their sensitivity, can reveal their suspicions and knowledge of a diagnosis through not only verbal but inadvertent, nonverbal communication as well. When becoming aware of a patient's risk or symptoms, providers may change even their tone of voice. "We saw the counselor's face, and knew in two seconds," Simone, the 29-year-old bookkeeper, said about learning that she had the HD mutation, "because she is a very 'la dee da,' very happy person." Simone felt immediate horror.

Genetic counselors may relay breast cancer information nonverbally, too. Laura, the symptom-free graphic designer whose mother had breast cancer and had tested to help Laura, who then did not want to know the outcome, said that the genetic counselor had a student observe the meeting. Laura then guessed the result.

> When I got there, the counselor asked if this trainee could sit in. That's when I knew — why would they ask somebody to sit in if the results were negative? She didn't beat around the bush. She told me right away—which is best. I started crying, and she talked . . . about plans. They sat there for

as long as I wanted. But I just wanted to go home. I get tearful even remembering it.

Genetic counselors may indeed have more time than physicians to handle the emotional issues that erupt.

Yet providers may be insensitive, informing patients of genetic diagnoses in inappropriate ways. Ron, the motorcyclist, said about his father's HD diagnosis:

> He was in a hospital, and wasn't told. All these students were brought around him, and the doctor said, "This man has Huntington's, which is yadda, yadda, yadda." My father didn't know . . . That wasn't very pleasant.

Given the terrible impact of learning one has a mutation, providers may not be as sensitive as they should.

However, with mutation-positive results, the process of giving the news can never be wholly positive, no matter what the process. Simone, the bookkeeper who only learned of HD in her family when she got engaged, and who deduced her mutation from her counselor's face, added:

> It was a horrible rainy day. I kind of knew, going in, because the weather was so bad: this is the day that you would get really bad news. We came in, and she handed us the letter, which we could open if we wanted to know the number of repeats [i.e., the extent of the abnormal gene]. We still haven't opened it. Then we left. There was no counseling. Nothing. She called up over the weekend. But it was such a definite thing: here are the results, thank you very much. See you later.

The counselor may have in fact provided additional support but, under the circumstances, it did not register. The fact that Simone had only recently learned of this disease made it even more difficult to accept. As she suggests, superstition (the rain as portent) can freight these interactions.

In contrast, other patients feel that the counseling process is too long and intense—providing too much information, cognitively and emotionally, with the result that they feel overwhelmed. Even Susie, familiar with medical information from working for an HIV organization, said about the counseling she underwent due to her family history of breast cancer, "I was given good information, but there was so much of it! My brain spiraled into what-ifs. I was in a total haze. At a certain point, nothing was going in."

Still, in the end, the "right" amount of information can vary—based on complex emotional and cognitive responses. Providers must gauge the appropriate amount of background, but may be inherently unsure. Given the ambiguity and incompleteness of information, a little knowledge can be potentially dangerous, fostering anxiety. "What's too much is subjective," Susie added. "When I got home, I was trying to figure out what it meant." Moreover, some information (e.g., the number of DNA base pair repeats) may simply constitute too much data, because the implications are not wholly clear. Simone, who sadly surmised the result of her HD mutation testing from her counselor's face, added, "She said they hadn't correlated the number of repeats with actual onset, so there was no advantage of us knowing that."

In this context, giving more *written* (as opposed to only verbal) information could be very helpful. When Carmen, the Latina former clerical aide with both breast and thyroid cancer, was told she had the *BRCA* mutation, "The counselor didn't give me anything written. I forget things. I could have given written information to somebody else to explain it to me in simple words." She underscores problems with educational levels, given the intricacies involved.

Counselors were often seen as playing the role of devil's advocate, repeating the same questions. Yet in retrospect, individuals generally came to appreciate why the process takes so long. "They kept asking the same questions," Karl explained:

> "Do you really want to go through with this? Why do you want to do it? What purpose can it serve?" When I look back, I understand why . . . But they were persistent and annoying . . . They might just say, "Look, you're going to get annoyed with us. We're going to ask some of these questions over and over again, but there's a reason . . . You just don't know it yet." They even may have said that, and I filtered it out.

Luckily, he found he lacked the mutation. Still, counselors could potentially establish expectations more realistically by more thoroughly describing the process in advance, ensuring that it is understood over time, and better preparing patients to expect this barrage of inquiries.

At-risk individuals with science training, in particular, felt that the process was not sufficiently flexible, given their prior understanding. Antonia, working in neuroscience, said about testing for HD, "the process can take six months . . . Most people would need that." But if someone like herself "wants to know in a hurry, and knows his or her own mind, and is able to tell them, they should do it quickly." Admittedly, if she had instead found that she had the mutation, she may have looked back at these practices differently.

Several lay people also felt that the lengthy procedure was not wholly applicable to them because they had already seriously considered and weighed the options. They felt that more flexibility may be needed. Tim, the successful lawyer who was asymptomatic for HD, said, "They really drill you. I felt I had a very good reason to get tested. I didn't waiver . . . The process was right for the *general* person, but was a little annoying to me." Nonetheless, in the end, he appreciated the rationale, in part because he learned he had the mutation.

For breast cancer, too, those who have had symptoms may have already strongly decided to proceed. Ori, the Israeli with breast cancer who underwent the assay to motivate her daughters, paid little heed to the genetic counselor. "I was very, very determined to have this information because of my daughters and granddaughters," she reported. "So I didn't care much what they said."

Yet as discussed earlier, it can be difficult to know one's own mind, and what is best for oneself. Indeed, with time, many who initially wanted to test immediately became aware, through counseling, of the complexities of these issues. Simone, the asymptomatic bookkeeper who learned about HD only when she became engaged, said:

> We wanted to know right away . . . I didn't need the counseling. But then, as it turned out, talking to staff here: "O.K., we're not ready to go through with this." The biggest question they asked us was, "What do you want to do if it comes back positive?" . . . That was the killer question. It took us a while to decide.

In this case, genetic counseling served its intended purpose well, prompting a patient to consider all possible scenarios, which turned out to be helpful as she subsequently learned that she had the lethal marker.

Simone appreciated, too, useful conceptualizations and metaphors that the counselors provided:

> They said to view it like a New York apartment: You have a tiny New York apartment, and are so tight for space, and spend ages organizing your closet, because you only have one. That's the same thing with HD: if you know this is the amount of time you have . . . make the best of it.

In large part, genetic counselors may be helpful due to innate empathy, not training per se. "She genuinely cares," Simone added. "It's not just part of her job or training."

But others resisted or discounted what a counselor said, though to do so could leave them ill-prepared for the results. Vera, the marketing executive who was offered the assay because she was Asian and turned out to have a breast cancer mutation, had not really paid attention to the genetic counseling. Though she had had breast cancer, she was convinced she would not have the mutation, since none of her family members had had the disease.

> The counselor went through the whole routine, explaining the conse-
> quences if the results came back positive, blah blah blah. I was like, "Well,
> I don't think they will. I'm just doing this as a lark." I didn't give it much
> credence. But when I walked in to get the results, and saw another doctor
> with her, I'm like, "Oh shit, something's up." Maybe I should have taken
> her more seriously the first time.

In fact, Vera feels she had been dishonest with herself.

> I thought I was up to hearing the results. But I wasn't. So I lied to myself.
> I was fine when she was telling me [the results], too. But I couldn't wait to
> get out of there. I went downstairs to a little piece of grass, and cried.

Certain other aspects of the counseling process proved very helpful—partic-ularly posing questions that clients had not considered, and providing concepts to help grasp the phenomena involved. Many liked that genetic counselors were straightforward and sensitive. Susie, who had benign ovarian cysts but no breast cancer, and worked for an HIV organization, reported that "the counselor said, 'I'm going to cut to the chase and tell you: you're negative.' I burst into tears out of relief."

Referrals to mental health services can be especially beneficial. The Huntington Disease Society of America recommends "psychological and/or psychiatric screening" for depression and emotional support,[24] and several individuals here were referred to psychiatrists who prescribed antianxiety med-ications as well. Hence, an added benefit of genetic counseling could be referral to mental health services that individuals do not otherwise access.

Psychotherapy can play key roles, and help in both making decisions about testing and accepting the results. Roger, who tested for HD after he veered his car off the road, can cope with the diagnosis in large part due to psychotherapy he began in conjunction with the testing process. "I'm really at peace right now," he said. "Ten years ago, I would have been bonkers about the thought of having a genetic disease. But I've been seeing my psychologist." Psychotherapy assisted him with acceptance, but can be helpful even if not leading to complete acknowledgment of one's risk. Roger added that his sister was untested but, due to psychotherapy, "it's not on her mind all the time like it was."

Hence, psychotherapy can help with the threat of disease and the uncertain-ties inherent in decision-making, lowering the *level* of anxiety involved in these decisions. Consequently, mental health treatment can be an important adjunct to genetic counseling. Linda, the art teacher, lacked the HD mutation, but thought that no one should test without closely consulting a mental health provider.

Genetic counseling aided logistically, too, in encouraging considerations and plans regarding future insurance coverage. Before undergoing the assay, individuals frequently bought health and long-term care insurance. Genetic counselors have helped patients handle privacy issues, too—suggesting, for example, that patients ask their physicians explicitly not to include genetic test results in the medical chart. Clinicians may also know of research studies that offer testing for free, with added protections of confidentiality. Overall such knowledge proved rare, but highly welcome. As Benjamin, an engineer, from Maryland said about such a study: "The results are kept confidential, and can be destroyed immediately, so there's no linkage back to you. And it's all free." Still, he lost his job because his company knew he could then go on disability due to Alpha.

IMMEDIATE POST-TEST REACTIONS

Responses to test results vary widely in both the short and the long term, depending in part on the disease and the results. Reactions can shift over time, from immediately learning the result until years afterward.

Those who tested negatively were of course relieved. For an individual who had children, or was considering the possibility of having them, the absence of a mutation was good news for not only him- or herself but for future generations as well. A mutation-negative result was especially welcome when it suggested that these children were not at risk. Cancer may still be in one's family, but the test offered reprieve, even if not absolute. Susie, with benign ovarian cysts and a family history of breast cancer, but no symptoms or mutation, concluded: "If I hadn't taken the test, I would have worried all the time."

Not surprisingly, those who learned that they had a mutation were deeply disturbed by the news. Yet individual reactions varied, based on the specific disease, and the presence or absence of symptoms. Those with Alpha generally felt relief: a definitive genetic diagnosis made sense of their prior, perplexing symptoms, and reduced uncertainty. For Alpha, a mutation-positive result also offered concrete benefits: reduction of stigma and initiation of treatment. Dorothy, a former TV producer, now had to wheel around metal oxygen tanks in a cart, and was awaiting lung transplantation. Learning she had the Alpha mutation "answers questions. Like: why I was sick all the time as a child? In my apartment, cleaning, I would wheeze, and not know why."

Those who smoked and learned they had the Alpha mutation found out that their symptoms were not their fault. Diagnosis reduced their perceived blameworthiness. Benjamin, the engineer, said about his test result:

I wasn't happy, but was relieved. Prior to that, I was diagnosed with emphysema. I smoked, and probably caused my illness, even with a genetic component. But it gave me a reason why I had emphysema at 42.

In effect, he traded one label for another that he saw as less stigmatized: "I was glad it wasn't *just* my smoking. I was now willing to tell people about my illness. I still felt *tainted*: I have this genetic stigma: I'm not a normal person." But he now felt able to tell people he was ill.

Indeed, Dorothy wishes she had tested *earlier*, because she is now seen as blameless for her illness. "Now that I've been diagnosed, I'm treated nicer: 'Oh, she has a *disease*!'" But in fact the difference may be due to the presence not of a disease, but of visible treatment and disability, and non-culpability.

Diagnosis with HD, too, can be a relief, though to a much lesser degree, reducing the uncertainty and constant worry of not knowing one's fate. "I expected the test would come back positive," Jim, a physician with the HD mutation, said. "When I actually found out, it was just such a relief to finally know, and not having to worry. Not knowing was scarier."

Shock and Disappointment

Despite these perceived advantages, knowledge of a mutation disappoints most people. Shock arose from the fact that the information represents the prospect of illness and death in a very real way. Before testing, risk can be seen as abstract. With a confirmed mutation, it becomes far more concrete. "That knowledge affects everything," Ron, the motorcyclist, said about receiving news of his mutation.

Many are shocked, too, because they are confronted with complex information concerning a disease about which they know little, or are confused. "We taped the meeting," Dorothy said about learning she had Alpha. "We went back to the house and sat down and listened to it several times, trying to figure out what it was all about."

Even those who said they had expected to test mutation-positive and had undergone genetic counseling felt that they hadn't sufficiently anticipated how they would feel. Many were devastated. "After I had given my blood, I had forgotten about it," said Laura, the graphic designer who deduced her breast cancer mutation from the fact that her genetic counselor had had a trainee join them. "The morning I got my results, I freaked out."

Such reactions may be inevitable. One cannot predict entirely the full range and depth of one's emotions. Those who had assumed they'd be mutation-negative and proved mistaken were especially upset, often completely shocked.

Even if one is intellectually prepared for the possibility of a mutation, denial and rationalizations can trigger surprise. Some thought they were too old to have HD. In the absence of symptoms, the diagnosis seemed even more abstract and surreal, and for offspring or kin, more frightening.

Over time, individuals tended to adapt to their diagnosis in various ways. Even with a mutation-positive result, most did not regret their decision to test. Generally, they felt that their choice was right for them. Still, retrospective assessment is difficult, and might be biased by prior assumptions, subsequent decisions, and cognitive dissonance—minimization of internal distress about past decisions, however painful the outcomes.

Not surprisingly, those who found they lacked a mutation had few regrets. But those who tested positive generally did not rue their decision, either. Oliver, for instance, was glad he learned he had the HD mutation, because it has helped him decide to do what he most wanted to do—continue to pursue a PhD. "The test itself has been an unambiguous, *positive thing* for me," he said. "It made me feel that the decisions I made in my life were good—getting a doctorate."

Yet even those who felt that testing was beneficial for them avoided recommending it for everyone. As Simone, the 29-year-old bookkeeper who only learned of HD when getting married, and then inferred her mutation from her counselor's face, said: "What we did was right for *us*, but may not be for others."

CONCLUSIONS

These men and women highlight several key aspects of decision making about genetic testing. Complex pros and cons prove hard to weigh. The varied contexts of these individuals' lives—including past personal and professional experiences and social interactions with, and pressures from, family members, clinicians, and others—profoundly shape these choices, yet can conflict.

Decision making about genetic assays involves a complicated series of interrelated processes, including pre-test assumptions and self-monitoring, which pose numerous challenges. Intricate issues also shape decisions of *when* to undergo the assay, and counseling and testing procedures themselves vary widely, and are generally experienced as overly long, but ultimately helpful.

Many decision-making theories have focused on individual cognitive and emotional factors, drawing on psychological models and emphasizing traits of seeking or avoiding information and being risk-averse;[30,33,34] yet the people here reveal how they make these decisions in the contexts of varied experiences, and dynamic relationships with multiple sets of others (spouses, siblings, offspring, and providers), and these *social* inputs can clash.

A few prior studies have mentioned perceived responsibilities toward others[37] as a factor in testing decisions. But here, interactions with others constituted not simply a dichotomy of paternalism and coercion versus autonomy,[22] but a broad and nuanced social terrain. An individual may be inclined to avoid testing, but overcome that tendency because the knowledge will help his or her offspring. Or, an individual may tend to seek information generally, but avoid *this* information because of fear of discrimination to one's self or family. Doctors' advice has been mentioned in two studies on genetic testing,[54,55] but only a few studies have probed physicians' rates of ordering genetic tests in general.[39,40] The men and women here illustrate how doctors can play key roles in these decisions. While theories on health information have described traits of monitoring versus blunting, the individuals here balance these tendencies against other—at times competing—issues, including family members' preferences. At times, individuals weighed the *strength* or *degree* of their tendency toward monitoring or blunting against the perceived degree of others' wishes or needs. These traits may interact with pre-test assumptions and self-monitoring. "Monitors," who see evidence of possible symptoms, may opt for testing more than do those who do not observe clear symptoms themselves—but not always.

While one prior researcher, Susan Cox,[7] thought that approximately one-third of her sample "evolved" in their decisions,[7] *all* of the individuals here engaged in a dynamic process in some way. Psychologists James Prochaska and Carlo DiClemente have proposed a "stages of change" model in which people go through four stages in altering health behaviors—from precontemplation to contemplation to action to maintenance.[21,22] The interviewees here provide important added details and dimensions. For example, the men and women here suggest a range of particular critical components of a pre-contemplation stage—specific types of self-monitoring and pre-test assumptions, and problems involved.

Individuals wrestle with questions of not only *whether* to test, but *when* to do so. Some individuals have been noted to delay testing,[22] but the people I spoke with illustrate specific medical, psychological, logistical, and interpersonal factors that interact and can shape timing decisions. Testing often occurred at particular junctures in one's life, when one needed to make a key life decision.

The reasons offered for and against testing both resemble and differ from those identified in prior research,[9,10,12] reflecting in part the fact that technologies have changed since several earlier studies were conducted. Since earlier linkage tests (in which labs test broader sections of DNA across family members, not single mutations in one individual) are no longer used, the difficulty of obtaining blood from relatives does not emerge here as a reason to avoid testing. Importantly, adults can also now undergo assays to decide whether they or their adult offspring should consider the expensive (and not entirely benign) procedure of screening embryos.[56,57a] Though in the past a leading reason to test was, "if my risk goes up, so does that of my children,"[9] PGD now enables mutation-positive parents to avoid passing on the gene.[57b]

Despite legislation to reduce discrimination, substantial privacy concerns still arise. Surprisingly, these fears have been mentioned in few previous studies of testing decisions, especially not those conducted in countries with national health insurance.[7] Certain factors mentioned in prior studies—"emotional reasons" and "other personal reasons"[12]—appear in fact to involve several complex phenomena. Many individuals test because they "just wanted to know," but that desire often in fact relates to other factors (e.g., professional experience), and some who thought they were the type who want to know in fact turned out not to be so.

Pre-test assumptions of being gene-positive or negative, based in part on fears, are not always correct. Assumptions of positivity can prompt decisions to test (to confirm suspicions) or not to test (fearing the result), depending in part on the role of these other factors. These pre-test assumptions shape individuals' decisions, but in turn also grow out of multiple factors: for example, self-monitoring, denial, misunderstandings of genetics, and varying levels of desire for information and of anxiety tolerance. Though one study in Scotland found that individuals at risk for HD felt *uncertain* about their risk,[58] most men and women here made assumptions, even if these later proved wrong. Uncertainty caused intense anxiety. Future studies can further probe whether those who assume that they have the mutation undergo the assay more frequently than do those who assume they lack it, and how often these pre-test assumptions prove right or wrong.

Similarly, yearnings to decrease anxiety can sway decisions either way. Individuals balance both present and imagined future fear against a range of other considerations. Significantly, individuals are forced to *predict their tolerance of future anxiety*, yet their abilities to do so can vary, raising questions of how at-risk individuals make these prognostications, and how accurately. With HD, anxiety can also result either directly as a symptom or indirectly from worries about the disease. Ego strength and denial of distress have also been suggested as predictors of distress,[59] but may in turn be related to other factors, and hence be difficult to gauge.

The need for certainty also appears here as a trait in and of itself, suggesting the theory of "negative capability"—that individuals vary in their ability to tolerate uncertainty and ambiguity. This phenomenon is described by the poet John Keats as "when man is capable of being in uncertainties, mysteries, doubts without any irritable reaching after fact and reason."[60] The individuals here tolerate uncertainty to widely differing degrees. Fear of a bad result usually outweighed possible relief from a good result—which is consistent with theories that individuals tend to be risk-averse.[33,34] Yet how individuals *perceive and interpret* risks vary. Hence, risk aversion may lead to decisions either to *avoid* testing, or to *seek* testing (to avoid the risk of later being surprised by becoming ill).

Clearly, balancing these competing factors is arduous. Indeed, dilemmas in medical ethics often entail weighing options that represent not good versus bad, but competing ethical goods.[61] While some ethicists insist that one should adhere to set principles, and that these will provide clear answers and approaches to problems, others argue that in moral decision making, principles can conflict, and that pragmatism is needed, paying close attention to interpersonal processes such as those here.[62] These men and women underscore, too, the need to assess social, historical, and geographic contexts, which have been underexplored. For instance, no studies on testing decisions have commented on possible differences among industrialized countries (Canada versus the United States, or the United Kingdom) with contrasting insurance systems. In a prior Canadian study, for example, some individuals never had any doubts or ambivalence about testing,[7] while almost all individuals I interviewed did so. Indeed, for HD at least, testing rates appear higher in Canada than the United States.[5] Such national and historical contexts are critical.

As we shall see, these highly personal decisions of whether and when to test, balancing desires and the need to know, probabilities of fate against fears of bad news and inputs from multiple other people, have profound implications. These conundra alter the lives of these interviewees as well as their family members— born and unborn.

CHAPTER 3

"Whom Should I Tell?":

Disclosures and Testing in Families

"As soon as they told me I had the mutation, I thought: now I've got to tell my family," said Carmen, the Latina with both breast and thyroid cancer. "That was one of the hardest things I've ever had to do."

People who learn that they have (or may have) a mutation face dilemmas of whether to tell others, and if so whom, when, and how. A person divulging his or her genetic risk to a family member is revealing that, in fact, both of them (as well as other family members) are at risk. Hence, the potential discloser must weigh whether this information will benefit or burden listeners, and how to proceed. Individuals must balance moral responsibilities to family members against potential stigma and misunderstandings of genetics, generating dilemmas of whether to tell parents, siblings, offspring, and long-lost relatives.

These disclosures are important, but have received little attention. Genetic test results, once divulged, can clearly affect families in many ways.[1] In general, family members do not always communicate genetic risks to each other,[2] but only a few studies have begun to probe these realms.

Many barriers exist.[3,4] Families are intricate social units, varying in norms.[2] Most people prefer to disclose genetic information to a family member themselves, rather than have it done by a doctor.[5] Yet individuals tell selectively.[2]

Overall, disclosure may be associated less with medical than with familial, psychological, and social issues.[6] Many patients do not inform all their at-risk relatives about chromosomal abnormalities,[7,8] breast cancer,[9] or cystic fibrosis.[10] With breast cancer, disclosure may increase with various factors, including age, past history of cancer,[9] motherhood, higher distress,[11] having older children, having more open parent-adolescent communication styles,[12] being a carrier,[5,13] and seeking support and medical advice.[5,13] Several obstacles may hamper disclosure of genetic risks to extended family members.[14]

But genetic disorders differ from each other in critical ways. One study explored disclosure among individuals with four genetic versus four nongenetic conditions, and found that these two groups generally did not differ—both groups objected to a doctor disclosing information without their knowledge to other family members.[15] Yet in this study, the conditions explored were heterogeneous. For instance, HIV was examined as a nongenetic disease, though it evokes strong privacy concerns that can make it resemble genetic more than non-genetic disorders.

Earlier research I conducted on disclosures of HIV found that individuals vary in *what*, *how*, and *when* they disclose. Some people disclosed indirectly or in code (for example, by simply saying "I have some problems with my immune system").[16,17]

Yet research on genetic disclosure has tended to examine *whether*, but not *what*, *how*, and *when* these divulgences occur. How individuals at risk view and experience these issues, and how feelings of guilt, fear, shame, or discomfort affect disclosures have received little attention. In contrast to many other disorders, genetic disease invariably affects other family members. These revelations may then have psychological implications that can shape subsequent health decisions. For instance, obtaining one's breast cancer mutation results can profoundly affect family members,[18] but psychological distress may decrease after disclosing to sisters and increase after disclosing to young children.[5]

The health belief model (which suggests that health behavior is shaped by perceived susceptibility, disease severity, and costs and benefits of the behavior[19]) may help make sense of decisions about genetic disclosures, but has not been examined in this regard. As we have seen, individuals often learn that they are at risk only when informed about it by family members also at risk. Thus whether, when, how, and to whom an individual discloses information within a family may shape whether, when, and how these members make choices about whether to pursue testing or have children, or disseminate the information further.

Erving Goffman has described how individuals with stigmatized conditions generally struggle to manage such information, which can be hard.[20] But with genetic disease, individuals manage *for* others, too, information *about* these others. The sociologist Talcott Parsons has also described the "sick role" as entailing rights and responsibilities, exemptions from certain duties, and obligations to get well.[21] People at risk for genetic disease must choose, through disclosure decisions, whether to put others and themselves into the role of being at risk, and what that means.

Overall, I found that every disclosure involves intricate decisions of what, how, when, why, and whom to tell. These issues arose across all three diseases.

WHETHER TO TELL

Individuals grapple with whether the inherent nature of genetic information mandates that they reveal this knowledge to others, and if so, who. Many feel that obligations exist to disclose to family members because the information affects these others as well. Yet this assumption that disclosure is necessary quickly leads to complicated logistical decisions and risk/benefit calculations.

At one extreme, a few people keep the information almost entirely secret—even from immediate family members. "I've told nobody," Simone, the 29-year-old bookkeeper with the HD mutation but no symptoms, said, "except my husband. Not my siblings." But such nondisclosers tended to lack visible symptoms. Visual evidence of the disease could itself reveal the diagnosis.

Many hesitate to tell family members, and would do so only if the latter specifically asked or wished to know. But questions then arise of how that desire for the information, if present, would be ascertained. "I would only tell my mother, father, and sister if they wanted to know," Karen, the lawyer, said about her potential *BRCA*.

Yet within a family, hiding information can be difficult, if not impossible.

Family members can also readily betray each others' confidences. In families, norms operate about both maintenance and betrayal of secrets. Information can also be considered highly fluid, and leak. Francine, an African American woman with HIV whose mother had breast cancer, but who has not herself had symptoms or testing, said:

> I have a family of big mouths—we're going to talk. We can't hold water for nothing. So I need to be very selective whom I tell. If we are told, "Don't tell that person," we won't tell *that* person. But we'll tell somebody else. That's just the way it is.

These norms can be powerful, and hard to change.

WHAT TO TELL

These men and women wrestle, too, with dilemmas of *what* exactly to tell their families—from suspecting that they might have symptoms or the mutation (even if they have already undergone testing), to admitting that they had begun genetic counseling, or gotten the result.

Not all told when they merely *suspected* symptoms. "Do I want to trouble my mother and sister if I have a little twitch in my hand?" asked Oliver, who decided to get a PhD despite having the HD mutation. "Probably not, unless I was fairly certain." He feared that such partial information could serve merely to unnecessarily frighten others.

Individuals may divulge only ambiguous or partial information. A person may say just that he or she had started the counseling process, or planned to do so. Though asymptomatic, Linda, the art teacher, had assumed she might have the HD mutation, and thus

> didn't tell anyone in my family except my little sister that I was testing. She knew I initiated the testing, but she had no idea how far along in the process I was. They thought I was still in the counseling session, though I'd had the blood drawn. I never told my mother or stepmother. The night I found out I was gene negative, I told them. I didn't want anyone . . . watching for signs of how I was doing. I had gotten good at obfuscating things, which I was never good at before.

She wanted to give both herself and others time to get used to the potentiality of a mutation.

Some revealed only that a disease was a possibility—even if it had in fact been diagnosed. They might admit that particular symptoms had developed, but not mention the diagnosis per se. For instance, some said "ataxia" (i.e., problems walking), which was nonspecific, rather than use the label "HD." Similarly, with Alpha, individuals may choose to admit merely to emphysema, rather than their genetic mutation, or they might mention the diagnosis as a possibility but not as confirmed. HD symptoms were purported to be due to multiple sclerosis, alcohol, or "nerves." Families may even encourage and defend obfuscation and deceit. Silence can in fact generate lies, since family members may ask questions. Evelyn, whose husband opposed her testing for HD, and who then consulted a psychic, periodically visited an HD clinic with her affected mother to get information and support.

> My daughter said, "Where are you going?" I said, "The hospital." My kids know I come here. They think it's for cancer: "I'm going on a test study for people who are caregivers for people who are sick." There is always that *little white lie*.

As she suggests, lies vary in size and degree—a "little" versus "a lot," "white" versus "dark"—with different moral implications. A "white" lie suggests innocence and innocuousness—ostensibly making it less ethically problematic.

Though at first many try to hide evidence of a disease, at a certain point visible symptoms can preclude concealment. Walter, on disability from the government because of HD, and going to the gym daily, said, "I try and minimize my movements, so people won't actually notice—so I can try and walk like *normal* people." His goal of being seen as "normal" underscores how HD can otherwise be viewed as "abnormal" and stigmatized.

Patients with Alpha also often wish to hide symptoms of their disorder, but are not always able to do so. The point at which one needs to carry oxygen can be especially troubling, as it publicly signals disease. For breast cancer, too, patients may disclose only partial information—for example, genetic assay results, but not treatments. As we shall see, women with the mutation must decide whether to discuss with others the possibility of prophylactic surgery to remove breasts or ovaries. Reticence can result from expectations of conflict about whether they should choose or decline these frightening procedures. Mildred, who works in finance, has had breast cancer and bilateral mastectomies followed by reconstruction, but has not told her boyfriend that she has the mutation, and that doctors are urging her to excise her ovaries: "I know he would make me go for ovary removal. So, I haven't told him. But the doctors keep asking me about the procedure."

Disclosures also vary in the degrees to which they entail discussions of relevant details. Patients can find longer discussions threatening and overwhelming, and hence eschew these. When Tim, the lawyer, informed his siblings that he had the HD mutation,

> They said "I'm sorry." That was the end of the conversation. There really isn't much left to say. They talk to me a little about getting tested themselves. But there isn't a lot of back and forth about it.

His perception that there "isn't much left to say" suggests not only the painful implications of the diagnosis, but the possibility of *mutual avoidance* of further discussion, given the pain it may cause.

HOW TO TELL

How to disclose proves difficult, too. These men and women have to gauge how to "prepare the ground" in advance, and over time, to minimize responses of shock. Disclosures can range from abrupt to gradual. People may find explicit conversation too threatening, and hence only discuss genetic risks indirectly or implicitly. Indirect discussion can manifest itself in nervous humor. As Bill, the asymptomatic, untested salesman who assumed he would get HD because he resembles his father, said:

> My sister and I never speak about it . . . We probably will have that conversation one day. But I guess *we speak about it without speaking about it*. She might even say, "You know, we can get that disease one day."

I'll say, "I know." But we don't get into details. We'll just talk about our brother [who has HD] . . . and laugh about some of the crazy things he does.

Bill felt they *should* discuss it more, but the topic was too personally threatening—even though doctors have told him that if he hadn't developed HD by now, at age 36, he probably will never do so. Still, given the threat, he saw his family as *delaying* conversations, rather than permanently preventing them. They communicate implicitly—for example, tacitly suggesting mutual anxiety and unease.

Familial reticence can reflect larger cultural or religious tendencies. For instance, taboos about disease and sex can impede discussions about breast cancer. "For my Catholic family out in the Midwest," said Joyce, a Catholic woman with breast cancer who works in a spa, "cancer is a bad word. Talking about breast cancer is like talking about sex. We whispered."

WHY TELL

Issues arise concerning *why* tell or not tell, shaped by *who* was being told. Separate though related reasons to tell or not tell emerge with siblings, parents, children, and extended family (cousins, aunts, and uncles). For many, the very meaning of genetic disease is that other family members are at risk, yet the issues involved in disclosure differ somewhat by categories of relationships. Still, certain questions and concerns are shared.

Once symptoms appear, patients may disclose because to do so has become both unavoidable and essential for coping. Georgia, a journalist with HD symptoms, was told only three years ago by her mother that the disease existed in their family. "I don't really think I can live a normal life," she said about her diagnosis, "unless a few people close to me know." She needed support for the multiple stresses the illness presented.

Generally, family members were thought to have a right to know if they were at risk. Hence, many people disclosed because of perceived responsibilities to the health of their family, to enable these others to pursue appropriate medical care and family planning, if desired. Disclosure could facilitate avoidance of potential transmission of the mutation to future generations. Adult offspring felt that their parents, even if not wanting to find out more about a deleterious gene and deal with it themselves, had an ethical duty to divulge it at some point.

Disclosure can also occur unhesitatingly because it is felt to be a cultural or familial norm. Family members may simply *expect* to be told. Though some families are taciturn, others are far more communicative. Pablo, the Latino artist, said about HD,

> We like telling people, especially in my country. Because one day my father will be dead, and why was he dead? Why didn't they tell us? The whole family knows. We have to be totally . . . honest, or they will never forgive us.

His lack of symptoms or testing also make disclosure easier for him.

For breast cancer, too, disclosure can occur to try to get used to and accept the diagnosis. Karen, the lawyer, revealed her breast cancer to others in order to remind herself of it, help her cope, and "normalize it for myself, and people I interact with. But sometimes, I get the heebie-jeebies around it, related to lesser life expectancy, and stigma."

Historically, over time, these cultural norms and taboos about discussing disease can shift. In the recent confessional culture of Oprah, Jerry Springer, and Facebook, openness may be spreading. An older generation may have kept mutations more of a secret, as these were less understood, and perhaps, as a result, more stigmatized. As Ginger, a 60-year-old medical secretary with Alpha, said, "My father's mother died in the early 1900s. My family doesn't know why. People didn't talk about things then."

WHY NOT TELL

Individuals may decline to tell others, particularly elderly parents, to avoid burdening them. But tensions can then surface. Desires to avoid encumbering others commonly stemmed from prior experiences and interactions, often tinged with guilt. The implications of a disease, since it is genetic, may already overwhelm elderly parents. Charles, an accountant at a large Chicago company and a former smoker, did not tell his mother he had Alpha, though she suspected it. Families may intuit a member's illness, but still not broach the topic—respecting the patient's privacy. He chose to hide the information, but doing so carried a large cost.

> I didn't want to worry her, so just kept silent. She was pretty smart, so I thought she eventually suspected. If it was a nice day, people would go for a walk. I usually wouldn't. She never asked me what the real problem was. She was very perceptive, but also very sensitive. I think she felt that if I didn't want to tell her, she wasn't going to pry. One time, I went to help her wash her windows, and got short of breath. She finally

said, "Look, that's enough." But we never talked about what really was wrong.

Fears of troubling parents may also reflect guilt over having disappointed them in the past. Charles did not want to disturb his mother, but also felt badly about his drinking, which had upset her. "I was a wild young man," he said. "She would never go to sleep until I was home."

Others fear that parents, if told, might also feel remorse—in part because of having transmitted the mutation. Such feelings may not be rational, but persist. Jim, the physician who described some relief at learning he had the HD mutation, nonetheless said:

> It was hard to tell my father, not because of privacy, but because he felt guilty . . . that he might have passed it on . . . the doctors [had] told them they shouldn't have any more children.

Shame, fear of stigma, and desires "to keep up appearances" can also impede disclosure.

Barriers exist not only to disclosure, but to ongoing discussions following revelations of family risk. Joan, the psychiatrist with a strong family history of breast cancer (including her daughter) who herself had no symptoms, but tested to "educate" her family, said:

> Our family doesn't talk about this. If I said to one of my daughters, "What are you doing about your increased risk? Your sister has breast cancer," she would say, "Shut up, Mom." My mother was farm family pioneer stock. I never saw either of my parents sick. If you were sick, you went away, and came back when you were better. You weren't paid attention to when you were sick. I saw that as "death with dignity"—stoicism.

She bemoans this reticence in her parents, but sees it in her daughters as well.

Histories of interaction in a family may also restrain disease communication. Certain family members may be estranged. Sarah, the computer programmer, has an extensive family history of breast cancer. If she had the mutation, she would tell most, but not all, of her family—since she hasn't seen her sister in five years. Several individuals feel that if their disease were not genetic, they simply would not contact estranged family members about it.

Due to long-standing hostilities, family members may interact but not be supportive, further undermining potential disclosures. Francine, whose mother had breast cancer and who has not herself had symptoms or testing, said that in general her mother communicates very little to her.

> She just doesn't talk to me. Because she knows I'm—I wouldn't say judgmental, but straightforward. I'll say, "Why are you telling me this now? Why didn't you tell me before?"

Family members may also announce that they don't want to know—for example, to avoid jeopardizing their insurance. Yet such mutually agreed-upon silence can be hard to maintain. The desire to not be told can also complicate communication and interpersonal dynamics. Family members may have difficulty censoring their conversations. Laura, the graphic designer who inferred her mutation from her genetic counselor's decision to have a trainee sit in, initially didn't want to know her mother's test result. That way, if an insurance company asked, Laura could honestly declare ignorance. Yet genetic results can become the stuff of family conversation in ways that are difficult to screen.

Dilemmas arise, however, of whether one should always respect others' wishes not to be told. Desires for silence can themselves vary from explicit to implicit, and from more to less legitimate. Laura added:

> My mom didn't want to know my sister's results. I thought, "Should I tell my mom that *I* have the mutation?" She never told me *not* to tell her. I didn't know if I was different. Or if she just didn't have the courage to tell me not to tell her. Or if she just assumed I would not tell her.

Laura struggled with these possibilities, illustrating how these decisions are shaped by perceptions of complex family histories. Slowly, she broached the topic with her mother, but highlights the intricate choreography involved—assessing only indirectly her mother's wishes regarding others' disclosures.

> I told her that she had never given me the direct impression that she didn't want me to tell her. I decided to take part in research—so *that* slowly opened the door for the conversation.

In the case of HD, psychiatric symptoms can further hamper disclosure. Individuals have to assess whether family members, because of age or psychological fragility—due in part to possible symptoms—can handle the information. Hence, within a family, certain siblings may know of an individual's test results while others do not, forcing those who know to maintain secrecy. Siblings can vary widely in their perceived emotional vulnerability and resilience, and coping styles—for example, taking more emotional versus rational approaches. Simone, the young asymptomatic bookkeeper who only learned of HD when getting married, said about her siblings, "When bad news comes, they cry and don't ask questions. Immediately, they think of the worst . . . I am definitely more organized and together." Nonetheless she, too, had been upset, surmising her mutation from her counselor's face, though presumably still better able to cope.

Even within a family, shame and stigma can decrease disclosure. Especially with HD, stigmatized psychiatric symptoms can perpetuate concealment. Even without symptoms, HD risk can be too troubling to discuss, in part since psychiatric symptoms can generate discrimination and fear. These symptoms represent loss of control, and are not fully treatable. Psychiatric symptoms can impede disclosure either directly (through symptoms) or indirectly (through stress that ensues). These problems can strain a family, further hampering openness, discussion, and the interactions of parents, spouses, siblings, and children. Consequently, family members may appear insensitive or not fully supportive. HD can also impede good parenting, compounding these difficulties. Parents themselves often encountered problems growing up because of HD in their own families of origin.

WHOM TO TELL

Whether, what, how, and why to tell can vary depending on *who* is told. Certain pros and cons are similar when one is deciding whether to inform siblings, parents, or children. Yet certain differences also surface.

Siblings, for instance, may immediately inform each other, since if one has the gene, the others are also at risk. On the other hand, obstacles related to the nature of the relationship could also block these divulgences. The most troubling disclosure could be to a sibling who might then have the mutation as well. At the same time, siblings may not fully grasp the information and its implications. Yvonne, who eventually had lung transplants and now wants to move to the South, initially understood little about Alpha. She thought that because she had it, her sister would automatically do so as well. Patient education about these issues can take a while: "I thought: now she's going to have it because of me. My sister and I are so close. I felt embarrassed—*that I was the one giving it to everybody.*" She feared being blamed as the messenger of bad news. She suggests here, too, a common misunderstanding that we will explore later: that a genetic disease in a family means that everyone in that family will get it, or have a very high chance of doing so.

Perceived vulnerabilities may also block disclosures to a particular sister or brother. Siblings may simply not want to know because of anxieties concerning their own risks. Simone, who deduced her mutation from her counselor's face, asked her brother, "Would you want to know if I'm positive? He said no."

Thus, a person who learns of a mutation might approach each sibling differently, based partly on perceptions of their resilience and possible early symptoms. Family members were felt to have a right not to know, if they so wished. Yet desires for such ignorance could verge on minimization or denial, which could pose problems, too.

When long-standing tensions exist between siblings, old resentments and hostilities have to be weighed against altruistic concerns for their health and that of their offspring. Yvonne didn't communicate with one brother, but had to overcome that estrangement to inform him and thus his children of her Alpha mutation. The medical benefits of the knowledge compelled her.

> I don't speak to him, but just had to call him: "You've got to get your kids tested." Just because he's a jerk doesn't mean that his kids don't need to find out. If they catch this disease early, they can control it—by never smoking, and by taking Prolastin.

Other siblings may be closer, but simply not feel much ethical obligation to each other. They may interact only casually, and disclose only incidentally, in passing. Charles, the accountant and former smoker who never discussed Alpha with his mother, did not think of telling his brother about it. Prolastin was not yet available, and his family rarely discussed the disease.

> I didn't tell him when I first knew. One day he mentioned that he some-times got short of breath when he played tennis. So I said: "Maybe you ought to get tested." That's the only time we really discussed it.

His brother turned out to have Alpha, too.

Importantly, lack of intra-familial disclosures may occur in part because physicians do not mention or encourage such communication. Charles contin-ued, "I started to see a specialist, who asked if I had any siblings. I never really focused on: 'Maybe my brother's got it, too.' I never really thought: 'Maybe I ought to tell him.'"

TELLING CHILDREN

Patients face troubling questions about disclosures to offspring who are young adults—from late teens to early twenties. Patients rarely if ever told young chil-dren, but had to balance protecting older offspring from the stress of the infor-mation versus helping them cope and possibly take preventive measures.

Disclosures to children can be the most difficult aspect of learning that one has a mutation—far more than one may anticipate. As Albert, the policeman, said about his HD mutation,

> The hardest thing was: how do I tell my kids? I didn't think it was going to be that hard. But I didn't know how they were going to react. I didn't want it to affect their whole lives negatively. One son dwells on it, and thinks he has it.

This son may or may not in fact be manifesting early signs of the disease.

For breast cancer, too, disclosures to offspring can be the most difficult aspect of learning one has a mutation. In general, parents want to avoid worrying young children about information that won't affect these offspring for a long time. Isabelle, as a social worker, is highly sensitive to these issues.

> My kids are 16 and 20, and know I had cancer, but I don't tell them, "Oh, I have this gene, and you might have it too." I haven't really discussed that with them. I try to be reassuring. I think they know I have the gene, but I don't think they realize that they may have it. At some point, I'll have to talk to them—that they should get tested . . . But why make them more anxious and have that hang over their heads—they're still kids, and there are no real benefits.

She made careful risk/benefit calculations about disclosure—the potential harm to them (i.e., anxiety) versus the lack of current benefits to them. She thus divulged to them her risk, but not theirs.

Parents also face challenges in disclosing even to offspring who are 18 years of age or older. After having breast cancer, Beatrice, the Latina math teacher, tested in part for her 18-year-old daughter's sake. But Beatrice, despite her matter-of-factness about medical risks, is less certain about the moral issues involved. She remains unsure how she would have informed her daughter if the test had turned out mutation-positive. "I've never lied to my kids," Beatrice said. "I knew I would tell her, but didn't know how."

WHEN TO TELL FAMILY MEMBERS

Decisions of *when* to tell these family members pose quandaries, too, and get shaped by varying time frames—for example, the life cycle of the family member who is told, and the medical course of the informer's disease. Within families, concerns about disclosure tended to increase at critical life junctures of at-risk individuals—at points of marriage, engagement, or having children.

Many wait to disclose until they have definitive answers to convey in order to resolve uncertainties and family members' consequent worry. As suggested earlier, disclosures to others can thus occur not at the initiation of the testing process, but at its conclusion—when the test result is available.

Others do not readily volunteer the information, but divulge it only if and when asked or forced to do so. Disclosure may occur only after symptoms or treatment become visible and nondisguisable. Ori, the Israeli woman with breast cancer, told her younger daughter only right "before she got home from college, because I was bald." Ori subsequently tested to encourage her offspring to monitor their health more closely.

Though careful plans may be made concerning *how* and *when* to disclose, advanced decisions can be hard to carry out. Instead, the information can simply leak or get blurted out. Ron, the motorcyclist, didn't tell his mother about his HD mutation, partly because his twin had committed suicide. But "then we had an argument and I told her, which is exactly what I did not want to do," he said. Especially without symptoms, the revelation that one carries a mutation can shock others who have seen the disease in other family members as well.

Patients encounter dilemmas, particularly with children, and have to assess the maturity of each child over time. Predicaments arise especially concerning the age at which adolescents should be told. Carmen, the Latina with both breast and thyroid cancer, decided that she would disclose her mutation to her daughter "as soon as she starts getting her own breasts. Sometimes she asks about my scars. I tell her, 'Mommy was sick.' One day, I'm going to have to explain it." Yet many parents continually seek to postpone that fateful day.

Relatedly, a patient may disclose to children in waves—often spread out over a decade or more—since offspring may be different ages. However, patients' perceptions of a child's ability and need to understand a genetic risk and its implications may not be wholly accurate, distorted by parents own needs or desires to minimize or deny the illness and protect their kids.

Though young children may feel overwhelmed by a parent's illness, utter silence can hurt as well. Ongoing concealment may end only inadvertently when children accidentally discover the information. At least initially, children may be too young to comprehend, but later might be able to do so—though parents might not recognize this change. Bonnie, the 24-year-old at risk of breast cancer, said that her mother had at first hidden the diagnosis, and discussed it only when Bonnie confronted her about this silence. Disclosure can be indirect and involuntary. "I was 12," she said. "I walked in while she was

changing and saw her scar. 'How'd you get that?' She was like, 'Well, you know
. . .' She tried to explain it the best she could."

Such leaks may be impossible to prevent. Joyce, who worked in a spa, resided
with her 8-year-old daughter and was receiving chemotherapy for breast cancer.
Joyce fears what would happen, if she dies, to her daughter. She does not think
her daughter would handle the information well (that Joyce, though without
the *BRCA 1/2* mutation, had breast cancer and a strong family history). But
Joyce realizes that the information may nonetheless be leaking out.

> I haven't talked to her directly. She might have overheard me on the phone.
> We live in a one-bedroom apartment, and there isn't tons of privacy. I was
> sleeping with my wig on, for fear that she would wake up. What if I die?

A few learned about their risk as relatively young children, and vary in
how they later viewed their parents' decision to disclose at that point. Certain
information can be helpful, even if frightening. Roger, who tested after he drove
his car off the road, said:

> I was 10 when I first found out about HD. I was very stressed out about it,
> depressed, unable to sleep . . . It was really tough, hearing that I was at risk
> for it. My mother told me that she had had children because there
> might eventually be a cure . . . it was very tough—the fact that I might get
> a disease like my mother . . . Me and my sister were able to understand
> at 10 . . . My mother first showed symptoms when we were eight or nine.
> My aunt also had HD, and was 15 years older than my mother, so they
> were able to tell us that "it's probably going to be like *that*."

He thinks it was appropriate that he was given information when he was.

> Looking back, it was right. She just told me about the disease so that
> I could understand. My pediatrician did the same. He could have told me
> all these facts. But he just told us in a way we could understand at ten: that
> there is a fifty-fifty chance, so we were able to understand about our own
> risk, and what to expect with our mother.

Here again, *who* is told can shape *what* is told (e.g., young children can be given
age-appropriate information). Ironically, the fact that the disease is genetic, and
thus visible in other kin, may make it less abstract and more understandable,
though still frightening.

In retrospect, others felt they were told too early—that they were too young
for the information they were given. They distinguished between knowing

about the disease in general (i.e., that it affected a parent) versus knowing that one was at risk oneself. "It was a lot to put on my shoulders," said Antonia, who learned about her HD risk at age 15 and subsequently became a neuroscientist. "But my dad thought I was up to the task. It made me older than I should have been. I grew up very young." She now feels that 15-year-olds should not be told. Yet the age at which one is old enough may not be clear.

For breast cancer, too, children may have difficulty comprehending the disease in a parent and its implications for them. Bonnie, who as a girl saw her mother's illness, reported:

> My mother had breast cancer when I was eight. Around 12, I started understanding it more, and coming to terms with it. As I got older, I learned in biology classes that it's hereditary.

To determine when one is "mature enough" is difficult since children vary widely in their emotional and cognitive development. For adolescents, the meanings of a parent's disease can also gradually change from a parent being sick to being at risk oneself.

In contrast, others felt that they were told *too late*. Disclosure may not occur until an offspring's marriage—transpiring only then so that prospective spouses might know about it before they consider having children. Simone, the book-keeper who only learned of HD when getting engaged, said:

> Growing up, I was aware that MS was in the family. Then, I got engaged to my husband. My mother said—like she had been keeping a family secret—that it wasn't actually MS, but HD. She wanted to tell me before we got married, because she didn't want my husband to marry into the family when *this* was there.

Parents might not tell adult children at risk who might then have children, unaware of the risk. Keeping HD secret, and then disclosing too late, can incur subsequent resentment. Simone was angry both at her mother's nondisclosure and view of the disease as shameful:

> Now, when we're 24, we find out that they've been *lying* to us our whole lives. I've been dating my husband since I was 16. So, if she wanted to make sure we didn't get serious, she should have told me way back then.

With breast cancer as well, offspring may be angry because they feel they were told too late. Due to long-standing family dynamics, parents may have difficulty resolving conflicts between protecting versus informing offspring, and do so poorly. Susie, who worked for an HIV organization and had benign ovarian cysts but no breast cancer or mutation, found out late about an extensive family history of the cancer: "My dad and his mother and sister never talked to me about it. That pissed me off. Maybe they were scared. I got an email from my cousin, who had decided to tell everybody."

FAMILY REACTIONS

As we saw earlier, responses to first learning one's genetic risk vary from fear and avoidance to acceptance, testing, and further disclosure. At times, the health threats that family members feel can limit their sympathy for each other. Families—themselves all at risk of the disease—may fail to support fully, and may even ostracize an ill member. The diagnosis can threaten and disturb other family members, distancing them from each other. Dorothy, wheeling a metal oxygen tank and awaiting lung transplants, felt that since being diagnosed with Alpha, she has received little comfort from her family. "No one has said, 'Gee, this is awful. I'm really sorry.'"

Children's reactions may be more complex, given various stages of cognitive and emotional development and dependence on parents. Offspring may range from angry and sad to appreciative and supportive. Yet adult children may react adversely to bad news, and simply not want to talk about it. Diane, the Spanish teacher who woke up to learn she had had a mastectomy, found that her 37- and 38-year-old daughters—for whose benefit she had tested for the breast cancer mutation after she had the disease—did not want to discuss it at all.

> They don't even want to approach the subject. I have tried. One said her life was stressful enough. She didn't ask me about the results. Since it was negative, I mentioned it. She said quickly, without wanting to discuss it, "Oh, good."

Diane's own stressful cancer and treatment no doubt frightened her daughters.

Since offspring may distance themselves, parents may simply not know their adult children's reactions. They just do not discuss these issues together. Albert, the policeman who tested to guide his children's reproductive decisions but was too late in doing so, said that his oldest son now doesn't mention HD to him. "We haven't talked about it in months. I don't ask him how he's feeling about it. He won't bring it up." The implications of Albert's test result—that his children may have already passed the mutation on to his grandchildren—are too disturbing.

Adult children may also hide their reactions from their parents—outwardly behaving supportively, while inwardly feeling distraught. As Sherry, a waitress with breast cancer but no family history or testing, said, "I told my oldest son, 'I was so happy the way your brother took it.' He said, 'The way he took it? He got off the phone with you, and called me, crying his eyes out, cussing.'"

TELLING EXTENDED FAMILY MEMBERS

Separate though related quandaries emerge of whether to contact extended family members—from cousins, nieces, and nephews to "long-lost" relatives who may unknowingly be at risk. Such contact can constitute the only notification these long-lost kin receive that they are in danger. Yet compared with immediate family, moral obligations and social rules here are often vague, since these relationships are more fluid and far less socially prescribed. Consequently, these decisions necessitate the complex weighing of one's own right to privacy versus one's responsibilities to these extended kin.

In general, ethical obligations are clearer to immediate than to more distant family, but ambiguities arise. Social obligations to distant families may be far less because, as evolutionary biologists point out, one shares fewer genes with extended than with immediate family members. Therefore, biologists argue, the bonds of responsibility and concern are diminished as well. The greater the genetic connection, the greater the social and moral bonds, since, as the biologist Richard Dawkins avers, genes seek to replicate themselves.

Yet here the presence or absence of one specific mutation, not the overall percentage of one's genes, is important. I may share only 1/16th of my genes with my first cousin once removed (my cousin's child), but that small fraction is critical if it contains a lethal or treatable mutation. Whereas I might otherwise communicate little if at all with these extended relatives, genetics heightens the reasons to do so. An individual may only learn of his or her risk of having a mutation after being informed of that fact by a long-lost relative. As suggested earlier, one person's disclosure is another person's initial discovery of risk. Such communication can be vital, if not morally obligatory.

The odds that such discourse occurs may be tenuous, due to a series of social and psychological obstacles. Surprisingly, disclosures to extended family members have received little if any attention. Yet these issues will be increasingly important as more genetic markers are identified—even if these have only partial penetrance or predictiveness. Indeed, the potential mixed and ambiguous meanings of markers—that they may have only limited clinical utility—can exacerbate difficulties in deciding about seeking, receiving, and interpreting such results.

Individuals here range considerably in whether they try to contact extended relatives, and how, what, and when. A patient may hesitate to inform nieces and nephews—who may be young adults, just starting their independent lives—and leave these disclosures to aunts and uncles. Many individuals thus tell their siblings, but not the latter's children, deferring to these parents' judgment. A woman may tell her brother about her breast cancer only because he has daughters (since their risk may increase as a result). But quandaries also arise of *when* exactly to tell such a brother or his daughters—whether and when to inform young adults. Generally, one feels more responsibility to one's own offspring than to the offspring of one's siblings (nieces and nephews)—for whom one's sibling has primarily responsibility. Mildred, who works in finance and had breast cancer, the mutation, prophylactic mastectomies, and breast reconstruction but had not told her boyfriend about her mutation, added:

> Someday, I'm going to have to tell my brother, because he needs to tell his daughters. It's not my place to tell my nieces. They are not even 20. I would wait until they get older. I don't have a specific date or time. It's pretty heavy to tell a young girl: "Have your ovaries removed."

Yet even if not close, extended family members may proceed to contact each other—despite obstacles of social or geographic distance. Altruism can prompt patients to go to great extents to notify long-lost relatives whom they know barely, if at all. Still, the information may not be acknowledged or well-received. Genetic information may get disseminated by email, and lack sufficient details or context. Susie, who worked for an HIV organization and had benign ovarian cysts but no breast cancer or mutation, described how she had learned about the disease in her family:

> My cousin in California emailed me, saying she had just found she had one of the *BRCA* genes . . . She talked about various surgeries, which scared me. I'm not used to getting medical updates by email. She's wonderful, generous, open. But I was shocked. I didn't know what it was, or what to do about it. So I sat on it for a long time—two years.

While Susie was glad to be contacted by this cousin, others do not even consider informing extended relatives who may be at risk. To avoid such contact can help one minimize the impact of the disease. Karen, the lawyer, has sought neither testing after her breast cancer nor contact with any relatives about the disease. "My cousins are all dead. There is a next generation, but I have not thought to find out about them," she said. "It's willful, reckless ignorance on my part."

Other individuals consider or attempt reaching out to distant relatives, but encounter obstacles. Patients may simply not be in close touch with such relatives, or know how to find them. These relatives may be hard to locate, which also thwarts the ability to obtain a complete family history.

Many people simply know little about their extended family, further justifing noncommunication. Geographical distance can perpetuate social distance. Conversely, geographic proximity can increase social closeness. But even after being contacted, additional communication may not occur. The phenomenon of long-lost relatives can be mutually fueled and reinforced. "It would be like contacting a *stranger*," Karl said, concerning HD in his family. "We're connected in having a family history, but I don't have an emotional connection to them." He underscored the distinction between biological versus emotional links— particularly concerning a disease with psychiatric symptoms that can impair interactions.

Similarly, some know of cousins, but simply do not feel close enough to warrant disclosure—raising questions of what determines this threshold of communication, and how one assesses it.

Individuals have to balance upsetting versus warning relatives. Genetic information, especially if it is not definitive, is often easier to not mention. Anna, for instance, a secretary in her forties, has diabetes and a strong family history of breast cancer, and a breast lump that turned out to be benign. But she did not tell her cousins about the lump, since the diagnosis was not yet clear. She valued not scaring them more than warning them.

Misunderstandings about test results can also mold these decisions. Samantha, the actress with breast cancer, lacked the mutation, but her doctors recommended that her cousins be carefully monitored. Still, she did not tell these relatives,

> because they're going to worry, and then *cause cancer just by worrying about it!* One cousin is a worrywart. Mammograms are full of radiation. And I don't think I got cancer because of genetics. If got a positive result, I would have told.

She balances here her sense of her cousins' emotional vulnerability, and her belief that her cancer resulted from the environment, not genes.

An individual may also avoid telling extended family members because of concerns that these relatives would then be too solicitous or overbearing, further reminding the patient of the disease and its worst possible implications. Vera, the Asian executive with breast cancer and a mutation, did not tell her extended family because she feared that they would all visit and be *too* present. Desires for independence can thus perpetuate silence.

Only my immediate family knows. Otherwise, everybody would have visited me in the hospital. It would have been crazy—too much to deal with. Everybody is calling my mother now every day. I need a break.

Those who decide to disclose to extended relatives then have to assess *how* to do so. Letters and emails can be troubling to both send and receive, because the information may be out of context and utterly unanticipated. The ideal tone of such missives can be hard to achieve. For conveying this complex and sensitive information, email is increasingly used, but limited. Face-to-face interactions may be best, but sometimes avoided because of upsetting emotions.

WHAT TO TELL EXTENDED FAMILY

People face dilemmas of *what* to divulge to not only immediate family, but more distant relatives as well. Social distance can lessen the amount of information conveyed. Moreover, concerns within immediate families that the information is too stressful may lessen with more distant relatives. Patients may expect, too, that distant relatives will provide less social support than would close family. Distance can thus be mutually reinforced.

Distant family members may also be unsure how to reply to the information, and what kind of support to offer. Given various obstacles, warnings to long-lost relatives may get ignored—letters are discarded or put away, all but forgotten. As Evelyn, whose husband opposed her testing, and who then had consulted a psychic, said:

The day I learned about HD in our family, my father gave me a letter from my mother's first cousin saying someone had HD, was there anyone else in the family showing signs? This letter had been written years before. It had been in his drawer three, four years. My parents had ignored it, and not gotten back to the writer, which I found appalling: someone in our family is reaching out for help! You knew this was in the family, and you just chose not to tell us!

This secrecy contributed to her desire for knowledge, and for getting tested despite her husband's opposition.

Disagreements can occur about not only whether to inform nonimmediate family members, but how to *reply* to the information once received. With distant (versus close) relatives, the social and hence ethical bonds are generally weaker, resulting from, and leading to, less knowledge of these relatives' reactions—even whether they then get tested.

Extended family members may simply not want such communication—refusing to deal with the information and not responding even when urged to do so. Roger, who tested mutation-positive for HD after his car swerved off the road, said, "My sister tried to contact our cousin three to four times, but he won't return her calls. He's probably scared."

Family members may explicitly instruct members *not* to inform particular relatives. Simone, who learned of HD in her family only when she got engaged, said that her uncle "told my mother, but didn't want his kids to know. I was not to speak to them about it." Simone railed against this restraint.

In short, while distance in the relationship may reduce the sense of responsibility to aid one another's health, genetic information often prompts reconsideration of these norms. With a mutation, which may be shared, many people feel that these social bonds should increase much more than otherwise.

TELLING IN-LAWS

Tensions emerge, too, in telling in-laws. Not at risk of the disease themselves, in-laws can nevertheless be emotionally affected by a mutation in a family. However, they may misunderstand, be prejudiced, and even disapproving of a family—and its genetics—into which they have married. The discovery that a daughter- or son-in-law has a mutation can prompt stigma and discrimination. Mary, the housewife, had early symptoms of HD and was terrified that her in-laws would find out and condemn her.

> Even before I knew I had this, my husband's family was very judgmental . . . Now, it's even harder. His father said, "I wish I had a daughter-in-law that smiled." Their house is spic and span. I don't clean. So I don't ever want them to know about the HD. If they found out, they would try to get my kids: "I knew she was crazy."

However, odd configurations of concealment and silence can then ensue. She didn't want to tell her in-laws, so she agreed with her husband that she wouldn't tell *her* family of origin either. Yet she then surreptitiously told her family.

Labyrinths of secrecy can result—as to who else possesses the information. Mary continued:

> If my husband knew that so many people in *my* family knew, he would be upset. I didn't tell him that I told my sister. He figured it out; and *I got caught in a web of lies*. I don't know whom I told and didn't tell. She was laughing at inside jokes—maybe I tripped, or did something wacko—that

she could only have gotten if she knew . . . He still thinks no one else knows. But my sister told her husband. He knows that my husband doesn't know that he knows.

Thus not only knowledge of a mutation, but also knowledge of who else has the knowledge, can be concealed. But such secrecy can be hard to maintain, necessitating further ruses. Mary tried to disguise her symptoms in part by smoking marijuana, and blaming any questionable behavior on the drug: "Everything HD-related I do—tripping or falling—I blame on pot . . . I can just say I'm stoned."

Yet as symptoms develop they can be hard to hide, making such silence increasingly difficult. In-laws can be unsympathetic. Patients may confront misunderstanding and judgment from siblings' in-laws as well. As Roger, who tested when he veered his car off the road, added about his HD:

My sister's in-laws don't know I have the disease. They're closed-hearted, and wouldn't understand. The last time I saw them, they asked me why I'm eating so much. My sister said, "Oh, his metabolism has always been high." But next time, my other signs are going to be much more obvious. I can't hide it much longer.

THIRD-PARTY DISCLOSURES

As suggested earlier, a patient's diagnosis might be disclosed not by that individual but by another, without the patient's permission. An informed individual may tell other family members, constituting "secondary" or third-party disclosure. Disagreements can occur as to who should or should not be told.

A few patients, in disclosing to others, specifically forbade the listener from spreading the information further. Evelyn, whose father had for several years hidden a letter from a relative about HD, and whose husband opposes her testing, described the continued secrecy in her family: "My aunt was adamant: do not tell my children." Evelyn agreed to keep silent, since she felt her relationship with these cousins was not close enough to obligate such communication.

Yet many individuals either fail to foresee or try to forestall such third-party revelations. Alternatively, such secondary disclosures may occur despite a patient's efforts to prevent these.

When such extended disclosure occurs, despite attempts to block it, patients, as well as those who were told by the patient and then informed a third party, have to decide how to react. Information, once leaked, can spread even wider, taking on a life of its own. The secondary discloser may have sworn the third party to secrecy, but in vain. Within families, the flow of information and knowledge of this flow can become complex. Trust has been betrayed, but the consequences may or may not be serious or harmful. As Sherry, the waitress with breast cancer, said:

> My oldest son told his father-in-law—a doctor, who then called me. Then my son called me. I told him that his father-in-law had phoned me. He said, "I'm so angry at him! *He wasn't supposed to tell you that I told him!*"

TESTING FAMILY MEMBERS

People face dilemmas about not only whether to disclose genetic information to family members, but whether to encourage these relatives to pursue testing, treatment, and prevention. A patient who discloses to relatives must then decide whether to push them to test, and if so, to what degree and when. As we saw earlier, in deciding whether to undergo an assay or not, individuals often confront family members' needs and pressures. Individuals tested not only because they perceived on their own that to do so would help kin, but because these relatives explicitly *requested*, and even pushed for an assay. While decisions to test oneself entail weighing altruism against autonomy, decisions to pressure others to test pose dilemmas about the degrees of responsibility, paternalism, and authority one feels towards others. Conflicts arise since decisions of how much to push vary with each disease, based in part on epidemiology, preventability, and treatment. Adults have to balance competing desires and responsibilities against perceptions of these others' rights. This pressure may prompt a person to undergo testing, or it may only trigger resentment.

At times, such encouragement could be straightforward and noncontentious. For HD, some want a parent tested so that neither they nor their kids will have to undergo testing themselves. Evelyn said to her mother, "I want you to be tested for *us*." If her mother was negative, Evelyn's kids would not be at risk.

For breast cancer as well, a mutation-positive test could trigger desires to test a parent—to see which side of the family the marker came from, and therefore who else might be in danger. If she had been positive, Beatrice, who assayed her genes in part because she had finished having children, would have tested her mother to know whether to contact cousins on the other side of her family: "If it's from her, then we don't go any further. She was an only child. But if she's negative, I have to call my cousins on my father's side." As a math teacher, Beatrice felt more comfortable than many other interviewees pondering these decision trees.

Yet these assessments of others' risk through third party testing can incite conflict. These third parties may refuse testing, viewing the risks and benefits of the information differently than do the two other parties involved. Given the tradeoffs, a relative may feel imposed upon, and have to balance his or her own rights and desires against perceived obligations to family members.

Contentious issues remain concerning how much to exhort adult offspring or family members to undergo testing. In part, the decisions hinge on what could be done if a genetic mutation were found. Yet even here, family members often dispute whether the advantages of knowing indeed outweigh the disadvantages. Many adult children choose, at least for long periods of time, not to be tested. Parents then have to decide how much to continue to push. Ethical quandaries can ensue in balancing one individual's right to postpone testing against another's desire to know whether the first individual has a mutation. Finances and differing insurance plans can impel a person to goad a family member to test. Yet usually at a certain point, when meeting with resistance or refusals to test, such pressure eventually ends, though both sides can remain bitter. Arlene, a nurse in her forties who had also studied religion, had breast cancer in her family—including her sister—but was untested and asymptomatic. She said:

> My sister chose not to do genetic testing. That's her choice, *but it affects the entire family*. It would have cost *me* $3,500. If she tests, then everybody in the whole family can test for $350. If she had been positive, and I had been negative, it would put my odds way down. I offered her the co-pay of $250. But she said no. It's a control issue. Some people would rather not know. *Yet you have to look at the overall good of the family, over the good of one person*. I had to respect her right. But, if she chooses not to have it done, I pray that my insurance company would either let me test, or just approve me to have a bilateral prophylactic mastectomy.

Those who already have had symptoms may face less discrimination, and have their insurance cover testing costs. Free and anonymous assays are often available through research studies, but family members may still refuse these. Other family members may feel powerless to alter this decision. Ginger, the medical secretary, had a son who was a geneticist and refused testing because of the emotional and logistical threats of having Alpha. "He's worried about finding out he's got an abnormal gene," she said. "I can't force him." In the end, the decision was his, but she continued to urge him.

A parent may push for offspring to test in part because of regrets over having transmitted or exacerbated the disease. Barbara, a part-time professor in her fifties, said that due to her Alpha,

When I see my daughter get a cold, I feel guilt. I smoked around her. I'm trying to be forceful, but the doctors are very aware that testing is not something to do lightly, because of potential discrimination. They think maybe we should wait, and let her decide for herself.

Despite the doctors' remonstrances, Barbara remains worried and pushes, in part because of her remorse about having exposed her daughter to harm.

In the end, many demur from trying to sway other family members—even adult offspring—because of perceived limitations in the ability to do so. Dorothy, the former TV producer, carting oxygen and awaiting lung transplantation, tried to persuade a male cousin to check for Alpha. But given the low probability of her success and possible negative repercussions, she ultimately gave up. "He's in denial," she said. "He just can't accept that a horrific genetic disease could be in his family. He came over with a book of Old Testament sayings and said, 'Pray for a miracle.'"

Questions emerge, too, of how much to try to affect the degrees to which others engage in preventative behaviors. With Alpha, an individual who learns that he or she is at risk or has the mutation can then avoid smoking and environmental exacerbants. For breast cancer, an individual with a mutation can pursue more vigilant medical follow-up, and consider prophylactic surgery. Adult offspring with the HD mutation can consider PGD prior to having children themselves.

For Alpha, testing relatives is important because of the rarity and hence low awareness of the disease, but dilemmas then arise of whom to encourage (cousins, nieces, and nephews) as well as when, how, and how much to do so. Some readily seek to test their offspring, who may then learn their gene status and make appropriate lifestyle choices (e.g., not smoking). A mutation-positive test result can potentially motivate prevention. Betty, the designer with Alpha who carries an oxygen concentrator, said, "It is good for a kid to know: if you're a chemist, wear a mask. Pollution makes things worse. When you have a bronchial infection, get antibiotics, so you don't have scar tissue." The burden and inconvenience of the disease impels her to urge others to engage in prevention.

"Whenever my granddaughter has a cold, I think she has Alpha," said Barbara, who feels guilty that she had smoked around her children. "When she was born, she had jaundice, which is an indication. I'm hyper-vigilant, looking at her." Conversely, a mutation-negative result can lower anxieties.

Yet testing children can lead to discrimination and distress. A child found to be a carrier for Alpha can do little about it, and faces potential stigma.

At times, an individual may seek to assay others against their will. Some patients quickly tested their offspring without considering the potential harms.

Many saw their decisions only in retrospect as premature or ill-advised. Testing of children can also result from lack of understanding or education about the genetics involved. Gilbert, an electronics factory worker with Alpha, said:

> As soon as I found out, I tested my children. I never gave a thought to privacy, or whether an employer could find [out]. It wasn't a conscious decision. Is it more important to know your status as an Alpha or to worry about privacy?

Given these disadvantages of directly testing children, other patients sought alternatives. With Alpha, labs can assess an individual's blood levels of the enzyme Alpha-1 antitrypsin directly, rather than the presence of the mutation itself. This phenotypic (rather than genotypic) gauge can help determine whether the individual has the mutation, and if so, whether they are homozygous or heterozygous. But this test is not necessarily accurate. Nonetheless, patients may analyze their offspring's blood for this enzyme. With Alpha, all of a homozygote's parent's children are by definition at least heterozygous (i.e., carriers), and hence at risk of symptoms themselves. Whether these children are homozygous or heterozygous depends on whether the patient's spouse has the mutation or not. (As described earlier, heterozygous carriers may have symptoms, though less severely than homozygotes.)

Some seek to test their offspring so that the latter will know before having children themselves. Benjamin, as an engineer, was very aware of the statistical odds involved:

> I had my kids before I knew. I tested their Alpha level. It was in the median range, so they're probably carriers. The odds are about 3% that their spouse is also a carrier, though neither of their spouses has been tested.

He checked their Alpha levels because they had asthma. Such a level may not lead to discrimination—even in their medical chart—since a carrier's level can still be normal. Nevertheless, it may signal that a person is at risk, and could thus potentially attract insurers' concerns.

To avoid the disadvantages of testing a child directly, others seek to test their spouses. For Alpha, as a recessive gene, if a homozygote patient's spouse is a mutation carrier, 50% of their offspring will be homozygous. If the spouse has no mutation, offspring will be heterozygote, not homozygote, and may have no symptoms. Therefore, some patients tried to assay their spouses rather than their children. Gilbert, the factory worker, added "I had my younger son test his wife for Alpha when he got married. She doesn't have the mutation. They will test the new baby and find out whether she's a carrier." His daughter-in-law agreed to test because she could do so anonymously through a research study.

Yet problems arise because parents may be divorced, and awkward scenarios can then ensue. Jennifer, the schoolteacher diagnosed with Alpha after her son was, does not want her grandchildren tested because of possible discrimination. Her daughter-in-law could be tested instead, but has divorced Jennifer's son. Jennifer now plans to test her grandchildren herself.

> For years I tried to have my daughter-in-law tested, so that we would have some idea about the children. But she doesn't get how serious it might be. They have now divorced. I had the children with me for a week, but was remiss, and didn't have the testing kits from the Alpha Foundation that are guaranteed private. I will have these when I see the kids at Christmas.

The fact that she wants to test them, and almost did so without their parents' knowledge and consent, is troubling. What exactly she would do with the information—whether she would tell the children the results, and if so, when and how—is not clear. Again, genetics creates difficult and unforeseen scenarios.

Community organizations may also make recommendations about whether additional people should be tested. One major Alpha organization at first advocated that everyone at risk be assayed, but then altered this position because of discrimination concerns.

Some people want to test *deceased* relatives. After his twin committed suicide, Ron faced this issue, which precipitated complex intra-familial tensions, anger, and guilt. Quandaries emerged over who had the rights to take genetic samples from the deceased, and what to do if kin disagreed.

> I managed to get a DNA sample off the coroner. I can't actually do anything with it because the sample is part of what my brother "is," so is owned by his wife. She's chosen not to have it tested. It's a difficult situation. If we knew one way or another, it would give us some indication of whether his children are at risk. They're nine and 11—getting to the stage where she has to make decisions whether she's going to tell them about HD or not. At the moment, they know nothing about it. She's remarried, trying to ignore the situation. She's a Baptist, and decided that God told her it was the right time to test the sample. But then she decided not to do it.

Guilt and complex family dynamics can complicate these issues. As Ron continued:

> She threw my brother out of the house. That's partly why she doesn't want to test his DNA. If he was positive, it's not only a problem for the kids, but also that he got sick and she threw him out.

These dilemmas of family testing and disclosure emerge prominently, too, with other disorders—for example, sickle-cell disease. For that diagnosis as well, testing can occur without disclosure. Roberta, the former nursing student with breast cancer, said that her daughter-in-law was a sickle-cell carrier. Roberta's granddaughter was tested for this blood disorder but not told the result.

> My daughter-in-law has the trait. My son does not. They wondered about my granddaughters. When one granddaughter was five, they found out she has the trait. Now, she's 11. It doesn't affect her health at all. When she gets married, if she needs to know, they'll tell her. But should she be told when she's 18, or wait until she's married? The family rule is always: if you ask a question, you get an answer. But if you don't need to know, we don't bring it up.

If the information can prompt prevention or treatment, testing and disclosure appear potentially important, perhaps even mandatory. Roberta also suggested here the presence of family "rules" concerning such openness and secrecy.

Yet degrees of biological and social closeness to a relative also shape degrees to which testing is encouraged—particularly with extended family members with whom obligations are less clear and strong. Dorothy, the former TV producer awaiting transplants, feels she has a responsibility to inform relatives about their Alpha risk, but not necessarily to follow up. Even with siblings, she feels she should encourage testing only slightly: "You just send them the information. That's the end of it. You can't push more than that." Similarly, Benjamin, the engineer, tested his own kids but not his cousins for Alpha, and accepts the latter's refusals.

Others, due to their own ordeals, do not contact or pressure relatives to test—particularly extended family members. Carol, who after having breast cancer and the mutation aggressively underwent prophylactic removal of her breasts and ovaries despite her boyfriend's objections, feels restrained in how much she can encourage others to pursue their own health:

> My cousins should be tested, but don't even go to the doctor. I should push more. I could wind up saving a life. But I haven't called. I have other things going on. Many of us could help save someone's life, but instead have this and that to do. At the end of the day, I'm tired.

OTHERS' PREVENTIVE BEHAVIOR

People thus face dilemmas about how much responsibility they have to aid the health of others—to push family members not only to test, but to follow preventive health behaviors. Since prevention can be hard, questions arise of how much to try to change others' lives and activities. Relatives may balance benefits and costs of prevention very differently, producing conflicts. As Gilbert, the factory worker, said about his brother's risk for Alpha:

> My brother quit smoking, but hangs out at a smoky local bar. God knows why he would risk second-hand smoke. But he wants to live his life and enjoy himself. If he loses a couple of years, so be it.

In the end, Gilbert disagrees with but accepts his brother's priorities: "His social life revolves around those bars. If you took that out of his life, it would not be a good life."

A consensus emerged that ultimately, relatives have a right to continue to engage in unhealthy behavior—but that the decision should at least be conscious and informed. Gilbert similarly tried to push his children to quit smoking, but to no avail.

> They are carriers and smoke. I talk to them until I'm blue in the face. They can't give it up. I finally decided to stop badgering them. If it costs them five years of life, they know the consequences.

Beliefs about the precise benefits and efficacy of certain preventive health behaviors may also vary. Individuals often confront difficult personal tradeoffs about their own mutation and that of others. Diane, the Spanish teacher who woke up from surgery with an unexpected mastectomy, hoped in vain that her daughter would follow more alternative treatments.

> I believe in a holistic approach, more than stuffing yourself with antibiotics. My oldest daughter drinks wine every day, which is really bad. She should abstain from dairy, chocolate, alcohol, smoking . . .

Yet generally, in the end, these interviewees concluded that they could do little to alter others' refusal or denial.

Parents may feel frustrated that their advice is ignored, which can be part of larger intra-familial tensions. A parent cannot control adult offspring's health decisions, and pushing too hard can prompt resentment. Kate, a former nurse in her seventies, said:

> I've been trying to get my two daughters tested for Alpha. They're not interested, and they smoke. I say, "Burning up those sticks again . . ." "Awww, mom!" My youngest daughter is now smoking *more*.

PROVIDERS' INPUT

Clinicians can also shape these disclosure and testing decisions. Yet while physicians may try to affect whether and what information gets disclosed, their perspectives may conflict with those of the patient. As Evelyn, whose father had hidden a relative's letter about HD in a drawer, said, "My doctor talked to my mother, grandfather, aunt, and uncle, and they all decided *not* to tell the kids. That was so wrong!"

But providers were often seen as falling short because they did not prepare patients to address disclosure decisions—that is, who or what to tell.

Questions also arise of whether providers ever have a responsibility to notify a patient's relatives about a serious genetic risk, if the patient refuses to do so. This scenario of pitting patients' rights to confidentiality against physicians' broader social obligations arose in the Tarasoff case,[22] in which a psychiatrically ill university student murdered his girlfriend after disclosing thoughts about doing so to his psychologist. The psychologist notified the campus police but not the girlfriend, and was found liable. Most interviewees in this book opposed a doctor breaching confidentiality, particularly with HD, and felt that physicians were obligated not to do so. "It's supposed to be confidential just like with a lawyer or a priest," Tim, the lawyer with the HD mutation, said. "I don't think doctors can do otherwise." Yet judges have ruled that physicians at times have a duty to warn third parties about genetic risks.[23]

A few individuals draw finer distinctions. Gilbert, the factory worker with Alpha, feels that doctors should tell siblings, but not spouses. He recognizes that doctors could still face challenges, however, concerning how they learned of the patient's risk.

> I would support doctors telling the siblings. The catch-22 is: if these siblings ask the doctor, "Why do you think I might have it?" then the doctor is faced with, "Well, I tested your brother, and he's got it." That's not kosher: breaking confidentiality. I think the doctor can only say, "Well, I have reason to believe you may have this particular problem, and I recommend that you get a test."

IN SICKNESS AND IN HEALTH: DISCLOSURES IN DATING

At-risk men and women who are single and seeking long-term relationships face added challenges. Dating is critical to establishing an ongoing supportive relationship and having children, yet in these contexts, disclosures of genetic information can be fraught. Painful rejections can occur.

Spouses are important sources of social support for maintaining long-term physical and mental health[24,25] and coping with diseases.[26,27,28] Unfortunately, not all spouses cope well with their partners' illness, and declining health can lessen marital quality, and thus social support.[29,30] How, then, do individuals pick a partner who will hopefully stay with them in sickness and in health?

Surprisingly, in general, little research has been done on whether health issues affect dating, and, if so, when and how. Several psychosocial studies have explored aspects of dating and spouse selection, suggesting the existence of "assortative" mating, whereby people tend to choose spouses similar to themselves. This research has examined sociodemographic factors in selection of prospective mates, focusing on age, race, social class,[31,32] and physical attributes such as weight, height,[33] and attractiveness.[34] Studies have suggested that premarital relationships may evolve early, or progressively over long periods.[35] But research has neglected the potential roles of medical or genetic issues.

In dating, two members of a couple decide whether to make unique and extraordinary investments into each other's lives. Unlike friendships, dating could lead to offspring, raising the stakes enormously. Yet in dating, at least initially, the two individuals are usually strangers. They then closely and carefully assess each other.

How do two such individuals broach the topic of genetic risks that may be stigmatized, and cause disease and death in themselves and potentially their future offspring? What challenges do they face, and how do they address these?

These men and women struggle with a series of conundra of whether to disclose to dates, and if so when, how, what, and why. Many fear or face rejection. Questions arise of what ethical obligations, if any, they have to disclose, and how to decide.

To avoid these dilemmas, some choose to forego dating altogether. Even in the absence of genetic risk, dating is difficult, involving fragile and confusing choreographies; mutual trust and social, and thus ethical, bonds develop to become the most important of one's life. Disclosures of mutations can exacerbate these challenges.

Whether to Tell Dates

Once these individuals decide to get married, they generally feel obligated to tell their prospective spouses. Many value privacy, but feet it is now limited, especially since their future children's health may be at stake. As Kate, the former nurse with Alpha and two grown daughters, said:

> If you're going to get married, your genetic make-up may affect not only your wife, but your children. You have an *obligation* to tell your wife— certainly if you're going to have children. A person is entitled to genetic privacy, except as it affects somebody else.

Kate's reasoning, though, implicitly raises questions of whether this obligation to tell is less if one does not wish to have children, and, if so, to what degree it is then lessened.

Moreover, in dating, before deciding to marry or enter long-term committed relationships, multiple other questions and uncertainties surface. People have to balance perceived obligations to disclose against potential risks of rejection. These individuals often debate what to do, gauging the long-term potential of a relationship against the risk of rebuff. According to Rhonda, the 31-year-old single nurse who at age six had seen her mother's breast cancer and later herself had the disease, a mutation, and a mastectomy,

> When you start a relationship, you think, "Now I'm going to have to tell this person. *Is this worth it?*" I dated men where it has come up very early on, and I realized this is not the person for me. That's fine. If I need to tell, I will. If not, I won't.

Genetic risk can thus force considerations about the seriousness of the relationship far earlier than otherwise.

Why Tell Dates?

Those who told did so primarily from a sense of ethical obligation to their prospective mate. Some readily told their partners because of having known and trusted them for a relatively long time—often, prior to the first official romantic date. As mentioned earlier, Tina quickly told her future husband about her HD risk because they had known each other for an extended period beforehand. The fact that he had revealed personal information to her, and that she felt asymptomatic, facilitated reciprocal disclosure.

> Within the first 24 hours after our first date, I told him, "You're going to meet my dad, he's a mess. He has this awful disease. So does my

grandmother. I could probably have it, too, and could maybe give it to my children." He had had a girlfriend who died in his arms of cancer a few years before. He had told me about that before we even got together.

Disclosures can thus mutually facilitate each other, and both result from and enhance trust. Similarly, individuals may disclose in order to avoid any perceived dishonesty or lack of trust.

Many think that divulgence is morally obligated because their future children's health may be affected. Conversely, several feel that disclosure is easier if the prospective spouse is uninterested in having kids. Ron, with the HD mutation, said, "If she wants children, then our relationship won't go anywhere. I've had a couple of relationships with women who had already had children—that's the simplest."

Similarly, for women, the pressure to disclose can diminish after their child-bearing years. As Patty, the fashion designer untested and asymptomatic for HD, said:

Because I'm 43, this weight is now taken off my shoulders. It's safer: when a guy meets me, he doesn't usually think of family. I wanted kids, but hit 40. Maybe HD pushed the idea of kids out of my life.

As in other kinds of relationships, disclosures may also occur because genetic risks or symptoms can simply no longer be concealed. Georgia, who has symptoms of HD, but no testing, told her boyfriend because she'd otherwise have "to lie about why I lost jobs." At a certain point, disclosures may simply be impossible to postpone, because of evident signs of disease or treatment.

Why not Tell Dates?

Given potential rejection, disclosure can be difficult even when one is in a relationship for an extended period of time. With romantic partners, disclosures can lead to painful emotional break-ups. In dating, rejection can be more painful than in many other types of social relationships—in part because hopes can be so high. As Ron, whose brother committed suicide, reported: "One girl simply said to me, 'I can't go out with you anymore.'" He felt "she was a bitch," and remained bitter because of both what she decided and how she told him.

Rebuff can result from not only symptoms, but treatment effects as well. Prophylactic removal of breasts or ovaries can engender negative responses.

Diane, the divorced Spanish teacher and mother of two daughters in their thirties who woke up to find she had had a mastectomy, said:

> I've had bad reactions from lovers. The mastectomy is hard for me to deal with. So naturally, it's going to be hard for someone else. I don't feel comfortable with it, even after all these years. So, I stay alone.

Rather than disclose, she chooses silence, and with it, singlehood. Individuals' views of their genetic risk or disease—particularly if negative or uncomfortable—can thus shape prospective mates' responses. Many (but by no means all) women undergo reconstructive surgery after mastectomies, but it can remain noticeable, affecting patients' views of themselves and fears of the reactions of others. Diane underscores, too, how issues of dating can be difficult for older as well as younger people.

What to Tell Dates?

As with other relationships, dilemmas surface of *what* exactly to tell dates—how much detail about the genetics or disease to provide. But whereas family members may themselves also be at risk, that is not the case with dates. Instead, many people try to minimize the potential risk to themselves and their potential descendants. Types of disease, degrees of risk, and likelihood of impact on future offspring can again play key roles. Alpha, for instance, which is treatable, may be easier to divulge than HD, which is not.

At times, people decide to offer only partial or incomplete information. For any given disease, it is easier to say that one is simply at risk rather than that one in fact has a mutation. The latter appears more frightening in its greater definitude. "I used to be able to say that I was merely at risk," Ron reported. "Now, I don't have that option. I still seem to be without any signs, but don't want to be dishonest." He wanted to provide the "whole truth"—that is, the most complete and up-to-date information.

Individuals might also say that a disease is "in the family," but not that it is genetic. An individual may disclose not that he or she is at risk, but that a relative is. Bonnie, who at age 12 saw mother's breast cancer, said about her sister, who had been rejected:

> Now she's seeing somebody who is crazy about her. But she still hasn't told him. She said to him, "My mom is a breast cancer survivor." So she

had relief that he would kind of understand. I don't know if she's going to tell him about her ovary and breast removal.

But does he ever have a right to know? One could argue that if they are about to get married, her continued silence could represent a lack of full openness and honesty, and thereby an implicit violation of trust. But at what point does she *need* to tell? When might her reticence undermine his faith in her? In developing relationships, perceptions of trust are crucial because they are seen as signs of larger issues. Arguably, assessments of trustworthiness are more critical than in other, longer relationships.

Individuals face dilemmas of exactly how much detail to provide concerning not only the eventual lethality of a mutation, but also the potentially long period of disturbing symptoms that can occur and burden a spouse. At a certain point, one may decide to instill a sense of these difficulties, but these harsh details can be difficult both to describe and to hear, and can impair a budding romance. Ron, whose brother committed suicide, continued,

> I've never gone out with a girl where I've thought: she understands what 20 years of me dying is going to be like. I've tried to make them understand: if I start exhibiting symptoms, all bets are off. I don't want to be in a relationship under those circumstances. I think I'd kill myself if I got sick.

He raises a question of how much one is responsible for conveying the harshness of the possible future, especially since it may not in fact transpire. These issues surface prominently for HD, but may appear with other disorders, too.

In particular, people must decide whether, at least initially, to provide information concerning reproductive implications, and if so exactly when, what, and how. Some, but not all, of these men and women were aware of the possible use of PGD to prevent transmitting mutations to offspring. Yet this procedure is expensive and complicated. Nonetheless, a few interviewees offered such information to dates. Simone, the 29-year-old bookkeeper who only learned of HD in her family when getting engaged, felt that at-risk individuals who were dating should tell prospective spouses about the technology: "You're going to have to take into account: you can have kids, but this is what you've got to do to ensure they don't have this disease."

Relatedly, questions arise of *how* to tell—for example, how best to frame the information. Many tried not just to give bare medical facts, but to cast the news as positively as possible, or at least to avoid presenting it entirely negatively. "Usually I email the girls I date *good* news," Ron said, "as well as bad."

When to Tell Dates

The extraordinary need for trust while dating also shapes decisions of *when* to tell. Many grapple with dilemmas of when to disclose particular bits of information. Fears arise of telling either too early or too late. But to gauge the most appropriate moment can be extremely difficult. Tim, the lawyer with the HD mutation but no symptoms, wrestles with this question.

> I wonder: when is the right time to tell them. I don't want to tell them right away, because it's just odd. But I don't want to get married to the person and they don't know yet—it would be a betrayal of trust not to tell them for so long . . . Since I found out, I've been on dates, but nothing has really developed such that I've felt obliged to tell them. It's an important moral issue: not to tell someone too late in the relationship. I worry about doing the wrong thing.

He struggles to avoid both the social awkwardness of raising the topic prematurely and the moral reprehensibility of unduly delaying. But ascertaining the right time is hard.

To make this decision, especially when it could in itself influence determinations of the seriousness of the relationship, some people develop their own set of rules. A few people establish predetermined periods after which they will tell. These rules may be firm or flexible, automatic or dependent on other assessments. Ron eventually concluded that for HD, disclosure within two weeks was appropriate.

> I don't want to get into a situation where somebody becomes attached, and doesn't understand the situation. The last thing I would want is: a couple of years into a relationship, turn around and tell them. I don't know whether my approach works in my favor or not. I started dating somebody last week. She's 32. I don't know enough about her yet to really know what she wants in life. The last woman I went out with was 37 and had children. That was a little bit easier.

To understand another person's desires and preferences requires time. However, prospective spouses may also not yet have figured out such long-term wishes regarding relationships and children.

While Ron usually waits two weeks, others establish more subjective benchmarks. Gilbert, the 61-year-old factory worker with Alpha, would tell if and only if the relationship appeared to him to be serious or have long-term potential.

I wait until I see whether . . . I might be interested on a longer term basis. I didn't bother telling anybody, until I met someone I wanted to date steadily . . . At that point, I would explain: "If this is a problem, then you should say so, and move on." I never had anybody back out because of it. Most women—maybe the kind that I picked—would be understanding.

He suggests too, however, that he chooses women who would be less likely to reject him.

Others vow to resolve these tensions by telling (or deciding they will tell) only if asked. Kym, the South Asian physician with a strong family history of breast cancer but without symptoms or testing, said she would tell a date if the topic came up, but would otherwise not volunteer the information. In part, the implications of her family history are less relevant than if the disease were HD. Thus, the degree of penetrance of the mutation can affect the moral calculus. She may also feel less obliged to disclose since she herself has had no evidence of disease. The imperative may hence be less than for those who have a mutation or symptoms.

Yet family histories can readily get discussed on dates, and include aspects of relatives' lives that can lead to or even necessitate these divulgences. Ron, whose twin committed suicide, said, "With the girl I've just met, the 'tell me about your family' discussion is going to be next. Unfortunately, with my family, it's messy: especially if I have to say I had a twin." One family fact can thus unspool others. Eventually, a significant other usually also meets one's family members.

Others simply resolve to avoid these revelations as long as possible, ending the relationship itself if the truth needs to come out. A few wait until after they break up, and disclose to these former partners only then, as mere friends. Patty, 43 and divorced, who pushed her HD risk "under the rug," added,

I can't tell guys I date. I won't let them know, unless I get very close. The topic of my mom doesn't come up. I just describe her as aging a little—forgetful. Not many people meet her. I just figured: if I ever get really close to someone, I'll deal with it. I have to make sure the guy falls in love with me first, before I tell him I'm defective [laughs]. I tell them after I date them, so that they stay my friends [laughs]. A guy I dated six years ago is one of my best friends now.

She disguises the truth—that her mother has HD, not just memory problems. Patty does not feel that providing only such partial knowledge is morally wrong, because she is not close or strongly bound to these men. Thus, she is able to obtain a degree of closeness and support, even if it limits the ultimate nature and extent of the relationship. Yet humor cloaks deep pain and moral uncertainty. She suggests that she will confront disclosure fully in the future if she needs to—thereby postponing decisions about these issues now. Thus one can date but remain somewhat distant, not wanting relationships to develop beyond a certain point.

Reactions from Dates

As mentioned, rejection does not always result, and in fact can be surprising and impossible to predict—coming at times from individuals who patients anticipated would be understanding. Bonnie's sister had been spurned by a boyfriend—a physician—because of the disease and a prophylactic oophorectomy and mastectomy. The *unexpectedness* of such rebuffs makes them even more wounding. This sister

> told a boyfriend that she had had cancer, and he flipped out. A week later, they broke up. He was a doctor, but doesn't know how to react to cancer! Here's a potential wife, but she's got cancer. He doesn't want to marry someone who's going to die. I said, "You're better off without him." But it was traumatizing to her.

When rejection happens, several factors may be involved. Perceptions of the severity and implications of genetic risks vary widely. Rejections occurred particularly with HD, and mastectomies and oophorectomies due to breast cancer. In contrast, being at risk but untested and asymptomatic can be less frightening than having symptoms, the mutation, or invasive therapies. Generally, individuals who appear wholly healthy find that their risk alone appears less likely to precipitate a break-up. Serious disease in a potential spouse's family can also potentially reduce the likelihood of rebuff. Such individuals may more readily accept disease, even HD, understanding and countenancing the risk—though not always.

Alternatives to Disclosing: Not Dating

As suggested earlier, potential rejection leads some to hesitate to date, or to avoid it altogether. Diane, the 66-year-old divorcee who had an unexpected mastectomy but no mutation, observed that "it's difficult enough to have a meaningful relationship, anyway . . . Some women are very brave; others are not. Some men are very compassionate; others not."

Not surprisingly, such avoidance of dating altogether transpires among individuals at risk for HD as well, and may be partially unconscious, or a manifestation of deeper anxieties. Tim, the lawyer, has not been in a relationship since he learned he had the HD mutation. The prospect of having to divulge his risk of HD appears to impede his dating, but he has difficulty acknowledging that that is the case.

> Since I found out, I haven't been intimately involved with anyone. I ask myself: at what point do I have to tell someone? I can't just lay this on someone on the first date. I've only been on a few dates, not anything that has developed into a full-blown relationship.

He cannot bring himself to go on more than a few dates with any particular woman because he would then feel obliged to tell her. He fears painful rejection. Rather than not dating altogether, he simply eludes going on more than a handful of dates with any one person.

Third-Party Disclosures in Dating

When an individual has not disclosed to a prospective mate, external others may wonder if they should intervene in some way—either pressing the individual to tell, or revealing the information to the potential partner themselves. At times, people feel that a sibling should disclose to his or her significant other. Antonia said that her brother's current girlfriend may know about their mother's HD, but not that these siblings are themselves at risk. "She's seen my mom, but I'm sure he hasn't said that *he* is at risk," she said. "She's only 21. I don't want to discuss it with her, and scare her off." But Antonia, a neuroscientist, remains uncomfortable with her brother's reticence. She feels he is embarrassed by their mother, and hence does not take his girlfriend to see their mother much: "He lives around the corner, but sees mom only once a month." Still, Antonia and others generally refrain from in fact divulging the information to a relative's significant other. But they ponder the possibility, and encourage relatives to disclose—though usually without success.

Interviewees thus face a series of dilemmas of whether to date, and if so whether, what, how, and when to disclose their genetic risks. They vary across a spectrum in what they tell. Disclosures could occur indirectly or inadvertently—for example, from seeing affected relatives, prompting efforts to prevent prospective mates from meeting ill family members. Other patients, particularly if affected by HD, vow not to date at all. Though these interviewees struggled to disclose neither too early nor too late, determining when to do so is difficult, and predictions of a potential's mate's reactions can be wrong. Rejection, though feared, does not always occur even when anticipated.

These dilemmas have no easy or ready answers, but heightened awareness of these issues among loved ones, physicians, genetic counselors, and others can help. Education about PGD can also be important to help reduce fears of children being affected by genetic disease, since these risks can now be lowered. Management of stigmatized information can clash with perceived ethical responsibilities to be honest. Degrees of trust, longevity of relationships, desires for children, and severity and treatability of the disease can all mold these decisions.

CONCLUSIONS

In disclosures of genetic information to a broad range of present and possible future kin, these individuals thus illustrate many complexities. While some readily tell their families, others provide only partial or indirect information. Disclosure decisions are based on several factors, including perceptions of others' ability to handle the information, intra-familial norms of communication, and at times one's own comfort with the results. While some make and carry out advanced plans for telling, disclosure is not always rational and controlled. Sometimes the information simply gets blurted out, or disclosed but then ignored.

Disclosure can also be difficult due to prior family communication styles and knowledge of the disease. The fact that this information can be stigmatized and changes perceptions of oneself and others, even in one's family, can further impede divulgence. Issues of disclosure to distant relatives also take on more importance than with other diseases that pose less potential danger to these extended family members.

These decisions represent *dynamic* processes. Distance, closeness, and silence can all be *mutually* reinforced. A mutation-free person may face fewer difficulties, but not entirely: when, for instance, disclosures to family members entail informing these others that they are still in fact at risk. Patterns of disclosure or nondisclosure can also stretch over more than one generation. People can have strong but complex feelings, too, about other family members' disclosure decisions.

While a study in Northeast Scotland[4] found that patients felt that the right time to tell children about HD was usually when they were potential parents (i.e., about to be married), parents in the United States generally appear here to face these issues earlier. Perhaps in part this is because in urban America, offspring may have children later. Health insurance systems also vary dramatically between countries in ways that can affect disclosure decisions. Yet such international differences have received little attention in genetics studies.

For these interviewees, the timing of disclosures was based not simply on "prevarication versus pragmatism," as in prior research. Rather, the information sometimes got blurted out. Though one prior study found that women more than men often served as gatekeepers of genetic knowledge,[36] that was not as much the case for the people I interviewed. In part, this difference may have emerged because the other study interviewed 50% more women than men, and included breast cancer—which affects primarily women. The data in this book suggest, too, that one's own specific mutation status can affect disclosure decisions. Past studies have not assessed all these factors. Future research should do so.

These individuals weigh not only whether to disclose but *what, how,* and *to whom,* and were not always rational. Individuals seek to manage stigmatized information about themselves, but feel moral responsibilities to their kin and to truth-telling. Sissela Bok, in *Lying: Moral Choice in Public and Private Life,*[37] held that essentially people should never lie. In contrast, David Nyberg, in *The Varnished Truth*[38] asked, "What's so good about telling the truth all the time?" and argued that telling lies is an intrinsic and necessary part of human life. Between these two extremes lie a vast range of possibilities that these interviewees charted. As shown, they navigate these conflicts between desires to conceal and perceived needs to tell the truth based on various factors (e.g., degrees of closeness and age of family members).

Clinicians rarely if ever discussed these issues with interviewees, especially regarding extended family members. Patients thus often wrestle with these complex and nuanced dilemmas without professional guidance. Yet genetic counselors and clinicians can potentially help at-risk individuals consider these conundra in advance.

Problems arise as well concerning secondary disclosure: one family member who is told, and then gives the information to third parties. Clinicians can help at-risk individuals anticipate these possibilities beforehand. Potentially patients, when telling someone, can state whether the information can or cannot be shared. Such a request may not be honored, but can at least be made.

Questions emerge as to not only *whether* clinicians should address these issues, but *how.* A patient may tell providers whether he or she disclosed, but it is important to discuss, too, *what* exactly was communicated—what precisely patients revealed or anticipate revealing (i.e., partial versus complete information). Providers and patients should also address obstacles to communicating information to extended relatives who might benefit from the knowledge. While patients may feel reluctant to communicate with these distant or estranged family members in part because of lack of prior contact, such information may be vital to impart. Providers need to help clients consider in advance what, how, and when to disclose results to these various kin.

Professional training and public education also need to increase awareness of these challenges—particularly when familial relationships are strained, in part because of genetic disease in the family. Mental health providers can also help address such tensions.

Individuals wrestle with these issues even before entering a genetic counselor's office. They may be at risk but not learn of that fact for years, even as adults, or they may receive the information indirectly, incompletely, or belatedly over extended periods of time. To understand these potential obstacles is vital to ensuring that those who might benefit from genetic information are made aware of their risk as best as possible, in order to help these individuals confront subsequent dilemmas they then face.

PART III

Genes in the Mind:

Understanding Genetics

CHAPTER 4

Genetic Tests as Rorschachs:

Questions of "Why Me?"

"Why did this happen to me?" These men and women have to decide not only whether to test and disclose, but how to *understand* these risks and results. These individuals struggle to make sense of this genetic information and its effects on their lives, and find meaning. People generally seek causes—especially for bad events. We tend to want to know why tragedy happens, and who or what to blame. Genetic disease is no exception, but the answers may not be clear. The stakes can be high: whether to fault oneself or others, and whether to avoid factors that may exacerbate disease.

Several researchers have suggested that people "personalize" risk by seeing it in very individual and subjective ways. But questions remain of exactly how people do so, and what patterns emerge across diseases. Given uncertainties about genetics, how do patients, family members, and providers all choose, construct, or view explanations?

Questions of "why me?" have been probed with regard to other disorders, particularly cancer, but have received far less attention concerning genetics. With other diseases, many patients may ask "why me?" and ponder spiritual issues,[1] often becoming fatalistic, or wrestling with questions of fate. In facing their own illness, both doctors and patients frequently ponder spiritual issues, including the role of "higher powers" in causing and curing disease.[1,2] Particularly for a disease with incompletely known etiologies, patients may seek "explanatory models"—ways of comprehending phenomena.[3]

But how patients confronting genetic risks view such issues remains unclear. Beliefs about free will versus determinism are deeply imbued in our culture; Greek, Hebraic, and Germanic mythology all speak of inborn character or external forces working in and through us. Scientists, too, seek causal theories to make sense of natural phenomena. Thomas Kuhn described how scientists historically shift their paradigms.[4] For a period, two competing conceptual frameworks may coexist, with some scientists trying to uphold one system until eventually abandoning it. But what do patients do? Do they act similarly or differently, and how?

Scholars have suggested several theories concerning understandings of disease in general. For instance, individuals may follow one of three main sets of explanations—environmental, behavioral, or hidden causes—with each set associated with different consequences and aspects of control and cure.[5] In viewing genetic versus other causes of disease, Bethan Henderson and Bryan Maguire[6] suggested that patients follow one of three "lay models" of inheritance: constitutional (that one's constitution is inherited, and may be "weak" or "strong"); genetic; and molecular (i.e., consisting of mere chemicals). Henrik Wulff described a spectrum of five categories of disease, based on the degrees to which they are genetic: from genetic in a strong sense, to genetic in a weak sense (i.e., as necessary, but not sufficient to cause a disease), both genetic and environmental (as in a genetic predisposition), partly genetic, and not genetic.[7] Jon Weil[8] writes about coexisting medical and personal "idiosyncratic" explanations.

Some investigators have suggested, too, that subjective feelings about a disease may affect patients more than objective data. When confronting disease, fear and avoidance can shape responses. When learning they have a threatening uncontrollable mutation, patients may become fatalistic.[9] Possible control over their disease creates tension between hope (being able to alter their illness) and self-blame (that they had failed to control it).

Yet, research on how views of illness and health behaviors affect each other have been inconsistent. Some studies, but not others, have suggested that genetic testing may increase fatalism. Other investigators suggest that individuals may fit risk information into their established views of the cause of a disease.[10]

Scientists still debate the etiologies of many diagnoses. Alzheimer's disease, for instance, has been explained in varying ways—from clinical to neuropathological to genetic. Neuropathologists view it more neuropathologically, and geneticists view it more genetically.[11] Ever since its initial description in the nineteenth century, controversy has existed as to whether this diagnosis is even a distinct disease. Alzheimer's may be more than a single disease entity, and the cause may be "constructed" rather than "discovered." In general, scientists may be shifting from monocausality to recognition of multifactorial causes for diseases.[12] But many questions persist of how patients, their family members, and others handle these ambiguities, and view these issues, and why—how they choose one or more explanations.

The past literature has also tended to focus on the outcome of genetic counseling, which not all at-risk individuals in fact pursue. Some may avoid testing altogether, due to their prior beliefs about these disease causes.

Though individuals may personalize genetic information in idiosyncratic ways, patterns and themes may nevertheless emerge, though in as yet unknown ways. It is unclear how individuals make sense of uncertain or inconclusive scientific data—how exactly people decide between competing theories, what they see as the pros and cons of conflicting explanations, what cognitive and emotional processes and factors are involved, and how they experience these frequently bewildering choices. To completely separate these multidimensional and overlapping queries is not possible. Hence, some overlap occurs below.

VIEWS OF FATE

These individuals often ask "why me?" and answer both physically and metaphysically. They encounter multiple conceptions of causes, and dilemmas of which to adopt. To see what part, if any, they might control, and to reduce stress and anxiety, they demonstrate deep needs to understand the roots of their predicaments. They approach these quandaries in various ways, balancing potentially competing views, and generally encountering difficulties. Though some people view these causal factors in binary terms—for example, as nature versus nurture, or genes versus the environment—others grapple with more complex interactions. Even those who have seemingly relatively straightforward situations—for example, both a mutation and the disease—confront ultimate questions of "why me."

The fact that genetic tests potentially provide information about one's future inevitably leads to searches to grasp what exactly that predictiveness means, and how to interpret and incorporate it into one's life and hope. Inherent uncertainties also lead to tensions and confusion, and questions of fate evoke complex notions of cause, blame, and luck.

On the one hand, genetics offers information about the future, even if only in the form of probabilities, and this perceived *predictiveness* invokes feelings that the knowledge is somehow being predetermined or preordained. For many individuals, this sense of *predetermination* suggests that an external agency must therefore have power and influence over them. Yet this idea challenges beliefs about autonomy and free will. Thus, individuals have to wrestle with the extent to which they are by-products of their genes and external forces versus autonomous agents operating solely based on their own volition.

In confronting these quandaries, genetic test results appear to function as a kind of Rorschach test that individuals interpret in a wide variety of ways based on broader psychological, cultural, and personal issues, needs, and beliefs. People struggle to fit the disease and its genetics into the stories of their lives— their ongoing narratives that give their lives a sense of coherence.

Yet while they try to integrate presumed genetic factors with their prior views about their lives, these efforts at synthesis prove difficult. These patients grasp for meaning and coherence, rather than chaos and chance. Genetic fore-knowledge of their potential death threatens their prior psychological refuge. Thus, these men and women struggle, seeking understanding and meaning, grappling with a range of beliefs related to cause—from physics to luck, blame, and metaphysics—and ways of coping with these possibilities.

THE MEANINGS OF FATE

Many believe that the disease constitutes their fate, yet the meanings and implications of that word vary widely. The term has a wide spectrum of philo-sophical, spiritual, and cultural connotations. Views prove fluid, and not neces-sarily consistent or logically coherent.

Many see a mutation as not only permanent, but inevitable. Yet in recogniz-ing the future implications, individuals often focus on particular aspects of this fatedness. For some, fate means ongoing symptoms—disease processes that, even if ameliorated by treatment, will ineluctably march on. "I've had other serious things happen to me in the past, but I got over them," Betty, the designer who carries an oxygen machine, observed. "But Alpha doesn't go away. There's a very real process of mourning my previous image of myself."

Individuals feel fated concerning a variety of other possible future challenges, such as ongoing insurance worries and/or needs for treatment. Many of these individuals then have to live with terrible awareness of the probable cause of their ultimate demise. Barbara, the part-time professor who feels guilty about having exposed her children to cigarette smoke, said about Alpha, "I live with knowledge of my own death. I've lost 40% of lung capacity. I saw a person at 40% two years ago, now at 15%. When you're below 20%, you have only one year to live."

A mutation can thus suggest not only the etiology, or cause of disease, but the *timing* of one's demise. Individuals then have to grapple with this predicament. "I'm not going to live to a ripe old age," said Charles, the accountant who still uses tobacco and hangs out in smoky bars, which could exacerbate his Alpha symptoms. "When you're pretty sure you're going to dead by 35, you have a different perspective." His genetic marker makes him fatalistic, which can in turn impair his health, and contributes to his continued exposure to disease exacerbants.

Though intellectually humans are all aware that they will eventually die, few confront this inevitability with the certainty of those who know they have or may have a potentially lethal mutation. This concretization of the threat and lack of time can itself foster stress. "Everyone says, 'I could die crossing the street,'" Charles sighed, "but for me, *this* is for real!" Definitive knowledge that one has a mutation or even a family history can suddenly make the risk of these diseases far less abstract.

This sense of fatalism can extend to not only oneself, but one's offspring. "The hardest thing about being at risk is knowing that your life may be *doomed*," said Antonia, the neuroscientist who eventually found she lacked the HD mutation. "That you may die prematurely at 50—and could pass this on to your kids."

Individuals must then decide how to respond: whether to accept, worry about, or deny this fate. The extent to which they adopt such options varies widely. Charles sought to avoid these painful ruminations: "I'm not spending a lot of time worrying about it."

Before undergoing testing, the assumptions many people make as to whether they possess a mutation or not can in fact verge on premonitions and reflect notions of fate. In looking back, many say that they not only felt destined, but foresaw their future. Either implicitly or explicitly, they invoke metaphysical notions of predetermination—that they *sensed* this future before it befell them. They desire coherence in the narratives and meanings of their lives, and often cling to these beliefs in death foretold. Such premonitions may arise because of perceived evidence—early possible signs or symptoms—but many believe that such premonitions are far less physical than metaphysical in origin. Arlene, the nurse who studied religion, said about her risk of breast cancer,

A lot of women told me they've known: they've had dreams, an intuitive knowing, that made them hyper-vigilant. If you're stressed and worrying about breast cancer, that is going to cause it: through ESP, the Holy Spirit, loose consciousness, whatever — that realm beyond clinical science. I've always been quite intuitive — I've kept a dream journal for 20 years. It made me sure I got a mammogram every year.

Others support the notion of such premonitions, though they did not have any themselves. Many wish they did, revealing the strength of underlying desires for certainty and prophecy in the face of deep ambiguity. Susie, who worked in HIV and had an ovarian cyst and a family history of breast cancer but no symptoms, and eventually tested mutation-negative, said, "My stepmom said, 'Do you have it or not? People can usually tell.' My cousin was sure she had it. I don't know. I wish I did." Yet such foreknowledge can cause difficulties—anxiety, and at times over-vigilance. Such beliefs also prompt dilemmas of how frequently to monitor oneself, and whether to undergo a genetic test.

VIEWS OF CAUSES: FROM PHYSICAL TO METAPHYSICAL

These individuals seek to understand not only *what* this fate consists of, but *why* it befalls them. Genetic assays provide a sense that the future is partially or fully predictable, and hence somehow preset. These notions in turn propel questions as to why and how that is the case. Answers vary as to whether this fate is due to physical or metaphysical phenomena.

In seeking such explanations, people draw on a wide spectrum of conceptual models: from purely physical to purely metaphysical causes to combinations of these. Yet while some prior scholars have offered schematic theories about such models, the individuals here revealed a myriad of complexities and nuances.

Persistent uncertainties, heightened fears, and realities lead to struggles with sweeping metaphysical questions—for example, whether destinies are predetermined, and if so, to what degree. Spiritual views can also reflect long-standing beliefs. As Kym, the South Asian physician, said, "I don't really know what I believe—somewhere between an actual God and an energy. It changes."

Some believe not in a specific preordained, individualized design, but in a potential overall *order*—rather than simply pure randomness and chaos. Reflecting on his HD risk, Karl, abused by his father, said, "There's not a plan, but certainly an order to things that's extremely complex and hard to figure out. I don't have a sense that there's a predestination." His experiences shape his sense of confusion about these realms.

Many go further, seeing spirituality as playing a role in their genetic risk. Spirituality can account for—or be affirmed by—one's disease. Illness may be seen not as punishment, but as proof of God's existence. Carmen, for instance, the Latina former clerical aide, felt that her breast and thyroid cancer and *BRCA* mutation were "proof that He gives you your life—that you have to go through this and deal with it." This Job-like sense helped her cope.

Physical Causes

Others look solely or primarily to physical factors as producing their disease. A few remain strict materialists, and simply reject all metaphysical notions of being "doomed" or "spared." They seek hope and acknowledge the mysterious, unknown processes involved, but ultimately see these as biological, not divine. Yet those who prefer biological understandings still confront and weigh a variety of possible physical explanations, influenced by a range of factors.

A few feel that larger metaphysical questions, while tempting, are too distant or unanswerable, and hence not worth pursuing. Karl wrestles with how much to blame HD for his father's abusive behavior.

> Everybody has the "Why me's?" But the world is just the way it is. Some people are born left-handed. There are biological reasons for it, but to try to figure out *the cosmic roll of the dice,* and why you ended up with one set of situations, and somebody else another, is not worth it.

In contrast, many of those with symptoms or mutations who have had less traumatic upbringings hunted for straightforward physical etiologies, even if these are still uncertain. They often select between, and interpret, multiple possible forces.

Yet physical factors still pose several unresolved questions: concerning how genes and the environment each contribute to a disease, and why some genes, but not others, express themselves. In response to these quandaries, individuals tended to focus on either genetic *or* environmental factors, or combinations of these two. Yet integrating these competing sets of explanations is not easy, as individuals grapple with desires for control, and prior views of themselves.

GENETIC DETERMINISM

Given the many unknowns involved, mechanical explanations are often pursued, but vary in detail. At one extreme, individuals answer broad questions of "why me?" in purely genetic terms. Jennifer, the schoolteacher who tested after her son did, was very matter-of-fact about the cause of her Alpha: "People say, 'Why me? Why did I get this?' Emphysema was in my grandmother's family: *that's* how I got it."

The type of disease influences these degrees of determinism. Overall, those at risk of HD appeared more likely to see their disease as the result of genetics (that their fate arose simply from a genetic mutation) while those at risk of breast cancer, where mutations were less penetrant and predictive, incorporated other factors more. But within these broad generalizations, key variations occurred. For all of these diseases, both environmental and metaphysical factors challenge wholly genetic etiologies.

A few rare individuals at risk for HD adopt purely genetic explanations, and actively reject alternative hypotheses. They accept the odds as randomness, without divine predestination. Antonia, in part as a neuroscientist, maintained such a matter-of-fact view: "You've either got a gene or not. So you have a genetic fate, one way or another." Yet the fact that she lacks the HD mutation made this view easier for her to adopt.

AGAINST GENETIC DETERMINISM

The notion that crucial aspects of one's being result simply from a dice roll—a mutation that one cannot remove—is difficult to accept. Most of these men and women thus resist genetic determinism, and adopt causal views other than the purely genetic. Even with HD, for which a "definitive" mutation has been identified, modifiers and indeterminate results leave room for doubt. These interviewees feel that other factors could affect when and how severely they become ill.

People resist genetic determinism in part because of its frightening implications—further onslaught of disease in oneself and others. Wilma, with bipolar disorder, refused testing after breast cancer, in part because "if my cancer was genetic, it would put me at higher risk for getting it in the other breast." The prospect terrifies her.

Genetic determinism also threatens experiences of free will, desires for autonomy, and beliefs that environmental and behavior factors can play roles as well. These men and women resist the notion that they don't wholly control their lives—or key aspects of it. They rail against threats to their sense of their own volition, wanting to feel that they are free, and experiencing themselves as such. Even with HD, knowledge of the mechanistics of genes does not completely answer questions of why one has received a mutation, and when and how it will express itself. In the absence of more scientific detail, myths and beliefs fill the gap.

Those at risk for HD also perceive gray areas and indeterminacies. Though HD has 100% penetrance, individuals confronting this disease often look to other disorders or behavioral traits to see how choice can in some ways modify genetics. A predisposition does not guarantee a disease, raising questions about definitions of this term. As Karl, unsure how much to attribute his father's abusive behavior to disease, said,

> In two different people, the same genes don't necessarily get expressed the same way. Even if you have a genetic predisposition, it doesn't mean it's *absolute* . . . Lots of things could happen along the way. There might be many other factors and interactions. Choice enters into it. The whole thing is muddled. You don't really know.

Yet views vary widely about how genetics in fact combine with other factors. Many feel there is "a mix of nature and nurture," but to distinguish between these is hard.

Individuals trying to untangle the relative contributions of different sets of factors frequently draw on analogies from behavioral genetics. But from the morass of observations within this nascent field, men and women construct varying understandings. On the one hand, some leaned somewhat, though not entirely, toward genetics. They cited behavioral and psychological traits as possibly genetic, reflecting in part certain popular beliefs. As Karl added,

> When you see things—like being obstinate, very free spirited, very self-directed, willful—in your parents, and then your children, it gives you pause. Maybe there's a little bit more of the genetics thing than we give it.

To grasp these complexities and variability, many people seek examples and metaphors. These men and women frequently see psychological and behavioral traits as passed down partially, but incompletely, and not wholly predictably. The specifics prove baffling. Antonia, a neuroscientist, feels that aspects of her personality come from her paternal grandmother, but that genes from each parent could somehow intermix, in not fully understood ways.

> Somewhere, the genes got muddled up. I resemble my dad's mom most. She was quite a dominant, forceful woman. My dad's sister is also quite like me. My parents and brother are not.

Individuals often cite additional, unknown biological variables as also molding gene expression. So-called *normal genetic modifiers* (genes that are not abnormal per se, but increase the likelihood of a mutation, if present, expressing itself) could be involved. But awareness of such factors appeared to result mostly from advanced scientific education. Shilpa, a Hindu medical student with a family history of breast cancer, though asymptomatic and untested herself, drew on her scientific training to reflect on this possibility:

> You could have the gene and, because of your mRNA, not get the disease. Scientists still don't know specifics behind that. Of 10 patients with *BRCA1*, only *three* get breast cancer. So there are obviously many variables we don't know about—proteins and hormones that might affect the splicing.

Environmental Factors

Patients also face questions about whether environmental factors are involved, and if so which factors and to what degree, and what, if anything, might reduce these. These factors may play particularly important roles in common, so-called complex disorders, such as heart disease. Hence, individuals often invoke these ailments as paradigms in trying to make sense of their own disorders. People often pick scientific findings concerning other diseases to shape or support their existing understandings of their own predicament.

Many believe in the involvement of environment factors, but struggle to identify which specific ones, and how. In promoting or preventing a disease, a wide range of environmental phenomena are suspected—from specific to broad, and from affecting a particular individual to an entire population.

In considering the causes of their disease, many draw on their observations of illness in themselves and their family members. Some believe their disease is environmental, not genetic, because they have no family history or they tested negative. Yet as discussed earlier, family histories may not always be fully known, recognized, or accepted.

Often, folk wisdom prevails that environmental factors cause and could potentially cure or ameliorate disease—particularly cancer. Shilpa, the medical student, and others feel that geographic regions vary—for example, that urban areas are more hazardous than other locales due to "toxins or cell phone towers."

The media may fuel such beliefs, which then become urban myths and the stuff of rumors. They may be incorrect, but nevertheless persist, reflecting suspicion of various environmental dangers.

To account for their own observations of who does versus who does not become ill, individuals also differentiate between specific regions as more or less deleterious. As Wilma—with breast cancer and bipolar disorder but no testing, in part because of her belief in environmental factors—reported:

> They say there's more breast cancer in Manhattan on the East Side than the West Side. That seems pretty far-fetched, but that's what they say in the news. Long Island has a lot of breast cancer. They are studying the soil and various factors there. I think it's a combination.

Subjective attitudes can mold such beliefs about the relative safety versus danger of particular regions. Desires to avoid self-blame can also shape these considerations. Joyce, with breast cancer but no mutation, working in a spa and living with her 8-year-old daughter, said,

> For a period, I thought cancer was caused by living in Chicago. At times, I thought living in New York was so punishing that it was like a charm against cancer. You have enough misery in your life in New York without getting cancer. It's a superstition.

The fact that she had the disease, but no mutation, made her more open to these ideas about non-genetic forces.

At times, individuals distinguish between genetic and familial disease, not necessarily seeing an illness that affects multiple family members as genetic. Rather, some feel that a diagnosis in the family is environmental, not genetic, if it results from environmental toxins to which family members have all been exposed. These beliefs can vary by disease. Families with breast cancer, in which no members have been tested or found to have a mutation, may have more latitude to hypothesize about nongenetic bases of their disease than do those in which a member has been found to have a definitive mutation.

Yet families with breast cancer histories who are mutation-negative may harbor mutations that scientists have not yet discovered. Still, as Roberta, the African American former nursing student with breast cancer but no testing, said,

It might run in families, but I don't think it's genetic. My cells go cockamamie for some chemically unknown reason. Everybody's got their own metabolism, and exposure to all kinds of stuff. Some people say if you live under the high tension wires, you're going to get it. Who's to say?

Individuals search for evidence to support their presuppositions. As Roberta elaborated, her family history of different types of cancers leads her to think that her cancer is environmental. In seeking evidence, she and others thus assess epidemiological data. Yet rumor and hearsay can also shape these causal theories. Roberta continued:

I think it's more environmental, because my family is originally from Louisiana, and during the 1970s and 80s oil boom, my mom went back down there and came back with breast cancer. I had cousins there, 16, 17, getting intestinal cancer, dying. Where's this coming from? Down there, they dump all this stuff in the Mississippi, from Chicago all the way to New Orleans, that they can't filter out. New Orleans has the worst water in the world! Toxic chemicals in the water do things to you. How do you get cancer at 15? Little kids with leukemia. My grandmother died an old woman, because of a bad heart. But now, everyone is showing up with cancer. You could say maybe it's genetic. But you can't really, until somebody proves it.

She felt that ultimately, disease in her family resulted from industrial pollution more than genetics. Her beliefs that she and her family were victims of powerful, harmful companies that she could not change may also have been partly shaped by her experiences as an African American woman, well aware of economic and social injustice in the United States.

Rising epidemiological rates of certain disease, too, can foster theories of environmental etiologies. Samantha, the 27-year-old actress with breast cancer but no family history or mutation, said, "Of people who get breast cancer, 99% don't have family histories! Seventeen-year-olds get it! It's become totally out of control!" Her own test result, showing no mutation, strengthens her view that the environment causes the increased prevalence of the disease among young women like herself.

Behavioral Factors

Others argue that behavioral factors as well such as exercise, diet, and mental state can affect whether, when, and to what degree disease develops. Yet individuals ranged in precisely how and to what degree they thought these behaviors have influence, and whether these operate in conjunction with biological components. Psychological and environmental factors—including stress—could interact and potentially be controlled. Wilma felt that "everyday stress and how you handle it does something to your hormones, playing havoc with your system." Her belief that such tension, more than genetics, caused her breast cancer resulted in part from her experiences with a psychiatric disorder, and contributed to her decision to forego genetic testing.

Combinations of Physical Factors

Overall, individuals tend to blame primarily *either* genetics *or* environment. To keep both in mind, with the ultimate etiology uncertain, is difficult. Usually, these individuals seek a "final" cause—a single culprit. In the end, even those who recognize possible gene-environment interactions tend to lean more toward one cause or the other. Most want to draw a line in the sand, blaming one side more, seeing their disease as *mainly* due to nature *or* nurture—but not both equally. Daniel Dennett and other philosophers have described "compatibalism" as somehow integrating views of free will versus determinism. Yet despite its potential benefits, this perspective is emotionally and psychologically difficult to sustain. This tendency may reflect how our brains work—how humans evolved, to look for a major cause, to organize a main response, and find something to control. Uncertainty and ambiguity appear harder to tolerate and address. In general, individuals at risk for HD tend to believe in genes as having more sway, while those confronting breast cancer see more mixed combinations of both genetic and environmental causes. Yet various factors could affect these beliefs. Shilpa, the Hindu medical student, said about her aunt with breast cancer,

> She grew up in a small mountain village—with no commercialism or phone towers. So, I think there is a genetic predisposition, but environmental factors are a *stronger* predictor of what she has.

Shilpa opposes genetic determinism on psychological and existential grounds. She feels that people commonly misbelieve that if they have the mutation, they will have the disease, and she fears such fatalism. She added, "I didn't want my family to feel: they have this gene, they're *doomed*, they have the disease—there is no in-between." Desires to reduce fatalism can thus shape views of disease etiology. She suggests, too, how degrees of genetic determinism can exist. Individuals can thus oppose strong or strict genetic determinism, but accept that genes are still somehow entailed.

Shilpa's scientific training does not prompt purely mechanistic beliefs. Rather, her religious beliefs also colored her notions about disease causation. She opposes genetic determinism, which she observes in many patients, and feels that even if she had the gene, her fate would not be guaranteed.

Yet she then faces questions of how to understand the relative amounts of different causal contributions, and is unsure of how to join these competing views.

> What are the odds of breast cancer for me, whose aunt has it? About fifty-fifty. Fifty percent there is a link. I do have control, through what I do. If my mom ends up having it, I'd think, "Oh my gosh, it's 75%."

In trying to parse the relative contributions of each set of factors, she offers percentages of contributions, quantifying the relative input from each set of factors, estimating these: "I feel like 50% is genetic, and 50% is your environment."

She thinks that since environment and genes are both involved, they must each contribute 50%—unless other relatives are also affected. These statistics are not scientifically accurate, but reflect her desire and struggle to make sense of her risk.

SEARCHING FOR METAPHORS TO CONCEPTUALIZE COMBINATIONS
To grasp these complex and scientifically poorly understood interactions between multiple genetic and environmental factors, individuals search for analogies. Particularly for complex diseases, individuals wrestle to understand

what having a mutation means conceptually, not simply statistically, in their bodies—how it interacts with the environment and behavior. Though scientists may be uncertain about mechanistic details, individuals nonetheless seek these.

In the end, many imagine that nongenetic factors (e.g., stress) stimulate the deleterious effects of mutations. But interviewees conceptualize such "triggers" in different ways. Some envision that more of something—added amounts— somehow tip the balance, or initiate a latent process.

Yet identifications of *which* specific environmental factors are involved, and how, is not easy. A few conclude that numerous phenomena interact to produce phenotypic results, and that attempts to parse these are futile. Karl, uncertain how much to blame HD for his father's abusive behavior, said, "A million things interact with each other, and stuff happens. Trying to figure out which stuff is going to happen when is impossible."

These concerns arise particularly for breast cancer. Some normalize the presence of this cancer—implicitly challenging its purely genetic basis, and seeing mutations as added, deciding factors. As Carol, who had breast cancer, a family history, and a mutation and who opted to have her breasts and ovaries removed, said,

> We all have cancer in us, it's just a matter of *triggering* it. Something starts it off. In my case, the gene is definitely an added extra. If everyone has X, I have X and Y to create Z: an extra component to exacerbate what's already there.

Several people try to conceptualize gene-environment interactions by supposing that while genes may determine *whether* disease occurs, environmental factors can control *when*. Despite her mutation and family history, Carol traces her onset of symptoms to particularly stressful situations.

> It was inevitable that I was going to get the cancer; it was just a matter of when. The trigger was there and got *pulled*. I know exactly when: I was going through a very stressful moment. A friendship was pulling me apart. I'll never know what happened, but I never heard from her again. It really upset me. I had never lost a friend. She didn't want anything to do with me. *That's* when I was diagnosed with breast cancer. I was diagnosed with ovarian cancer right after 9/11, and had gone down to Ground Zero the day after. They're talking about pollutants in the air down there. The cancer could have been festering, but *the stress completely blew it wide open.*

She draws on metaphors of weaponry: guns ("the trigger got pulled") and bombs. She suggests, too, a main *mechanism*—stress made her more vulnerable to genetic factors and determined when the disease occurred.

These triggers can be genetic or environmental, direct or indirect, and proximal or distal. For example, Laura, the asymptomatic graphic designer with a family history of breast cancer and a mutation, wondered whether toxins mutated her parents' or grandparents' gametes. She resists assigning full blame to genes alone, seeking to hold environmental poisons culpable at least in part for her risk. "My condition may have nothing to do with the environment," she said. "But it's possible that something in the environment mutated my grandfather's sperm."

Even if they have the mutation, individuals ponder the mechanisms of not just genes, but cells. Many *BRCA* mutation-positive women see the development and spread of cancer as involving more than genes alone. They feel that they can not alter their genes directly, but can affect their cells. Rachel, with breast cancer and the mutation but little sense of her family's medical history, since many of them died in the Holocaust, said, "Once I *replenish* what's been taken from me, in terms of cells, I'll be at a better point than before, mentally and emotionally. Perhaps the cancer will never resurface."

Even HD triggers thoughts that environmental factors may have important temporal roles. Some see stress as precipitating or increasing symptoms, though they recognize the ambiguities involved in these scenarios. Evelyn, asymptomatic, who consulted a psychic when her husband opposed her testing, said, "I've read that symptoms came out after a stressful experience: After the death of so-and-so, we noticed the disease. Or maybe that's when the family just *happened* to notice."

Others think that a genetic basis of an illness does not make it inevitable, but simply advances the disease process in time. Other aspects of one's body or behavior could precipitate the disease as well. Joyce, who worked in a spa and had blamed her cancer on the stress of urban living, said,

> My understanding of how cancer works is: you may have a genetic predisposition or damage, so that compared to other people, you have *a head start* on having cancer. It doesn't necessarily mean it is inevitable.

The fact that she had breast cancer but no mutation reinforces her belief in the role of nongenetic factors.

Still others seek more complex conceptual models, differentiating between active versus passive, or outer versus inner processes. Individuals attempt to grasp interactions between genotype and phenotype. Environmental factors, for instance, may increase the probability of genes going from an inward to an outward state. Kym, with no symptoms or testing but breast cancer in her family, draws partly on her medical training: "You can be genetically predisposed, but environmental factors can make you more likely to express it."

Similarly, in trying to grasp these processes, many invoke metaphors of infection, conceptualizing these more easily than genetics. With infection, external agents are definitely somehow culpable. Hence, mutations can be seen as lying dormant—as if they are potentially invasive life-forms. Bonnie, who as a girl had seen her mother's breast cancer and is asymptomatic and untested, struggled to understand her own risk: "If you're genetically prone, maybe you have the genes, but don't know if they're dormant, or are going to react to something in your body, and you then get the disease." She gropes for analogies from particular kinds of infectious agents—for example, prions that can have decades-long incubation periods and "stay dormant in the body for 30 years, and then be like Mad Cow disease." The fact that she is at risk but has not had cancer bolsters this view, which in turn helps dissuade her from testing.

Infectious agents are also viewed as possible triggers themselves. Isabelle, the social worker with breast cancer and a mutation but no family history, feels that mildew in a moldy apartment may have stimulated her gene. Absence of the disease in relatives can thus both shape and confuse these calculations. Yet as we have seen, family histories may be inaccurate or incomplete. Isabelle struggled to understand why she got sick.

> I come from a family where the gene hasn't been expressed. Why did it happen with me? Would this have happened if I lived where the air is fresh and the water's clean—if I moved out quicker from that apartment with mildew in the wall?

Yet though she at first said she had no family history, she later mentioned an aunt who had had breast cancer. Individuals may also selectively recall and consider such information.

Even with a mutation, some conceptualize the disease they confront as infectious, not genetic, highlighting questions about the definitions and meanings of primary versus secondary (or proximal versus distal) "causes." Sarah, the computer programmer, thinks that ultimately, cancer results from viruses, not genetics—partly reflecting that fact that she has a family history of the disease, but no symptoms or mutation herself. She feels that *BRCA1/2* mutations are in fact merely "suppressors."

> I assume they're all going to turn out to be viral carcinogens—insults to your immune system that set you up. I learned from the genetic counselor:

> BRCA1/2 don't *cause* cancer. They're actually tumor suppressors. If they
> are not functioning properly, or are mutated, you don't get cancer suppres-
> sion. But they're not *"the cause."* The cause is elsewhere. Every cancer for
> which they've found a legitimate cause turns out to be viral—*H. pylori*,
> and papillomavirus. Maybe people live with viruses without a problem
> unless they have a big enough insult to their immune system.

She looks for a single culprit but suggests that multiple factors may in fact be
involved, suggesting how confusing casual definitions can be. Searches for such
triggers arose with breast cancer far more forcefully than with the other two
diseases examined here, since the mutation is the least predictive of the three.

Physics versus Metaphysics

Many look to physical causes as explanations for their predicament but
ultimately find that the answers are not fully satisfying. Consequently, they seek
to *integrate* these ostensibly competing world views. Metaphysical factors
thus prove appealing to some degree. A mutation may explain why one has
symptoms, *but why does one have the mutation*? Larger metaphysical questions
persist of what causes the mutation in the first place. Some people implicitly or
explicitly blame God or "the great beyond" for the gene. Peter, a former
California businessman who now leads an Alpha support group, expresses
agnosticism consistent with his sober view of humankind and insurance companies: "I don't know if there is a God. But if there is a God, he fucked up."

Others argue that God is the *ultimate* cause of a disease, but that one's
behavior, particularly diet and exercise, could nonetheless alter the course of
the illness as well. Even if the underlying cause of the disease lies beyond one's
control, one could potentially affect when and how extensively the gene
expresses itself. Anna, the African American secretary with diabetes and a
strong family history of breast cancer but no symptoms or testing herself, feels
that God has plans, but that people can nonetheless affect these.

> God has a plan for everyone. He ain't sending me to the doctors for no
> reason. So, if there's anything wrong, there's a reason why I went to the
> doctor: to find out. It can't be prevented, because it's inherited. But it can
> be helped: morally and physically.

She feels that full prevention is impossible, but that she can ameliorate
the disease. Even if genes control *whether* and *when* a disease manifests
itself, many patients feel they can nonetheless potentially influence to what

degree it does so. Anna's spiritual beliefs also dissuade her from undergoing testing.

Yet these spiritual beliefs cannot be willed. Isabelle, the social worker with breast cancer and the mutation, feels that her intellectual skepticism impedes her ability to benefit emotionally from spirituality. Her doubt outweighs her desire to believe. She does not wholly understand her inner obstacles to faith, but has to accept them.

> The first time I ever wished I was religious was when I had cancer. We're Jewish, but I was not brought up in a religious household. Jewish identity was always important to me, but not in terms of the religion—going to temple, believing in a God, or praying. I've seen people have tremendous strength from believing in God, praying, worshipping, and going to church or temple. I'm almost envious: to have something you can focus on, and really feel there is a Greater Being that can sort of make it all O.K. I don't have that. I wish I could. But at this point in my life, *I guess I'm too skeptical*, for whatever reason.

She has difficulty grasping even her impediments to faith.

Given the vagaries, and shifting symptoms and possible evidence, many individuals also waver in their views. Beliefs do not necessarily exist a priori, but respond to evolving personal needs. These desires for belief can thus shape the nature and the content of the beliefs themselves. As Kym, the South Asian physician at risk of breast cancer but without symptoms or testing, said, "I am *undecided* whether things are predestined or not. Sometimes I think it's all just chaos. Other times, I think we're given what we can deal with on purpose, and there are reasons."

Worsening symptoms can spur searches for a larger purpose, while improved health may reduce concern about these issues. She continued,

> I believe what I need to at the time. In very difficult periods, I feel there has to be a bigger picture, and someone actually looking out for me: that this is happening for a reason, and I'm going to learn a lesson from this, find inner strength. *There's a purpose to all of this happening—there has to be.* I can't just be randomly put through this for no reason. When things are going O.K., I think about it less, and don't have as strong a need to reach for something.

Especially when ill, she feels a larger meaning is imperative. Though she is not religious per se, life would simply be too painful without such a greater purpose.

FACTORS IN DECIDING

Several other factors shape these causal beliefs. Education can play a key role, though often tempered by other circumstances. Higher levels of education, and in particular training in science, can help in comprehending certain aspects of genetics. Shilpa, with a family history of breast cancer but asymptomatic and untested, was persuaded by her medical training more than her Hindu background, largely because her aunt in a rural Indian village, far from industrial carcinogens, developed cancer:

> My science background helps. Most people think that if they have this gene, they have the disease. Society has that misconception. I say to them: no. You have a higher predisposition, but other things are involved: your body, proteins, hormones, and many unexplained variables.

Yet she sees these more complex conceptualizations blocked by societal needs—for example, psychological desires for certitude, and discomfort with ambiguity. "People want a full definite answer," she said. "Maybe doctors don't have time to explain all these things. But also in society: there is no in-between." Individuals may cling to a definitive answer, even if it is incorrect.

Similarly, many feel they have not had sufficient scientific education or input to know how to judge these issues. Diane, the Spanish teacher who had an unplanned mastectomy but does not have a *BRCA* mutation, concluded that she simply does not know whether her cancer is genetic or environmental. She feels that the question is not for her to answer, as she lacks an adequate scientific background. Her self-perceived ignorance reflects a lack not in her education, but in existing medical knowledge. "I really don't know if there is a genetic part of my cancer," she said. "I don't think it's for me to decide, not having that kind of [scientific] knowledge. I don't think anyone knows." Her past experience also makes her appreciate the uncertainties involved in medical care.

Levels of education may in turn correlate with other factors, such as social class and ethnicity, but large amounts of information can also prove overwhelming and confusing in and of themselves. Beatrice, the Latina math teacher, felt that she had been given too much information, and expressed concern for other patients whose primary language is not English:

> I was trying to decide whether to have radiation treatment. The doctor went through this whole explanation. I was trying to remember college biology. I have a master's degree. But how do other patients deal with all this information coming at them? It must be incredibly scary. I felt like

I had just taken a test in Biology 101. Suppose somebody didn't understand English well?

A master's degree does not necessarily provide genetic knowledge, and
science advances swiftly. She highlights needs for increased public education.

Psychological Factors
TOLERATION OF AMBIGUITY

In viewing causes of disease, psychological factors, such as ability to tolerate
ambiguity, can be critical, but also vary widely. People range considerably in
their ability to cope with gray areas. As mentioned, the poet John Keats described
this capacity by his term "negative capability."

It can be hard to grasp these notions of risk—for example, that a mutation
may only occasionally be present or manifest itself. Vera, the Asian executive,
said about her *BRCA* mutation,

> My boss said, "The reason you're having a hard time with it is you're not
> good at dealing with gray areas. You like knowing what the problem is,
> figuring it out, and fixing it." But this is *very gray*. So I can't say, "Oh, I'm
> going to do this," and it's a done deal. *It's not*. And doctors could be
> wrong.

In part, as an immigrant, Vera's background and experiences and those
of her parents may have contributed to her vigorous search for surety and
security.

> It had to be hard for my parents to leave Asia, go to a country where they
> didn't speak the language, accomplish something there, lose it again, and
> start all over. They just dealt with whatever was dealt to them. They kept
> going. Those are my examples.

She also did not at all expect the test result.

Others tolerate little ambiguity because they are by nature skeptical and
cautious. Francine, with breast cancer in her mother but no symptoms or
testing herself, felt she simply did not know the root of the cancer and was wary
of commercialism, media, and hype.

> I don't know the cause. They say that specific brands of soda will sterilize
> you. But *show me on paper*. I'm the type of person who believes nothing
> that you hear, and only half of what you see.

An African American woman from a disadvantaged background with HIV, she felt disempowered, and mistrusts institutions and sources of power. She wanted proof.

This ability to tolerate ambiguity may itself not be fixed, but shift over time. Psychotherapy, maturity, and other factors may enhance capacities to accept uncertainty, rather than require definitude. Karl has altered his view, in part since learning he lacked the HD mutation:

> Recently, I'm able to sort of accept the cosmic ambiguity and nuance of things. Part of that is maturity. Psychoanalysis has also made me much more flexible. I used to be very anxious, and didn't like uncertainty at all. Now, I think more, "let's see what happens."

CHOOSING EVIDENCE: PERSONAL EPIDEMIOLOGY

These interviewees also frequently try to develop personal epidemiological theories, assessing possible evidence over time. Learning that one possesses a mutation can lead one to reject prior nongenetic theories and epidemiological views. The discovery of a mutation can help one understand family history, alleviate self-blame, and alter prior causal views, even in the face of folk wisdom and media reports about perceived environmental dangers. Mildred, in finance, with breast cancer and a family history, said that before she learned she had the mutation, she thought the disease

> was environmental: Long Island, or red wine, or going to the beach. Everyone was coming down with cancer: lung, breast, prostate . . . We all said, "It's in the water" or "some sewer pipe." Now, I think about it differently. Someone might say, "Maybe it was a mixture." *But no.* I keep reading: those who carry the gene are more likely to get cancer in middle age. I fit that perfectly. I got it in my left breast, then my right one. Someone said the odds of that happening were like getting hit by lightning. *That* is genetics.

Her mutation-positive test result and two consecutive bouts of cancer led her to alter her views, and eventually undergo prophylactic mastectomies.

Yet in contemplating their prognosis, others reject the ostensible epidemiological data and feel the statistics do not apply to them. Many think that compared to the population average, they are healthier or younger, or have different sociodemographics. They seek to sustain hope.

Rachel, for instance, whose family died in the Holocaust and who now has breast cancer and the mutation, feels that the statistics don't apply to her because she has a healthy diet. She thinks her diet improves her prognosis, bolstering her optimism, and avoidance of depression.

> The fact that I'm vegan should lower the risk. I don't expose my body to most toxins. So, I don't think an individual like me is *in* those statistics. Someone may say, "Yeah, but it's a gene—black and white—there it is." But I *still* don't think I'm part of those statistics. If I had controlled my environment *more*, maybe the breast cancer wouldn't have expressed itself in the first place.

She suggests regret, and possible wishful thinking. The mutation already expressed itself, but she seeks to believe she can still somewhat control her fate.

Young women with breast cancer (e.g., in their twenties and thirties) can encounter difficulty identifying an environmental factor to which they may have been exposed, having lived fewer years. Thus, these women face added stresses in trying to grasp the reasons for, and future course of, their illness. Rhonda, the 31-year-old mutation-positive nurse who had seen her mother's death due to breast cancer, and was diagnosed at 23, acknowledged that genetics is important. But she feels that other factors could shape her precise clinical course. As a nurse, she is able to critique extrapolations from the medical literature. She thought she differed from older women, and that past studies thus did not really apply to her, either.

> The statistics were all about women in their forties. Articles said if you drink too much, or eat too much red meat, you'll get sick. But I've only been drinking two years, and don't eat meat. At the time, there were no statistics about women in their thirties—never mind their twenties! Doctors said to me, "Put yourself in with the 40-year-olds."

Yet she resists deducing her own fate from these other probabilities, seeking reasons to support her view. She doesn't want these lower rates of survival to apply to her. In fact, she underwent aggressive prophylactic surgery based on her assumption that her disease is genetic.

Those with cancer but no mutation tend to look more to environmental sources, developing theories based on observations of broad epidemiological trends. As mentioned earlier, they cite ostensibly rising rates of cancer as evidence of such environmental effects, even if the specifics remain unknown— as do some individuals who in fact have a mutation.

People may also look to environmental factors to explain why only certain members of a family get sick. Vera, tested because she was Asian, said that she was the first one in her family to develop breast cancer, and she blames cultural factors: "I am the youngest one in my family, and the most Westernized. Cancer struck me, and not my siblings. I eat more fast food, and sit in front of my computer all day." Though she has the mutation, these personal differences make her downplay the role of genetics.

Many individuals struggle to judge precisely *which* possible environmental or behavioral factors are involved. Yet to do so can be hard. Carmen, the Latina former clerical aide with breast and thyroid cancer and the *BRCA* mutation but no known family history, does not have much education, and faults environmental factors.

> I live near a power plant, and my daughter gets sick from asthma. I don't know if that's *from* the plant. A lot of people say it is. I'm not sure. I smoked and took birth control pills when I was younger. I think *that* contributed to breast cancer.

Particularly as a poorer minority woman, she feels impotent to reduce these possible environmental factors. To her, the disease and industrial contaminants all feel beyond her control. As will be discussed later, larger political beliefs can thus affect these calculations as well. Many poorer women of color, especially, feel powerless to alter larger economic and political forces.

Politically based beliefs can be strong, and persist in the face of possible alternative evidence. For instance, Laura, the graphic designer who surmised her mutation from her genetic counselor's request to have a trainee sit in, said that her family initially thought that their cancer arose from local industrial pollution. But now, knowledge that she has a mutation is forcing her to reconsider. She illustrates how families can ponder these etiological puzzles as a whole.

> My mom and her sister have had cancer three times, whereas their other two siblings never did. Everyone says: "Probably pollution. They grew up in a big refining town." It has always been fascinating that two siblings would be so hard hit, and the other two wouldn't.

Yet the disease could potentially still result from genetics, since not everyone in a family may inherit a mutation. Laura highlights a common misunderstanding that a genetic disease would invariably affect everyone in a family.

Over time, further observations, testing, and diagnoses can challenge such logic. But political views and ideologies die hard. Countervailing pressures can block changes in etiological beliefs, even in the face of data. For example, when Laura subsequently found she had a mutation she minimized the impact of environmental factors somewhat, but not entirely. As she contemplates the etiology of her disease, her political beliefs as an environmentalist still linger.

> I'm thinking more that the chemicals in the area didn't really have anything to do with it at all. *But I'm such a big environmentalist that I can't let that go completely out of my head*—though genetics people pooh-pooh the idea.

She and others thus attempt to integrate their medical history, epidemiological observations, and political views, shaping causal theories of their disease.

Those who had breast cancer but lack a mutation also face complexities and ambiguities. Some have a strong family history, and conclude that additional mutations, not yet discovered, have to be involved. Others look more to environmental phenomena. With cancer and a mutation-negative test, Denise, the banker with a master's degree, chose bilateral mastectomies rather than a lumpectomy simply because of her family history:

> I bet there *probably* is a gene—they just haven't come across it yet. Sometimes I think: could it have been the radiation? I've had more radiation to my breasts than the average person. I wonder if I have too many mammograms. But my gut feeling is that it is genetic.

She speaks of "betting" and her "gut feeling," grappling with the inherent uncertainties.

Samantha, the actress, also had breast cancer and lacks a mutation, but her prior narrative of her life—especially a recent personal trauma—molds her theory. Diagnosed after a horrible breakup with her boyfriend, she feels that personal, not wider environmental, stress is relatively more responsible for her disease. In defense of her causal theories, she, too, engages in deductive reasoning, providing arguments. For instance, she wonders why, if environmental factors are the cause, breast cancer is not more common.

> The environment is significant, but then why wouldn't *everybody* be getting cancer? I wasn't exposed to a ridiculous amount of radiation, but was very susceptible, because I was constantly stressed-out my whole life. My immune system is probably shot.

She challenges the environmental hypothesis, suggesting counter arguments. The philosopher of science Karl Popper[13] described such an attempt at "falsifying" a hypothesis (i.e., asking why, if the cause was environmental, the disease wouldn't be more widespread) as an essential characteristic of scientific, as opposed to "pseudoscientific," thinking. Samantha's reasoning here is valid and impressive.

NEEDS TO ASSIGN AND AVOID BLAME

Not surprisingly, genetics poses conundra of whether and how much individuals themselves or others are at fault for a disease, and what such attributions mean. Desires to avoid such blame and assign it elsewhere often shape these causal theories.

Popular beliefs, promulgated in the media, and at times bolstered by scientists themselves, have ascribed various illnesses to poor health habits—from smoking to unexpressed anger. Patients may thus be seen—by themselves or others—as being responsible for their illness because they practiced, and did not stop, these behaviors.

According to the Oxford English Dictionary, "blame" is derived from the Greek word for "blaspheme." The word came to mean "revile" and "reproach" in Latin, and now also means "to find fault with, to rebuke, scold, accuse, and fix responsibility on," and as a noun means "responsibility for a bad result or something wrong." Thus, while "cause" may refer to both good and bad events, blame carries a moral sense of something "wrong." Issues of blame for illness have been explored with regard to other kinds of disease, but much less with regard to genetics. The anthropologist Evans-Pritchard described how the Azande tribe in Africa desperately sought to assign blame for illness and other calamities, invoking a certain logic.[14] In the case of HIV, Paul Farmer and others have examined how blame can exacerbate stigma.[15] The American public may be more likely to stigmatize individuals whom they see as blameworthy for their disease.[16] But questions arise of how individuals who have or are at risk for these diseases themselves in fact see and experience these issues.

A few individuals blame themselves for their illness. Past traumatic experiences (e.g., history of incest, other stigmatized experiences, being a teenage mother) lead some to fault themselves for their disease. Those who have always felt that something was fundamentally "wrong" with them often see a genetic diagnosis as somehow confirming these feelings. These individuals also generally appeared somewhat depressed, which could result from, or contribute to, these views.

Most individuals struggle to avoid such self-blame—not just stigma that might result, but feelings that they somehow deserve their disease. Both internal guilt and fears of outward stigma propel efforts to eschew self-accusation. Instead, the men and women here generally seek to blame their disease on other factors, not themselves. Yet conflict can ensue.

GENETICS AS GETTING PEOPLE OFF THE HOOK

As suggested earlier, for good or bad, genetic explanations can be seen as reducing personal or social responsibility. For breast cancer, some thought that a positive genetic test would mitigate their own self-blame. Joyce, who worked in a spa and had attributed her cancer to the stresses of living in Chicago and New York, said that if she had been mutation-positive, "I'd feel devoid of all responsibility for my cancer." Instead, without the mutation, she is left chiding, in part, herself.

Blame becomes burdensome because it can imply that one then *deserves* a disease as punishment. Prior to genetic testing, other people may have blamed a patient for his or her cancer—implying that his or her poor diet, limited exercise, or misbehavior must have merited punishment. The presence of a mutation can potentially remove that onus.

THE ROLE OF LUCK

While some individuals see God as the cause, others look to fortune. In the face of unknown scientific factors, apparent randomness and potential blame, many invoke notions of luck. These beliefs have important implications for concepts of both cause and responsibility, and allow individuals to think that they might somehow defy the odds by being lucky.

Notions of luck persist in science, usually as metaphors. But the concept has received little attention in the medical literature, and its meanings are not always clear. I searched Medline and found that the word appeared in the titles of 183 articles (in English) since 1948. But none of the articles in medical science appeared to define it. Most of the manuscripts used the word "luck" in the title, and nowhere else. Luck is also mentioned in patient surveys, but the meanings are hazy.

According to the Oxford English Dictionary (OED), "luck" derives from the Low German *luk*, and later the German *Glück* (meaning "good fortune, happiness"), and probably originated as a gambling term. The OED proceeds to define luck as follows, suggesting several related but in fact somewhat distinct phenomena:

> The effect of . . . uncontrollable events; the sum of fortuitous events affecting (favorably or unfavorably) a person's interest . . . a person's apparent tendency to have good or ill fortune . . . Chance regarded as a cause or bestower of good or ill fortune (sometimes personified [as] Lady Luck).[17]

Though little studied in medicine, philosophers and psychologists have recently examined the concept. But between these two disciplines, perspectives, contexts, and priorities differ. Philosophers have generally appeared more interested in how luck may serve to limit moral responsibility. If one is unlucky, then one is less responsible.[18,19] On the other hand, psychological research has tended to explore several other dimensions of luck—whether people can or cannot *control* events—for example, how everyday intuitions about luck may be contradictory in referring to external events (which the individual cannot readily control) or people (who presumably can potentially control aspects of their behavior). "Luck" can refer to a person, while "chance" may refer more to external environmental events, and represents an external or unstable and uncontrollable cause.[20] People may be seen as having skill at somehow manipulating events (i.e., to have great luck). Individuals may also have an "illusion of control."[21] In addition, events may be seen as lucky if they could have been worse (i.e., compared to counter-factual possible events).[14] Malinowski[22] and anthropologists have also described belief systems concerning luck and magic as providing religious or other culturally sanctioned explanations of natural phenomena.

But as a whole, the medical, psychological, and philosophical literature have generally paid relatively little attention to these notions of luck, magic, and beliefs in controllability. Key questions thus remain as to whether insights from psychology, philosophy, anthropology, and medicine can be integrated, and if so, how.

The men and women here often referred to luck in attempting to make sense of the presence or absence of mutations and phenotypic variations. The concept arose spontaneously as widely used and culturally embedded, with many interviewees saying they felt either lucky or unlucky.

On the one hand, some people spoke of luck to suggest that they were not responsible for events that happened to them, and that an external agency was somehow instead involved. This notion jives with that of many philosophers. Karl, partly due to his childhood abuse, saw people invoking both genetics and luck to reduce their own responsibility for problems:

> People don't want to take responsibility for their own behavior. "We're not responsible for the failure. That was just bad luck." Or "we're not responsible for your success, that was just good luck": The cosmic has reached in.

Individuals may ascribe genetic events to luck, rather than attribute responsibility for an illness to the person. Karl feels that bad luck results from bad judgment. In the end, he holds people, including his father, as responsible for their behavior and its effects, including harmful repercussions. Yet Karl suggests that luck provides not only freedom from responsibility, but a sense of order and explanation as well—a source—"the cosmic." He thereby echoes the perspectives of philosophers, psychologists, and anthropologists—though these disciplines have tended not to address or include each other's views.

Perceptions of luck can also be fluid and dynamic—not static. Individuals may shift, not taking responsibility for baleful effects of their decisions, and seeing the denouements as misfortune rather than as their fault. Conversely, individuals may be seen as creating their own luck, through good choices. Karl felt strongly:

> People make their own luck: It's how you take advantage of situations. You can take advantage of all opportunities that come along, and later on, weed them out. You go through a learning period, when you make some stupid mistakes: "Maybe I shouldn't do that next time." People who refuse to learn, or don't take advantage of opportunities, have lousy luck. People who learn from their mistakes and accept new situations tend to have good luck.

But in any particular situation, individuals can disagree about whether luck is involved, and if so, how. Patients and external observers may conflict in whether they think luck has played a role. Karl continued, "A friend thinks he has terrible luck: permanently stuck in this place. But, he is not a guy with bad luck; he is a *shlemiel* who doesn't make very good choices for himself."

Still, whether an individual can wholly control these actions is disputable. Observers may perceive the extent of a person's good or bad luck differently than that person does him or herself.

As anthropologists such as Evans-Pritchard suggest, luck can be particularly invoked when other causes are unknown—that is, as a "stand-in" for as yet unidentified causes or contributory factors—in this case, as-yet unidentified genes. Invocations of luck may thus reflect residual gaps in scientific explanations. For instance, Benjamin, the 54-year-old engineer, considered himself to be fortunate since despite his Alpha, he still had health and thus, he believed, "better" genes than many other patients with his condition.

> I consider myself lucky: A lot of Alphas die younger than me. If there are such things as milder forms of the disease, and better genetic mixes, I must have ended up with them. I even smoked for 20 years!

His comments parallel scientific notions of so-called modifying genes that can alter the impact of a mutation on an individual, but are not deleterious in and of themselves, and may result in individual differences. However, scientists have not yet elucidated the details involved, leaving room for these perceptions of chance.

Luck arises, too, as an explanation when an individual defies the odds—going against expected disease progression, without other explicit physical explanations. As Gilbert, the factory worker with Alpha, whose children smoke, said, "People smoke, but haven't shown any signs yet. They may just be plain lucky."

In facing the vast uncertainties involved, Benjamin and Gilbert, with Alpha, hesitate to take (or be given) responsibility for good events in order not to "jinx" their luck. In contrast, Karl, who is healthy, described a man who sought to eschew responsibility for bad events in order to avoid being blamed. Painfully aware of the fragility and potential instability of their health, Benjamin and Gilbert choose modesty over tempting fate. Both these stances assume some larger order in the universe.

Others perceive God's favor, or lack thereof, as luck beyond their control. Carmen, the Catholic with breast and thyroid cancer and a mutation, said, "I guess He does it for some people and not others. It's just luck." She looks to God as the final mover of events. Individuals thus differ in how, and to what degree, they believe luck is related to spirituality.

These men and women highlight how disagreements and negotiations about assessments of luck occur. Individuals at times disagree as to whether luck is involved in a particular situation, and if so, to what degree. While one person may argue that he or she simply has bad luck, others may think that that he or she has simply made a series of bad choices.

Surprisingly, the OED does not comment on how and when luck is invoked. In the face of uncertainty, scientists and patients may do so when they don't know why a medical event has occurred—for example, why a person has deviated from the expected norm, becoming ill earlier or later than expected. The OED also does not mention the notion that luck alleviates responsibility. If luck exacerbated symptoms, then the individual him or herself did not do so—that is, bad luck, rather than poor diet and lack of exercise, is responsible.

Luck thus emerges here in the absence of a clear cause, as both a causal explanation and a moral excuse—a combination that serves to lessen responsibility—for illness, rather than immoral behaviors. These men and women view luck as an external and/or internal force. Hence, these interviewees invoke and combine philosophical, psychological, and anthropological approaches to luck—as explanations and exculpation in the face of scientific uncertainty. Yet they also indicate how this concept can be highly contested, which has received little attention heretofore.

EFFECTS ON COPING

These multi-faceted issues of cause and blame can affect coping in several ways. On the one hand, the discovery of a genetic cause of one's disease can help one accept one's disease. When initially learning that they have a mutation, some individuals feel relief, since it means that they are not to blame for their symptoms. For Alpha in particular, a mutation-positive test can reduce responsibility, since this diagnosis is viewed less negatively than emphysema, which results from smoking. Therefore, whether the discovery of a genetic mutation lowers perceived "taintedness" depends on what this new level of stigma is compared to. Alternative diagnoses or explanations for a patient's symptoms may have more or less stigma. As Betty, the designer who carries a bag containing an oxygen concentrator, said, "I feel less stigma with Alpha than I did with emphysema, because it's not necessarily pinned as being *my* fault. It was just the *luck* of the draw." For her, too, luck means the disease is not her fault, and is thus less stigmatized.

With HD, a mutation can explain frightening or stigmatized symptoms, particularly cognitive and psychiatric problems otherwise blamed on the individual. Acknowledgment that a disease is not self-willed or voluntary, but instead beyond the patient's control, can help a patient establish more realistic expectations for him or herself. Before her HD diagnosis, Mary, the housewife and mother, would

> feel bad, and think, "I'm so lazy. I should be doing this or that." It ripped me apart, not reading to my kid, or doing the laundry. Now, I feel better, and give myself more of a break. I know: I'm not really that lazy. I used to forget things. Now, I know I'm not going to remember. So I write them down.

Patients may be particularly faulted for psychiatric symptoms. Wilma views her bipolar disorder as genetic, and her breast cancer as caused by environmental problems. She sees the psychiatric disorder as more tainted than cancer, and wants to disallow any responsibility for the former. Partly as a result, she has refused genetic testing.

A genetic cause can reduce stigma because this explanation suggests not only that the individual did not cause the symptoms him or herself, but that the disease is not infectious, either. Fear of contagion can prompt ostracization. Strangers who observe HD and do not know the genetic basis of the disorder may irrationally fear that they can catch it. Roger, who tested for HD only when his car swerved off the road, said, "I have to explain that HD is genetic, not airborne. A friend was scared because he thought it was airborne. Once you say 'disease,' some people think you're going to kill them!"

People who do not yet understand the cause of HD can not only hold a patient responsible, but treat the patient harshly, or even abusively. For HD, blame can thus be particularly harmful, serving to justify anger at the patient. Genetic testing can potentially reduce such misunderstanding and frustration. As John, who dropped out of graduate school because of the HD in his family and later found he lacked the mutation, explained,

> My sister's symptoms brought out the worst in her husband. He'd humiliate her. For a long time he thought she didn't have HD, and that all these symptoms were her fault. He'd get mad. I thought it would be better for her to be in "a home," even though she really wanted to be at home and be his wife.

A mutation-positive test also can alleviate fault for not only current symptoms, but prior lack of prevention. For example, Anna, the African American former secretary with diabetes and a family history of breast cancer, felt that if her ailments were genetic she could not be blamed for her past behavioral lapses—poor diet or exercise. The fact that a disease could have a genetic basis was comforting, since it would mean that "it didn't come from me doing the wrong thing."

Anna is untested, but rejects the possibility that her behavior may have played any role in her disease—she does not want to admit any culpability whatsoever. Here, again, given desires to assign blame outside oneself, interviewees tended to see these diseases as purely genetic or not, rather than as having mixed etiologies.

Genetic information can not only remove negative images, but offer positive ones. For instance, a mutation-positive result can provide validation and vindication for individuals who develop cancer despite healthy living. For an individual who tried to follow a healthy lifestyle and nevertheless got sick, others may see the diagnosis as ironic justice. To reconcile one's diagnoses with one's self-image as "healthy" can be hard. Others who scoff at preventive behaviors may feel vindicated. Learning that one has a disease due to a mutation can thus re-instill a sense of cosmic "fairness." Rachel, whose family died in the Holocaust and who now had breast cancer and the mutation, said,

> I was a completely healthy eater. I don't have a lot of junk food in my house, and have always taken vitamins. When kids come over, I have ice cream or cookies in the house, but no Cheetos and Doritos. So, jokingly, other mothers would say I was a bad mom. When I learned I have this mutation, some people felt, "Well, even *that* didn't help save her"—all that health food stuff I've been saying. They felt there was some poetic justice

to the fact that after all of these healthy behaviors, I got breast cancer. So, when I found out it was a gene mutation, I felt better. It let me say: "It wasn't in my complete control."

A mutation-positive result can thus reaffirm one's sense of both self-esteem and justice in the universe.

Conversely, a mutation-negative test result can potentially increase blame of the patient. Failure to find a mutation leads some to feel that their illness must have been self-initiated. Joyce, the spa employee with cancer but no mutation who attributed her cancer in part to difficulties of urban living, continued:

Sometimes I blame myself for this cancer. I think it was stress-related. I had this messy divorce, and was a single mother, struggling financially. A month before 9/11, my grandmother and my father died. Then 9/11 happened. Then I got diagnosed.

In part, since she lacked the *BRCA1/2* mutation, she felt that genetics was not at all involved, and she thus faulted herself even more.

Yet in addition to reducing possible stigma, a genetic explanation can also enhance social support and entrance into the sick role. Patients who learn that they have a mutation may thus feel more relief. As Roger, tested after having problems driving, said about his HD mutation,

If people understand what's going on, they help you out. I say, "Do you mind getting a plate for me?" "Sure. No problem. Do you want me to cut the food for you? Do you want me to write your checks for you?" That's why I explain what's going on. If they didn't understand, they'd say, "Write your own checks, lazy!"

Lowered blameworthiness can also facilitate further disclosures of the disease to others. Bill, the asymptomatic, untested salesman who resembles his father, and now cares for his HD-affected brother, thinks the disease is easier to divulge than others—even HIV—because it is genetic, and hence not the patient's fault.

A lot of people hide AIDS, because they got it from doing something dangerous or illicit—being homosexual or a drug user—practices not acceptable to society. But if you're *born* with something, you've got no control over it. Why hide that? It's not your fault.

The fact that he has no symptoms also makes it easier to be open about his risk. Disease etiologies—genetic or otherwise—have critical implications for the empathy patients may receive.

The possibility of decreasing self-blame can also prompt genetic testing. Jan had breast cancer and turned out to be mutation-negative, but wanted to have the mutation, since it would have reduced her personal responsibility for her disease. She would also then have had a genetic explanation for why she was different from the rest of her family.

> It would have given me peace of mind that there is a link, and a reason why I'm the only one in my family with breast cancer. People with no gene link still don't know the reason. At least I would have known.

Indeed, others blamed her for her illness, saying, "Maybe if you weren't on the pill, this wouldn't have happened." She thus felt that the pros of learning of the presence of a mutation would have outweighed the cons.

Others see mutation-positive tests as both an advantage in reducing stigma, but a disadvantage as well. Knowledge of a mutation can be a mixed blessing: it reduces blame, but still constitutes bad news. Nonetheless, at least for Alpha, given that treatment is available, the good news often outweighs the bad. As Barbara, the part-time professor who feels guilty about having smoked near her daughter, said,

> The diagnosis both relieved and traumatized me. I was relieved because I found out what it was: this mysterious thing I kept blaming myself for. I had thought: maybe I hadn't eaten right, or my heart was closed. But the doctor put his hand on mine and said, "No, you were *born* this way." I learned that a lot of my problems were related to the disease: being tired, anxious, short-tempered. If I can't breathe or get enough oxygen, I get irritable. The diagnosis helped. Now, I pace myself.

The fact that she had smoked contributed to her sense that she had exacerbated her symptoms; the discovery of a mutation eased her regret.

Problems if One May Have Contributed to One's Disease

Patients who feel that they may have contributed to their disease even in some small way thus face added dilemmas of how to make sense of that possibility. Given remaining uncertainties, they are often not clear how to parse responsibility, guilt, and self-blame. Combinations of genetic and nongenetic (behavioral or environmental) factors can be hard to grasp, integrate, or accept. Many desire a black or white, all-or-none answer—whether they are responsible or not. Yet quantifying responsibility is difficult, if not impossible. As Benjamin, the engineer, said about his Alpha, "People ask: 'Did you smoke?' I don't like

that question, because the answer is 'Yes.' Or I say, 'Yes, but I had a predisposition that caused my disease.'" He admitted to his behavior, but still sought
exoneration.

Patients may wish to excuse themselves on the grounds that they were
unaware at the time that they were contributing to their eventual illness. Charles,
the accountant and former smoker, felt that "a good part" of his Alpha was
"self-inflicted, *though I didn't know I had the disease then.*" Yet even after learning of their genetic predisposition, he and many others continue to engage in
risks, still frequenting smoky bars: "A bunch of us have been going there for
years." He justifies this behavior by pointing out that going there is a tradition,
and that he is not the only one. To reduce hazardous behavior can be hard.

The Politics of Environmental Factors

As suggested earlier, broad political views can also affect beliefs about the nature
and impact of environmental factors. In particular, those who feel disempowerment and discrimination sense that capitalistic greed generated both known
and unknown environmental harms. Hilda, the African American health aide
with breast cancer and a family history of the disease but no testing, felt that she
received lower quality health care because of her race, and that her cancer
resulted from industrial disregard.

> People in the Bronx have more cancer and breathing problems. A lot of
> things go on in the Bronx that don't in Manhattan. I know that for a fact.
> The water, everything. There's more garbage and garbage dumps and
> landfills. That's what co-op city is built on. I think about it a lot. More
> people are catching cancer than ever. I don't believe it's from God, or
> genetics. *It's from the environment.*

She feels that corporate indifference (things "they" do) endanger marginalized
people, including her. Yet this causal belief also diminishes her inclination to
undergo genetic testing.

Moreover, political disempowerment can make one feel unable to counter
these forces, or even acquire much information about them. Bonnie, the asymptomatic, untested 24-year-old who had seen breast cancer in her mother and
sister, was concerned about the environment. "We just don't know anymore
what's in the air or our food," she said.

In part due to underlying political views, beliefs that environmental factors
contribute to disease can foster anger that ostensible genetic explanations are
receiving too much attention. Several men and women argued that focus on

genetics decreases attention to politically important environmental harms. As Bonnie continued,

> Genetic testing makes people too relaxed. Maybe I'm O.K. genetically, but going to get breast cancer because of my environment. You always have to be aware of what's going on environmentally, or something will happen, and it might be too late.

Having seen cancer in her mother and sister, she fears it, and advocates heightened political action. She cannot control what genes she has, but she can potentially improve her environment.

Broad societal questions surface as well concerning the degrees to which certain groups of individuals have a role in causing or curing their disease. Karl, abused as a child and lacking the HD mutation, felt,

> Genetics is a way of people avoiding responsibility for things. For example, "Society didn't create alcoholism. It happens to people because they have the wrong genes." It's a *genetic* problem. It isn't even society's problem."

He spoke with irony, believing that social forces in fact played key roles, too. He sees genetics as unjustifiably exculpating social processes and policy makers for responsibility for social problems. The specific boundaries between these alternative sets of forces may be unclear. Yet integrating these competing beliefs can be hard.

Lack of Control: Fatalism and Depression

Desires for hope and avoidance of despair both result from and lead to these causal views. Often, fatalism appears to exacerbate depression, while beliefs in metaphysics offer solace.

Regardless of the causal theories they adopt, these patients then wrestle with questions of whether they could affect their fate, and if so, how. Many want to believe in controllability, yet empirical evidence may not support this possibility—certainly not as much as these individuals wish. Desires to prevail over disease can prompt incorrect beliefs. Even those who favor physical explanations still often seek to view these causes within larger cosmological frameworks in order to regain some sense of control. Individuals frequently conceptualize forces in the universe beyond our influence as randomness and chance. Harriet, a schoolteacher with an extensive family history of breast cancer, no symptoms, and an inconclusive test result, felt that ultimately she could not alter her fate: "Why me? It's just beyond our control. When the cells are multiplying, *something just went whack.*"

Yet perceived lack of control could make individuals feel stuck and depressed. Diane, who had an unanticipated mastectomy, felt she had *no* control over her fate. The trauma of unexpected surgery left her feeling helpless. Since then she has come to feel more stoical, but remains unsure of the relative advantages and disadvantages of these various views.

> Since the operation, I've become more *fatalistic.* Before, I had much more trust in life. I felt that things were more up to me: you decide the life you make. Then *this* happened, totally unpredictable and unplanned, and changed my outlook. Maybe it's more realistic. Who knows?

LESSENING THE IMPACT OF GENES: SEEKING CONTROL

Individuals often hope they can control their fate, but vary widely in whether they feel they are indeed able to do so, to what degree, and how. They yearn for control, but are unsure whether they in fact have any, or whether God alone caused their illness. In general, amounts of control vary with several broad types of non-genetic biological factors: those over which individuals readily have some sway (e.g., diet and exercise), have no influence (air pollution), or can affect only with difficulty (staying in a stressful job that, in retrospect, may have contributed to disease).

In confronting their genetic risks, many who oppose genetic determinism believe they can alter the course of their disease through the power of positive thinking. These views partly reflect wider beliefs and popular psychology, and can reduce the harsh inevitabilities of genetic determinism. Thus, these notions can take on metaphysical overtones, including countercultural New Age ideas. To support these views, some look for scientific grounding as well. Shilpa, the Hindu medical student at risk of breast cancer without symptoms or testing, tries to integrate physical and metaphysical beliefs. "Quantum physics believes we have control of our destiny by the power of our thinking," she said. "*Your reality is what you believe to be real.*"

Though many think that behavioral factors at least contribute to disease, and conversely can reverse a certain amount of it, questions remain as to when, how, and to what degree. Many believe or wish to believe that they can control certain realms of their lives, and look to extend such self-determination to their health as well. Karl said, in part due to his abuse:

> I don't believe we're just a bag of genes, and walk around, doing what our genes tell us. There's a lot of will involved in our lives. Behavior, feelings,

experiences are defined by a multitude of things. Genetics is part of it. You have an effect over plenty of things. I taught myself to play music, and got good at it.

Yet the fact that he lacks the HD mutation also helps mold his attitude. His and others' own medical status and experiences can thus guide their theories about genetics versus freedom.

Many feel that spirituality, too, may have a role—though the specific mechanisms vary. Such beliefs are thought to reduce disease either directly or indirectly. Spirituality may not eliminate a disease, but it can decrease stress, which can in turn affect the illness. Individuals often thought that specific, concrete behaviors that contribute to cardiac and certain other common diseases could also affect genetic, additional disorders. Others feel that simply learning about their disease risk and potential prevention options can reduce perceived impotence, and consequently enhances coping. Bonnie, who had seen cancer in her mother and sister but is untested and asymptomatic, said, "I educate myself, so I feel more empowered. If I wasn't educated about available testing and medicine, I would feel *helpless*. My craving to know everything makes me not feel helpless."

In seeking to support their beliefs that behavior and free will could overcome or affect genetics, many draw on folk mythologies that offer models and analogies from behavioral genetics—for example, regarding homosexuality. Antonia, the neuroscientist, said,

> Ultimately, someone's will is stronger than their genetics. You're born with certain genes which predispose you to whatever. Gay people are born gay—it's genetic—but you can choose to suppress it, or go with it.

Though homosexuality has not yet been show to be genetic, she and many others suspect that it will eventually be found to be so.

Reducing Stress

Most people pursue these ideas further, adopting behaviors that they feel can be beneficial—such as lowering stress. They believe that a gene-positive test does not constitute their utter fate because they can still control their destiny through certain actions. If stress can exacerbate symptoms, then decreasing it can help. Some blame stress and invoke New Age or Eastern philosophies, holding quasi-religious beliefs that a lack of bodily balance, induced by stress, causes disease. Diane, the Spanish teacher with the unplanned mastectomy, looked to psychological factors in part because she tested mutation-negative.

Many things in my life that were not harmonious might have been precipitating factors. If your body is imbalanced, there are consequences. My childhood was not very good. My parents didn't get along. My mother had seven kids. It was after the war—not easy. My entire childhood caused stress.

Whether childhood stress in fact contributes to later breast cancer is not clear, but the larger point here is that she and others seek to understand their disease in this way, drawing on their former beliefs about themselves. They try to fit genetic information about themselves into their prior ongoing narratives about their lives. Genetics can thus become part of this life story, rather than radically disrupting it.

Yet others who have mutations nonetheless look to non-genetic factors as also having roles—at times citing physical mechanisms through which they feel these factors operate. Triggers (which, as we saw, could serve as ways of integrating genetic and other factors) also provide room for beliefs about control. Some think their disease is activated by stress, citing a weakened immune system as the mechanism. They feel they can thus reduce their disease by lowering these pressures. Rachel, whose family died in the Holocaust and who now has breast cancer and the *BRCA* mutation, struggles to grasp the causal roles of genetic versus nongenetic factors. "My gene would not have expressed itself had I been able to control the way I processed stress," she said. "Stress lowers your immune system. It killed my father. It's the antioxidant supreme!"

She invokes popular myths about antioxidants that have been hypothesized to play roles, but have not yet shown to be effective antidotes. Nonetheless, the firmness of her convictions reflects the strength of her underlying need to believe that she has some influence over her destiny. In trying to view stress as a factor or "cause," she sees it as operating by shaping not whether, but *when* and *how* severely her disease may affect her. "I have control to some degree over how long I'll live," she said. "The control is in how I eliminate stress. I think more positively, and as a result, am happy. That is one of the largest predictors of life."

Yet decreasing stress can be hard. The psychological pressures cited as contributing to cancer ranged from specific to general, and are not always readily avoidable. Many tensions of modern living can be involved. Ori, the Israeli with breast cancer, came to the conclusion based on her lack of mutation or family history that

I can't pinpoint one particular behavior that can be removed. I don't think it's genetic. Maybe it's from not sleeping enough, taxing the body, being stressed, not letting the T-cells do their thing. I'm guilty of not allowing them to patrol well. I'm always under some stress. It's the life we live: everything is a deadline!

Diet and Complementary and Alternative Medicine

Many believe that eating poorly can exacerbate disease, and eating well can be therapeutic, and they consequently try to alter their diet. Bonnie, having seen her mother's and sister's breast cancer, became an organic vegetarian as a result. "Our family's been meat eaters, and all have cancer," she reported. "More processed, genetically modified and improved food will hurt us. I eat less processed foods and feel much healthier." Though no evidence yet exists to support the notion that genetically modified foods harm consumers, she suggests a strong and persistent desire to blame at least something, or find an alterable factor.

Whether they felt that their illness resulted from genetics or environment, individuals had to decide whether and how much to try to lessen versus continue these perceived behavioral risks.

Conversely, discovery that one has a mutation can reduce preventive behavior, which may then seem superfluous. The presence of a mutation can make some individuals more fatalistic, and less inclined to alter their diet. Mildred, who works in finance, underwent genetic testing to see if she could avoid prophylactic surgery. Sadly, she turned out to have the mutation, and chose surgery. "After I had breast cancer, I started to eat organic eggs and organic chicken," she said. "Then, once I got tested genetically, I said, 'Well, that's out the window.'"

Some acknowledge genetic factors but feel that environmental and behavioral variables can still nonetheless play important roles. Given the desire for control, many think that willed behaviors can potentially modulate genetic factors, and that genetic testing is thus superfluous.

Physicians generally failed to support beliefs in complimentary and alternative medicine (CAM), and at times were even antagonistic. Some patients feel that physicians frequently conspire against such alternative approaches, and that much of medical research is misguided in dismissing these purported therapies. Samantha, the actress with breast cancer and no family history or mutation, said,

No one told me to change my diet. During my chemotherapy, I was drinking Pepsi. The doctor said *that* was fine. Now, they don't want me to take herbs. I'm doing a lot of alternative therapy, but I didn't tell my doctor. A woman gives me colonics. She cured herself of uterine cancer.

Holistic approaches are often seen as challenging and threatening the medical model. Samantha thought that diet, CAM, and spirituality were all closely related.

There's a whole cancer *conspiracy*: books about how they know a cure for cancer, but are not saying it, because many people would be out of a job—the pharmaceutical companies. I don't think people are *that* evil. But things are overlooked. People are against this whole *emotional dimension, because they're scared.*

At times, medical and political beliefs blur together—for example, that capitalist society stresses people in ways that precipitate cancer. Samantha added,

This society is very screwed up. There's too much about the way people look—too much pressure on women. Maybe that's why everybody's getting breast cancer. Half of America is constipated!

She believes that doctors overemphasize genetics, and she cites rising rates of breast cancer as evidence of environmental rather than genetic factors. She argues that as a result, her doctors missed her diagnosis: "I went to four different doctors and they didn't pick it up at all. They totally disregarded other possibilities."

Samantha remains biased against the medical model, as she feels it overemphasizes pharmaceuticals. Similarly, she takes an antidepressant, but attributes her improved mental state not to it, but to CAM. She feels that holistic practices have in fact made her healthier than ever before. Several nonscientific and antiscientific attitudes—reflecting views about politics, economics, psychology, and spirituality—can thus mold beliefs about etiology and treatment. She continued:

Two different psychics, who don't even know each other, saw toxicity in my colon. Everybody says, "You've never looked better." I'm still on the Zoloft. But this drug thing's getting a little out of control.

Yet even she and others who feel that they can alter their destiny face questions of to *what extent* they can do so. Individuals struggle with how much they can reduce a disease with strong genetic components, and how so. Many believe that a degree of influence was possible, but they then grappled with judging the amount, nature, and scope of this control and free will. Kym, the South Asian physician with a family history of breast cancer but no symptoms or testing, feels it is still worth trying to alter her fate, even if the change is small.

I try to maintain a positive attitude, a healthy lifestyle, and stay active. There's something to mind/body medicine. You *can* affect it—maybe not completely prevent or change something 100%, but maybe change the outcome a little. Maybe some things are loosely in place for us, but can be manipulated a little bit. Destiny is probably already mapped out: getting it or not. But I can maybe affect that *a little bit.*

Others are far less sanguine about their capacity to affect their genes. Kym feels it is never too late to engage in possible prevention, even if such efforts have not been proven to work—the costs can be relatively low, and the benefits high. But other interviewees find even these costs too high. Beliefs that altering behavior can reduce disease do not always sustain these changes over time. Nonetheless, the utter bleakness of a fatalistic stance propels attempts to seek some positive frameworks, despite lingering doubts. Diane, who had the unexpected mastectomy but no family history or mutation, said, "I'm fully aware the cancer can happen again, but *que sera, sera.* Perhaps there is some kind of a renewal thing—like the Indians believe." She muses about spiritual beliefs concerning reincarnation, but remains unsure. Her unexpected surgery, and the fact that she lacks a mutation or family history heighten her belief in the unpredictability of fate.

Others, who think that etiological factors can potentially be altered, nonetheless do not always feel *able* to affect such change. Logistical barriers can loom. Environmental factors can be too widespread, and thus difficult, if not impossible, to eliminate. For example, urban pollution may exacerbate Alpha, but not enough to justify relocation to a rural area. Charles, the accountant who still frequents smoky bars, said, "My wife and I really like New York. But pollution is part of life here." He resigns himself to the risk.

Elimination of environmental factors can also compete with other desires or needs. Patients may confront difficult choices, and not sufficiently want or be able to lower these factors. "I'd rather live a day in New York than the rest of my life anywhere else," said Barbara, the part-time professor and former smoker with Alpha. To enhance the quality of her life, she is willing to take certain risks.

Most people want some control, but in the end, feel they have to accept certain restrictions. They perceive limits to the "fairness" of the universe, though to accept these can still be hard, fueling fatalism. "I may not agree with destiny and fate," Bonnie said, "But I have to accept it. Some things aren't fair. I'm not powerful. I can't change destiny. I'm not Superman." She could potentially change some things, but not genes. "It's the deck of cards I was given," she sighed. "It's not like I can just *trade in* the gene at any time." This metaphor of a card game suggests both fixed rules and randomness. Bonnie is pessimistic, thinking that given "bad genes," healthy living can accomplish only a little: "If it's genetic, it's going to come out."

Others feel that they could alter potential environmental and behavioral factors, but that doing so would cause other stresses that could negate the advantages. They thus actively choose to stay in particular jobs that generate certain tensions, rather than embark on potentially disruptive change. A new position could increase stress, and hence illness. But consequently, they feel stuck. As a last resort, when they feel they can do nothing else, some turn to spirituality. A genetic diagnosis can prompt a spiritual quest that can, in turn, provide reassurance and spiritual healing. Such a journey can help in coping with both disease and other aspects of life. "When I was tested," said Jennifer, the schoolteacher who was tested for Alpha after her son, "I entered a church: a tremendous growing experience. I used the Bernie Siegel tapes a lot—part of my *spiritual journey*."

Beliefs about metaphysical connectedness can help, in part, by enhancing social support and assisting with psychological problems, such as poor self-esteem. She continued, "I can almost hear a tape: 'You are a worthwhile person and deserve to be well.' I began to create people around me that supported this. I now do a healing circle." She highlights how deeply issues of deserving versus not deserving punishment and disease can run.

Some individuals feel that spirituality can potentially control even HD—that they can mold their destiny, and should eschew "negative thinking." These views often reflect wider cultural beliefs. Sue did not have HD symptoms or testing, which helped her to think that spirituality—not genes—could play a decisive role. "If you lead your life in a spiritual way, you can have control over the situation," she said. "But, if you chose to be in denial, or not talk about things, it could get the best of you."

Denial versus Acceptance

Minimization and denial can also fuel and be propelled by metaphysical views, and impede pursuit of treatment. Joyce, for example, the spa employee who blamed her breast cancer on urban living, did not think that breast cancer in her maternal grandmother and aunt might increase her own likelihood of disease.

I was in incredible denial. From the time I was diagnosed, I just assumed that everything was going to be O.K. if I had breast cancer, which I *refused* to have. *I just thought some miracle was going to happen*, and I wasn't going to have chemo or radiation. Then, when it did hit me, it hit me like a ton of bricks. I was a wreck, angry, frightened, crazed. A sibling said: it's good you're having aggressive treatment because of the history of our family. I was startled. I had never thought of it that way. I didn't think my positive nodes were related to *their* brain tumor or cancer.

Even in the face of disease in the family, denial of genetic risk can exist, perpetuated by uncertainties about penetrance and predictability. Her beliefs also furthered her decision to avoid testing for a long time. New Age beliefs in the power of positive thinking can potentially impede or delay follow-up treatment in oneself and one's family.

Individuals vary in how much they consider these ambiguities concerning causality and controllability. Some remain unsure how to answer these questions—even whether these quandaries are in fact answerable—and try to accept equanimity and the lack of answers. They acknowledge limited control and try to move on. Rhonda, the nurse who at age six had seen her mother die from breast cancer, reflected: "You don't get an answer, but you get *past it*. You move on to acceptance, and do what you've got to do about it." She thought that the best one can hope for is treatment, prevention, and increased awareness.

For HD, too, the intrinsic irresolvability of these questions lead many to try simply to cope as best as possible with current realities. "You have to deal with things pragmatically," Karl concluded. "My brother has problems. How do I help now? How do I deal with this situation now?"

These views of causality can potentially affect other health behaviors, too, including testing, disclosure, and treatment. Those who viewed their illness as more environmental and less genetic were generally less likely to test.

Blaming Parents

Individuals wrestle with questions of blaming not only themselves, but their parents. Though seemingly illogical, quandaries persist of whether to blame their mutations on a parent, and whether one would be blamed by one's offspring, or should feel guilty about possibly transmitting a mutation. Some past research suggests that patients may blame mothers for a disease.[23] Yet such faulting, guilt, and fear in fact arise, too, among mothers themselves. Indeed, many parents feel responsible or fear being blamed for their children's disease. Parents could thus face not only anger about having been *given* a genetic disease, but guilt over giving it to others. Isabelle, the social worker with breast cancer and a mutation but no family history who blamed her cancer on her mildewed apartment, said,

> It's a totally illogical guilt. But I have it. Logically, it's ridiculous—most guilt is, anyway. But it's there. I don't think it's that uncommon: we're responsible for our children. My mother would feel the same way if she had this gene, knowing that I got it from her. It's difficult to know that your children may have this gene. We pass other things on to children, but having *this* mutation, with a 50% chance that they may have it, is *horrible*.

At one point, she wished she had not had children. As we shall see, she also thought they had a 50% chance of getting cancer—a misunderstanding.

Uncertainty hovers as to how future generations will indeed view the fact that tests existed today, but were not always used. Though illogically based, the possibility that children *could* blame parents for having passed on the gene leads some adults to decide not to reproduce.

Parents blamed themselves for not only genetic but environmental causes of their offspring's possible disease. Guilt can persist despite the potential ubiquity of certain environmental factors. Ginger, the medical secretary with Alpha, reported, "I worry: my husband and I both smoked when my son was young. Did that affect him?" She feels guilty about possibly having exposed her son to smoke, and feels frustrated and angry at him for exposing his own kids to it as well.

Parental guilt and responsibility can be particularly fraught for parents affected by HD, since the disease can undermine parenting. As we saw, HD can prompt emotional, physical, or other abuse. Though a genetic diagnosis can explain and make sense of these psychiatric symptoms, to know whether and how much to forgive an ill but abusive parent is difficult. Ambiguities here about the degree to which mutations alone can kindle symptoms have crucial implications. Offspring struggle with whether a mutation condones harmful behaviors; and to attribute such abuse wholly to HD is hard. Karl wants to avoid ascribing his father's behavior solely to this disease. "People do bad things to their children for lots of reasons," he said. "I wouldn't attribute it to HD necessarily. A lot of people have difficult, unpredictable parents."

Yet he has trouble sorting through these complex and conflicting issues. HD can impede parents' ability even to discuss past egregious behavior. Symptoms can make it difficult to understand the degrees to which the abuse was controllable. Karl continued:

> I finally felt strong enough to talk to my father about the sexual abuse. He said, "I don't remember anything." He might have been honest. Maybe he's not ready to cave in, or he buried it. Who knows? Maybe when he abused me, he was crazy. But maybe not. Plenty of people with Huntington's don't

have sex with their children! I was never going to get over being angry with him. Regardless of the reasons, once he died of the disease, I felt "maybe my anger is slightly misplaced." Maybe his behavior was beyond his control. Maybe my judgment at the time was harsh. That's difficult.

To understand and reconcile these complex issues of uncertainty, causality, anger, and mourning can be formidable. Karl struggles to figure out how incensed to be—how much his father's possible lack of full volition reduces culpability. Karl wrestles with ambiguities concerning the extent to which genetics represents an exclusive cause versus one of several contributory factors.

The difficulty of discerning what inappropriate behaviors result from (and can thus be blamed on) HD rather than on individual free will frustrates him.

I can't just say, "This part is from the HD, and this part is from something else." *That's the most confusing aspect of the whole thing*—the inability to separate what aspect of his behavior can be attributed to HD. *There's just no way to know.*

Even this disease, with a dominant and penetrant mutation, poses ambiguities. In the absence of certitude, only time—specifically the development of other physical symptoms—may be able to resolve these questions of causality. The fact that symptoms may fluctuate makes it hard to pin behaviors wholly on the mutation.

Desires for attribution of blame can also clash with difficulties in establishing definitive causes. As Karl added: "I want him to be responsible, but I don't think that's fair." Belief in even a small amount of volition—as opposed to a wholly biological cause—can impede forgiveness, relationships, reconciliation, and acceptance. "When he refused to talk to me about the sexual abuse, I stopped talking to him," Karl said. "I didn't even ask where his funeral was. He had left my life a long time ago." Still, such distance can prove highly discomforting. Many eventually resign themselves to uncertainty and to tempering their anger and blame, but doing so is hard.

Some people feel uncomfortable even considering parents' culpability for transmitting disease because of the logical absurdity involved. Charles, the accountant who still frequents smoky bars, joked about his Alpha: "I don't blame only myself. It's my parents' fault, too." He half-jests, but it is unclear to what degree; his humor reveals underlying ambivalence.

Other parents acknowledge the *potential* for a child to blame them for not having prevented gene transmission (e.g., by adopting, engaging in prenatal testing, or screening embryos). Yet parents and other family members may resist and feel defensive about having such responsibility. Even if illogical, stigma and guilt can hamper confrontation of the possibility of passing a mutation to future generations. As Jennifer, the schoolteacher with Alpha, reported:

> My aunt said: "You didn't get this from *us!*" I said, "Your mother was always short of breath!" Her sister died of emphysema. Everyone in her family had it. But she didn't want to talk about it—she would be ashamed.

For others, blaming parents is conceptually impossible—without one's parents, one simply wouldn't exist. These offspring know that parents would never have desired to transmit a mutation. As Betty, the designer who totes an oxygen machine for her Alpha, said, "They wouldn't have wished this on me, and they did enough other things right."

CONCLUSIONS

These individuals struggle to understand the causes of the genetic diseases they confronted. Their previous personal and political beliefs both shaped and were shaped by views about the causes of these diseases. Prior beliefs about oneself, larger political and social issues, and psychological needs (e.g., denial or hope) can result from and lead to causal theories. These attitudes can in turn affect coping, treatment, testing, disclosure, and reproductive decisions.

Scientific explanations remain limited. Scientists may accept this constraint, and anticipate answers from further research. Yet in the absence of objective fact, many patients (and perhaps some scientists, too) turn to metaphysics and luck.

The forecasts of genetics and of Greek mythology clearly differ—genetics is based on biology, and mythology on metaphysics. But they spark similar paradoxes and problems. To the Greeks, our fate is fixed. We can rail against it, but are condemned to it. Cassandra, who foresaw the future, was ignored. Oedipus tried to escape his destiny but couldn't. As with the Greeks, the people here commonly misinterpret, ignore, and deny information about their future, and try to avoid it. Humans often think they can dodge it, or rationalize it away.

At the same time, the prophecies of Greek mythology differ from those of modern genetics in that genetics can make certain predictions more accurately—even if not absolutely. Yet these modern predictions still contain ambiguities, and usually involve only slightly increased probabilities of certain events transpiring. Whereas Greek prophesies were linguistically murky, genetic forecasting is vague statistically. But both contain inherent uncertainties.

For millennia, philosophers have pondered conceptions of causality—how unseen forces yield observable phenomena—and tensions between free will and determinism. The men and women here reflect these underlying conflicts— the degrees to which humans are truly free agents, unrestricted by their bodies. The philosopher Daniel Dennett has explored the polarized debate between free will versus determinism, and described a third, middle path of compatibalism.[24] These patients highlight similar tensions, wrestling in their everyday lives with the haziness and complexity involved. Genetics prompts these patients to try to integrate free will and determinism in varying ways—by differentiating whether, when, how, and to what degree these opposing notions interface.

People appear hard-wired to seek knowledge of the future—because it is valuable to do so, to plan appropriately for potential perils, reducing anxiety about the unknown. But prognostications are often wrong. The drive to know the future poses advantages, but disadvantages, as well. It can stimulate deep foreboding.

At the same time, these men and women suggest tendencies toward what I call "single causalism"—that an outcome results from *one* cause. To fathom how two or more factors interact proves difficult. People seek to assign blame and responsibility, yet to "share blame"—even to grasp what that means—is difficult. It is easier to fault a single culprit, focusing one's anger on *one* target, rather than spreading it out, and having to decide how and to what relative degree to apportion it.

Yet in reality, many disease phenomena are multi-causal. Desires for simple understandings clash with more complex realities. Patients struggle to navigate these tensions. Barbara Katz Rothman and certain other scholars criticize over-attention to genetics as a cause of disease. Interestingly, the men and women here often reveal needs to find such a simple responsible force. They do not all opt for genetics. But when they don't, they nonetheless hunt for some other single cause, and find combinations of these hard to grasp. They may bring together explanatory theories in various ways—different factors determining when versus whether a disease will occur—but in the end, tend to focus on just one. To integrate two or more explanations, each with inherent ambiguities, poses challenges concerning the borders, interactions, and boundaries of each that are exceedingly hard to untangle. How they choose evidence varies widely, due to a range of factors. Many individuals here avoid evidence, or grapple to embrace it, based in part on their prior causal views.

While scientific understandings have generally shifted from monocausality to recognition of multifactorial causes,[11] patients still tend to seek single causes. In part, patients have more at stake—their very lives. Hence, these questions are not merely of intellectual interest, but have profound emotional implications as these individuals seek to exert some control, avoid helplessness, and find hope.

While scholars have often argued that avoidance of *fear* is the central psychological state that motivates humans in confronting disease,[9,25] in this case, needs for hope shape these issues as well. These men and women try to eschew not just anxiety, but also despair and depression. Testing can be beneficial as well, leading patients to feel less stigmatized, enter supportive communities, and find new sources of meaning in their lives. Particularly with genetic markers with unclear meanings, individuals may try to view the threat in ways that reduce it—by seeing it as controllable. Individuals can blame—but not change—genes, and thus look for ways of potentially improving their fate.

In deciding about the cause of complex diseases that are in fact of mixed etiology, interviewees often choose theories and narratives based on the relative strength and salience of prior personal, social, or political beliefs, and psychological needs. People tend to seek a cause—whether a person, a corporation, a god, or luck. Though some psychologists[26] have argued that individuals see a disease as less preventable when its genetic source is emphasized, the individuals here look for ways that a disease may in fact still be preventable even if it is associated with genetic markers. Moreover, the degrees to which the cause is indeed seen as genetic can be fluid, and open to subjective interpretation. Though a few scholars have suggested that individuals see a genetic disease in one of three ways—as environmental, as mystical, or as a puzzle[27]—individuals here in fact frequently combine these and other views. They integrate elements of different theories, each explaining aspects of the disease process—for example, whether versus when versus how severely one develops a diagnosis.

Though some researchers have argued that individuals see a disease fatalistically when a test detects an uncontrollable and threatening genetic marker,[9] in fact the perceived controllability and preventability of a disease are not necessarily fixed, but can be subjectively constructed. Even in the face of a genetic marker, individuals seek "wiggle room," assessing whether, when, and how severely they may become ill. These patients seek to avoid fatalism, and to view these diseases as alterable in some ways. They display a range of attitudes and decisions as to what factors are relevant, frequently constructing their observations of their own and others' experiences in such a way as to fit their prior beliefs about a particular factor.

Several social scientists have suggested a tension between seeing control as a source of hope versus a reason for self-blame (i.e., that individuals had failed to prevent a controllable problem).[9] Yet the individuals here differentiate between these two views of control. For example, they distinguish temporally between being able to have an impact in certain ways *now* versus not having been able to do so in other ways in the *past*. Prior feelings of self-blame mold these perspectives as well. People select objective data based on subjective predilections and, at times, palpably undeniable facts. Individuals integrate these subjective versus objective inputs in part by conceptualizing different realms or functions for each set of data or beliefs (e.g., perceiving "triggers," or differentiating between inner versus outer, or proximal versus distal effects of genes).

While a few scholars have argued that subjective representations of disease affect patients' behaviors more than objective data[28] and that if representations are invalidated, individuals change these, the men and women here illustrate the complexity of these processes. Patients struggle to construct understandings that feel satisfactory. At first they can deny evidence and maintain certain beliefs even in the face of potential counterevidence because they seek and perceive other facts as supporting their ideas. Moreover, individuals may choose not to undergo genetic testing in order to evade a sense of fatalism if they find they have a mutation. Instead, they may feel that metaphysics or environmental or behavioral factors are involved and can shape their risk of the disease, or they may blame bad luck rather than seeing themselves as somehow responsible. In this way, luck is often given agency (in other settings, it is even personified as "Lady Luck"). In order to maintain these beliefs in nongenetic factors, individuals may choose not to get tested, thus also impeding receipt of counterinformation.

Over time, people may challenge, question, revise, and adapt their causal views based on events. While prior researchers have argued that threat without control leads to stress or nontesting,[9] the men and women here suggest that they also change their beliefs about their potential influence over mutations. Desires for control can affect views of reality, even if because of misunderstandings of genetics.

Illness representations may affect health behaviors, but not always,[29] and this lack of correlation may be due to the intricacies of these issues involving denial, miscomprehension, and belief in luck and metaphysics.

Earlier researchers have also suggested that genetic testing may increase fatalism, though that was not found to be the case in at least one study exploring perceptions of alcoholism.[9,26] But these issues may vary for every condition, based on differing patterns and views of genetics. One cannot lump all genetic diseases together. Rather, diseases with genetic markers range in penetrance, complexity, and treatability. Genetic bases for a disease may not mean more fatalism if at-risk individuals perceive control in some way.

A "genetic-risk role" emerges here that resembles the "sick role" (as described earlier, in which patients have certain rights and responsibilities),[30] but with key differences. The genetic-risk role does not necessarily involve the presence of symptoms. In addition, the sick role assumes that individuals do everything they can to get better. But with a mutation, an individual may be able to do little, if anything. Individuals confronting a genetic risk may as a result look to behavioral changes, and perhaps emphasize these more. But these efforts may not in fact be effective. Nonetheless, such searches for a cause, or at least a sense of order, can abet coping.

As mentioned above, these patterns differ somewhat between these diseases. Genetic tests for breast cancer are less predictable than those for HD or Alpha. Yet with all three disorders, individuals try to wrest control from the specter of fatalism. Overall, many similar themes and issues between these diseases clearly emerge.

These men and women shed light on broader questions of what is a cause versus a contributory factor, and how we decide this. Individuals seek a cause, and do so based on combinations of perceived salience of evidence, psychological needs, and prior social and political beliefs. Unlike scientists, these patients have deeply emotional desires to escape despair and find hope, shaping these decisions. As we will see, these choices have powerful implications for many other aspects of these individuals' lives as well.

CHAPTER 5

"Am I My Genes?":

Genetic Identities

"Sometimes I think of myself as *healthy, but doomed*," Isabelle, the social worker, said. "Healthy, but with a curse."

In trying to make sense of genetic risks, these individuals struggle with questions about not only the *cause* of their predicament, but their very *identity* as well. Genes may be said to "form us"—but to what degree exactly do they do so, and how? Where and how do we draw the line between the genetic and nongenetic aspects of ourselves? For millennia, these issues have plagued philosophers and theologians, but how do men and women in their daily lives make sense of these tensions?

Other kinds of disease have been found to alter patients' self-views,[1,2] but genetics can pose particular challenges. Though identity has been mentioned as a possible factor in prior discussions of genetic risk assessments,[3,4] many questions remain of how exactly individuals decide whether, how, and to what degree genetic risks affect their identity, and what processes and factors are involved. Gender, social class, and particular aspects of a disease can affect how patients integrate chronic diseases such as multiple sclerosis and cancer into their lives,[5] renegotiate their identity, and construct their biographies.[6] Perceptions of illness-related stigma, in particular, can profoundly mold individuals' self-perceptions.[2] Illness identity can affect coping, views of and adherence to medication,[7,8,9] attendance at follow-up appointments, and the return to work.[10] Treatment can influence self-views as well. Radical surgery, for example, can alter both private and public social identities.[11]

Research has been divided on whether or not genetic risk information harms "self-concept" and self-views.[12] Scales have purported to assess self-concept and "illness identity."[8] But disagreements in findings suggest broader questions of what exactly constitutes self-concept, how learning one's genetic risk can affect one's identity, what challenges individuals face, and how they deal with these. For example, studies have found that the self-concepts of individuals who are carriers, noncarriers, and at risk for a disease may all be threatened (e.g., in terms of personal, physical, genetic, social, and family identity),[12] but in what ways and how remain unknown. From a theoretical perspective, concepts of genetic identity may be multilayered, and can refer to different properties of a person over time.[13]

Still, how individuals confronting genetic risk actually approach these issues of identity and incorporate these risks into their sense of themselves remains unclear. As a framework for conceptualizing genetic counseling, self-regulatory theory has been suggested, whereby patients actively process information. In this model, identity—impression of and experience with the illness—is one of fourteen sets of factors involved in genetic counseling.[3] But broader questions arise of what factors in fact shape this "identity," and how and why. Similarly, with familial risk perception, individuals may assess the relevance for themselves of a newly affected relative and develop a personal sense of vulnerability that affects coping and control, and further molds this relevance. But here, too, issues emerge of how individuals incorporate this personal sense of vulnerability into their identity and sense of themselves—that is, how their notions of vulnerability alter how they see themselves. A chronic disease involves a readjustment of one's previous self-concept and a negotiation between new and old identities. However, genetic disease may entail not a "new" identity but a "revealed" underlying one (i.e., one's genetic risk) that in fact was always present, if unknown.[14] Alternatively, a genetic disease may already have caused symptoms, and thus already constitute or create a new identity.

Attention has also been given to how genetic markers may influence racial and ethnic identities. Several so-called ancestry genes have been identified, and differences have been probed between genetic and public identities.[15] But the precise meanings of these markers remain ambiguous. An individual can have multiple such markers, which may not coincide with his or her own view of his or her identity.[16] Genetic markers have been found for diseases far more than for ancestry. Hence, genetic identities related to disease can potentially shed light on how individuals try to make sense other kinds of genetic data and integrate this information into their views of themselves more broadly.

Crucial questions thus persist of how these individuals approach issues of identity, what challenges they face, and whether and how these identities might affect health decisions.

CHALLENGES IN INCORPORATING GENETIC STATUS INTO ONE'S SENSE OF SELF

The men and women here wrestle with numerous challenges concerning their views of themselves. Given the fact that genes in many ways shape who we are, people face quandaries of how, to what degree, and with what implications. Individuals see these issues highly subjectively, differing in what aspects of their condition they focus on, and how and to what degree they do so.

These issues arise with other diseases as well, but genetics poses added problems in part because one can have a mutation without symptoms, or, in the case of breast cancer, can have not only a disease that can be treated, but also a mutation, which can predispose for future symptoms.

These interviewees draw on a spectrum of genotypes and phenotypes, interpreting these in various ways. They differ in phenotypes (i.e., whether they have had symptoms, and if so, whether these were mild or severe). Yet across these spectrums, similar questions emerge in seeking to interpret and understand these states.

At one extreme, merely a family history of a disease, without any symptoms or known mutations, could shape one's identity. Susie, who worked for an HIV organization and has an extensive family history of breast cancer, but no symptoms or mutation, said, "I think of myself now as 'someone at risk.' That's how most people in my family die. That means, unscientifically, that it's 'in my family', so I should pay attention to it." Even in the absence of a mutation, risk based on family history alone can thus mold identity.

Trying to Fit into Pre-existing, Social Categories

In attempting to grasp genotypes and phenotypes and the vagaries involved, these men and women frequently look to other socially established classifications. They grapple with whether they are "predisposed," "sick," "diseased," "healthy," or "disabled," and if so, how—that is, what these various categories mean. But these pre-existing disease-related categories often prove inadequate or problematic. With Alpha, many wonder if they even have a disease, and instead feel that they have a "condition." Yet they then struggle to distinguish between these terms. Support groups encouraged them to avoid the label "disease" since it could carry negative connotations, but patients are often hazy about the reasons for this distinction. Charles, the accountant who hangs out in smoky bars, said,

> I don't know what the definition is, but I always think of "disease" as something you contract, not are born with. It's the seriousness of what it is. Diseases can be self-inflicted.

He grapples with several possible distinctions here, based on the mode of transmission, severity, and patient culpability. In contrast, Gilbert distinguishes between these terms differently: "The disease is emphysema, but the *condition* is Alpha."

Others feel they have a predisposition, which they then seek to differentiate from a disease. But the definition of predisposition can also be fuzzy, with varying physiological, clinical, and pathological implications. Benjamin, the engineer and former smoker, challenged this term because it is not fully predictive, and suggests a lack of control. He felt that his behavior could potentially influence his risk of Alpha.

> If I create risky behavior, I'm more likely to succumb to that disease. The risky behavior is smoking. Drinking might be risky because of liver disease. Other risky behaviors might be working in a chemical factory, or with perfumes . . . Risky behavior doesn't necessarily mean "bad" behavior. It just puts you at risk for lung or liver disease. I wish I hadn't smoked.

He wrestles here with the meanings of predisposition, seeking a modicum of power over his fate to avoid despair. Moral issues arise, too, as he seeks to distinguish between risk factors such as smoking, which he sees as self-inflicted (and hence "blameworthy") versus occupational exposures for Alpha (in which the patient is implicitly "innocent"). In so doing, he seeks to distinguish between two different definitions of "bad"—as morally wrong versus physically harmful. He sees himself as having predispositions, but maintaining ultimate control. He also seeks innocence, wishing that he had not smoked—because of both the health reasons and the implicit culpability (i.e., that he had therefore contributed to his own problem).

Individuals differ, too, in the degrees to which they see themselves as fitting the categories "sick" versus "healthy." For example, despite having breast cancer and the mutation, several interviewees, including Rhonda, the nurse who had seen her mother die of the disease, still perceive themselves as healthy.

> I don't feel I'm a "sick person." I feel I'm very healthy. I know women who say, "I have cancer." I never thought like that. I don't look at myself as being "sick." I go for my check-ups but it definitely doesn't affect my everyday life.

She implicitly adopts functional definitions of "sick" versus "healthy," based not on whether she has a disease but on whether *she feels her state affects her daily life*, and hence her sense of identity.

The temporal and medical precariousness of being at risk also motivate searches for alternative terms and categories for the self. Various characteristics of specific diseases can help shape these categories. Thus, those with Alpha may think of themselves as occupying intermediary positions on a spectrum from sick to healthy—underscoring how Alpha can be more of a chronic illness. Yvonne, who had lung transplants for Alpha and now wants to move to the South, thinks of herself as ill and still "vulnerable," but improved. "I think of myself as sick," she said. "I'm better for now, but could crash tomorrow . . . If I have organ rejection, and we can't get it to stop, you're gone." She acknowledges the precarious and ephemeral nature of these states, focusing only on the present moment. Here, too, she switches from the first person ("I") to the more general second person ("you"), distancing herself slightly from the full threat.

Related questions arise of whether and when a mutation is "normal" versus "abnormal"—with all the possible implied moral and other implications of each term. For so-called complex genetic disorders (such as hypertension or depression), genetic predispositions may in fact be normal variants of genes. Individuals also pursue new phrases to grasp these murky, diverse states. For instance, Jennifer, the schoolteacher, described herself as "a healthy Alpha."

> I think of myself as healthy for my age and disability. That doesn't make a whole lot of sense, but that's how I think of it. We have a disease. But a lot of Alphas rarely present symptoms. So symptoms don't necessarily define illness.

She still views herself as part of the disease community, but as healthy, in part because she has not yet needed portable oxygen or lung transplantation. These identities are thus not simply binary, but nuanced across gradients, with individuals at times seeking to straddle several categories that may seem, from afar, conceptually distinct.

Still, integrating the diverse characteristics involved in these predicaments poses considerable psychological challenges. As noted earlier, Isabelle, the social worker, thinks of herself as healthy for the present, but doomed. She reflected on the persistence of uncertainty over time.

> I don't think of myself as sick, or as a mutant, but as healthy, and on the edge. There is a high risk of another cancer . . . It doesn't enter into everything I do—all of my functioning or everyday life—but just sort of *hangs* there. There's probably about a 65% chance I'll get it in my other breast. Then, I read studies that say 50%.

The fact that researchers dispute the exact probabilities exacerbates her sense of uncertainty. She struggles to find a degree of surety, seeking scientific data but seeing the ambiguity metaphysically—that she is "cursed," though she is not entirely clear by whom, or how.

Certain individuals see themselves as "disabled" more than diseased, suggesting how functioning (what one does, or can do) also molds identity. The fact that a disease has a strong genetic basis can shape identity less than the fact that the illness results in particular functional disabilities. "'Disabled' is a good way of looking at it," Jim, the physician with HD, said. "I can't do everything. Some days . . . I'm just not going to feel up to doing anything."

Yet meanings of "disability" vary, too. To some, it is merely a financial rather than a psychological state—an economic situation (i.e., receiving disability benefits) and not an identity per se. Benjamin, the engineer, does not work due to Alpha, and thinks of the category as merely bureaucratic more than based in reality. "I don't think of myself as 'disabled'—that's a whole political game," he said. "I think I could still now do the job I did, but I don't know that I have the mindset."

How much an individual fits into this category of disability can also fluctuate over time—even daily, depending on how one defines the term. Not surprisingly, many people then struggle with how to define the word, and how and when to apply it to themselves. Barbara, the part-time professor and former smoker with Alpha, mused:

> I now think of myself as *borderline*: I can pass for *not* being disabled. But I *do* get tired and irritable, and a lot of times just don't want to do things. People say, "Oh, let's do something on the 26th. Are you free?" Well, maybe, maybe not. I get a lot of infections. I am less disabled than before, because I am now getting the right dose of medicine. My health has improved. I'm thinking of getting a job. But it is hard to do things. If I meet a new person, I'm cautious in telling.

Disease fluctuations over time can thus complicate identities. She suggests that degrees of disability can be impossible to predict. She is concerned, too, that other individuals may or may not agree with her own assessment—which can add stress. These questions about identity can also prompt dilemmas about disclosing one's condition to others.

A successfully treated disease that can recur poses additional questions. With breast cancer, for example, individuals may see themselves as survivors if they have been asymptomatic for several years. But they may still face uncertainties. Even if a tumor is entirely removed, cancer can still reappear. After no longer being acutely ill, dilemmas about identity linger—how much to consider oneself to be a patient in some way, and what to do or not do as a result. Many people feel uncomfortable with the phrase "cancer survivor," since it suggests an inherently unstable state, though the popular media and many patient advocacy groups commonly invoke the term. Mildred, in finance, said that despite breast cancer and prophylactic mastectomies,

> I don't look at myself as a breast cancer survivor: "I'm a survivor, let me proudly wear my hat and pin." There's nothing wrong with that . . . I do hotline work. I don't do the Walk-a-thon, but do cancer runs—for cancer research in general, not just breast cancer. I don't look at myself as a "gene-positive person." I always say "I'm a *BRCA1* carrier." I would say I'm outgoing, athletic, enjoy people, and am sensitive. But I don't describe myself as a "cancer survivor."

In part, to do so would be painful. She suggests several alternative, competing ways she would describe herself. She prefers the term "carrier," since it suggests a less definitive disease, and perhaps less stigma than "cancer survivor" or "gene-positive person." She illustrates as well the multiple activities in which one can engage within the breast cancer community, all of which (as we will see later) can reflect and shape one's sense of self. Yet she has also not disclosed her mutation to her boyfriend or brother.

Time frames concerning one's disease and life are difficult to establish because of the unpredictability of both psychological sequelae and future events related and unrelated to the disorder. Whether the disease will return, and whether various nonspecific symptoms signal recurrence, remain unclear. The questions of when a disease "ends" depend partly on definitions of the disease and what the endpoint is considered to be. Language itself falters in providing accurate and appropriate terms for such inchoate states, involving uncertain prognoses. Yet these temporal issues (i.e., whether certain phenomena constitute a state or trait) frame questions of who one is. Karen, the lawyer with breast cancer but no testing, said,

> I consider myself a "survivor," but hate the term. It indicates that something's done and over, and to me, it's not. I occasionally use that word. I haven't found a better one. When I talk about it, I have varied between saying "I had breast cancer," or "I've had breast cancer," or different things indicating that it's ongoing. If I had to fill out a form, there's a fifty-fifty chance I would use that term. It is not done and over, because of childbearing decisions, medical things: I have osteopoenea, I'm going through perimenopause. My right hip was troubling me: "Could this be related?"

The presence of familial or genetic risk can thus resemble a ticking time bomb, continuing, ever-present, though whether one is sick, healthy, a survivor, or none of the above can remain unclear.

Diagnosis as Part versus Whole of Oneself

Individuals have to decide not only what terms to use in describing themselves, but *to what degree* to do so. Genetic risk can constitute a small or large part, but generally not *all*, of one's identity. People then struggle to gauge the actual extent of this identity. The relative amounts, boundaries, and relationships between this versus other parts of the self can vary widely between people, and over time for any one person.

A few individuals feel that the presence of an illness or a mutation altered their identities only minimally, if at all. Some of these men and women see themselves as being at risk, but feel that this state does not affect their core identity. "I am who I am," said Vera, tested because she was Asian. "I had breast cancer. I beat it. I may get it again. I'll deal with it when I get it again, if I get it again." Despite having had breast cancer which could recur, successful treatment lowers the impact of the illness in her ongoing life. She appears driven to succeed in her career, and does not want the disease to interfere. As mentioned earlier, she also has difficulty coping with uncertainty.

Yet far more commonly, these genetic risks shape individuals' views of themselves in important ways. "Genes make me who I am," Bonnie, the saleswoman who had seen breast cancer in her mother and sister, sighed. Without genes, she would not exist. The fact that she is untested makes it easier for her to accept the role of genes in her life, and not feel fatalistic about that notion. At the far extreme, patients with Alpha even call themselves "Alphas."

But she and others still seek to circumscribe the impact of genes on their lives. This restraint might be easier for individuals who have not had symptoms or mutations. Bonnie continued,

> I don't want to be identified solely as "I have relatives who had cancer," because that's just placing myself in one situation. There's so much more to a person than just being a cancer survivor, or having relatives who had cancer.

The fact that she does not have symptoms or the mutation limits the role she sees genetics playing in her life. But these interviewees vary in how they conceptualize their risk—to whatever degree they feel it exists—in relation to the rest of themselves. Many see it as one part among many. "It's a piece of who I am," Arlene, the nurse who studied religion and had a strong family history of breast cancer, but no symptoms or testing, said about her risk of the disease. "I'm pretty diversified."

Others try to quantify this portion more precisely, varying in the specific degree or size. Even HD, though it may seem all-encompassing, can be viewed as simply a part of one's make-up. Roger, who tested mutation-positive for HD after he swerved his car off the road, explained,

I have a genetic link to Huntington's, but it's not my entire being—just *one part* of me. I have 150 characteristics. This is one of many. So, I'm very good about dealing with it like that. I'm obsessional, funny, nice, a hand-washer, a hoarder, a checker (I do a lot of checking).

He attempts to quantify the diagnosis informally as one of 150 features. Yet in fact, many of the other characteristics he mentions—for example, his obsessive-compulsiveness—may be manifestations of HD.

Others also seek to assess and describe the degrees to which they accept, embrace, or deny this risk. Kym, the 32-year-old South Asian physician with breast cancer in her family but no symptoms or testing, does not worry about her risk "*that* much"—suggesting an objective correlate: the amount of time one spends thinking about it.

THE SELF AS "MUTANT"?: NEGATIVE VERSUS POSITIVE IDENTITIES

These men and women have to decide not only whether and to what degree to incorporate their condition into their sense of themselves, but how to do so—with what moral valence (i.e., from positive to negative). They often attempt to gauge whether, and how much to view this genetic identity as negative or neutral. A few see themselves as "mutants," "evolutionary errors," "mistakes of nature," or "freaks." They feel they have a "bad gene" or "flaw," and try to understand it, stumbling to find appropriate terms. The fact that a mutation can be viewed as tainted can impede one in constructing or embracing a genetic identity. Benjamin, the engineer and former smoker with Alpha, said,

There's something wrong with me: I've got this *bad gene*. I don't know how to explain that. You just feel you're not . . . I don't want to say you're not per-fect, but . . . there's "an identifiable flaw" in your genome. The first thing you think about is: I'm *flawed*, dirty. I've got this weird disease, this crazy gene.

Laura, the graphic designer and environmentalist with no breast cancer symptoms but a strong family history, seeks metaphors to conceptualize this gene, and remains unsure:

There's something wrong with me that's not even physical . . . the blue-prints of my body don't work well. The computer that determines the functions of my body, the central processing unit, doesn't work right. At any time, something can go wrong. It's like I'm walking with one leg. I don't have the checks and balances most people have.

She draws on metaphors from different fields: architecture (blueprints), information technology (computers), medicine (physical handicap), and politics (checks and balances). She and others grope for concrete mechanisms to understand and explain these genetic problems.

Many try to resist potentially negative connotations. Benjamin, the engineer, cited the theory of evolution and said that he did not mind being a "mutant" because scientifically, mutations are ubiquitous and thus normal.

> I don't call it a "disease," because it would then be worse for me. It's a genetic condition, a mutation. I don't have any qualms with the word "mutation." A lot of people do, but I don't. I believe in evolution: We're all mutants. Mutation is the way things change.

He sees his very existence as dependant on such genetic errors. Trained in science, he accepts the harsh realities of the disease more than most people, yet at times also wavers, trying to make sense of it. He struggles to balance the fact that epidemiologically, he is one of relatively few individuals in the population as a whole who have been diagnosed with a potentially fatal disease for which a mutation has been identified. He faces a more severe genetic problem than most people, though some others are sicker than he. He feels he has also been lucky, having only relatively mild symptoms.

> They claim that everybody has something, but that's just bullshit. One scientist says everybody has four or five flaws that might in the end kill them. But that doesn't *really* mean that everyone has something.

FACTORS INVOLVED

Several factors can clearly shape these views—for example, scientific education and genetic states, alternative ways one defines oneself, and degrees to which one does so. Roberta, the African American former nursing student with breast cancer but no testing, who blames her family's cancer on Louisiana water pollutants, described her identities: "Who am I? I'm a grandmother, a woman, a mother, and a human being. I'm pretty intelligent, because I'm always looking for new information. That's basically who I am."

She also sees her illness as reflecting social, more than individual, medical problems, and ascribes her breast cancer to environmental factors—for example, industrial pollution. The fact that she has not been tested helps decrease the impact of the disease on her sense of self, which in turn makes her less inclined to undergo testing. In addition, the mutations for breast cancer, compared to those for HD or Alpha, are less predictive of disease, allowing more leeway in beliefs about the degrees to which genetics (versus other factors) shape oneself and thus one's identity.

A mutation can also reinforce prior social identities as a member of a group that a disease commonly affects. Those with breast cancer symptoms or mutations, for example, may attribute the illness partly to being a woman. "Having this gene makes me feel more female," Laura said. "Women have to deal with special things, having this biological clock, bleeding every month, menopause. It's not a self-pity thing, but an added female thing."

Past traumatic personal experiences can affect these issues as well. A few individuals had particular past psychic trauma (e.g., mental illness), and now see themselves negatively as "mutant." Laura saw herself in this way due to having *BRCA1/2* and a history of depression and suicidal tendencies. "When I was 14, I 'cut' myself once," she said. "Sometimes I wonder whether I should even have been born. If I weren't here, there would be no difference." The fact that she now knows that she has a genetic mutation confirms her sense that there is something intrinsically wrong with her.

Improved treatment and symptoms can facilitate adaptation to a disease, particularly a chronic one, altering attitudes. Benjamin, the engineer and former smoker, said about his Alpha, "What helped me change was just living with it. I didn't have this big flashing light or something." Yet even with effective treatment, ambiguities persist. With Alpha, questions arise of whether, despite getting a lung transplant, one continues to possess the disease. As Yvonne, who had lung transplants, said, "I've still got Alpha." She thus wants to move to the South to abet her health.

The degree to which a patient's symptoms are localized to a particular organ or body part can also mold the impact of illness on a patient's sense of self. Patients may try to circumscribe the illness to only a specific, diseased part of the body, seeing the condition as involving that part alone. With disease only in her lungs, Dorothy, the TV producer who carries metal oxygen canisters while awaiting lung transplants, said, "If I didn't have these two lungs, I'd think of myself as healthy."

Views of identity can also depend on who one is with at the time; other people can either support or challenge one's own self-perception. At times, one's own and others' perspectives on oneself can coincide. As Betty, the designer who carries an oxygen concentrator, said about her Alpha,

Whether it is part of my identity now depends on the crowd I'm in. When I'm in an Alpha group: I'm one of you. It's part of me, a description of me, like having brown hair, or being this size, or whatever I am. But it's not a *total* focus.

Depending on social context, disease can constitute part, though not necessarily all, of one's identity. However, outsiders may identify a person as having a disease, while the individual resists it. Patients may welcome or fight an identity as "ill" in others' eyes. Entering and exiting the sick role can thus be contested, and negotiated.

An individual may define him or herself in genetic terms, depending on temporal factors as well—doing so only when the topic comes up. Harriet, an African American schoolteacher with an inconclusive genetic test for breast cancer and no symptoms, said, "In terms of who I am: I just say I had a history of cancer in my family. But it was not there every day—just when we're having the discussion." She frames her identity in familial, rather than personal ways (having had the disease in her family).

Yet over time, both community involvements and identities can mold each other. Karen, the lesbian lawyer, said about her breast cancer,

> In the group, we talk about: once you've been diagnosed, you cross a line
> . . . once you've had metastatic disease, you cross a different line. Part of my
> struggle is accepting that—not fighting to get back over to the other side.

In part as a result, she decided not to test. Yet seeing oneself as being at risk or having a disease can affect whether and to what degree one even enters a disease community in the first place. Similarly, the degree to which one confronts versus minimizes or denies one's risk can influence one's readiness or resistance to pursue testing or treatment.

IMPLICATIONS

As suggested earlier, these issues of identities can shape disclosure decisions, testing, treatment, and coping. For example, individuals' sense of their genetic identity can shape decisions of whether, when, and to what degree to tell others about it. "Do I tell people that I have a disease?" Barbara, the part-time professor, wondered about her Alpha, "Should I go on job interviews? Do I tell them I'm disabled? Are they hiring a disabled person, or an able? They get some perks for hiring disabled people."

Whether one is specifically asked about oneself, and by whom, can affect how one then presents and sees oneself in that context. Genetic risk or disease can mold one's private (but not necessarily one's wider) social identity. "I am a person at risk," said Kym, the South Asian physician. "But if someone outside were to say, 'Tell me about yourself,' that's not what would come to my mind." Since she is asymptomatic and untested, genetic risk may affect her less than those who have symptoms, ongoing treatment, or mutations. These individuals tend to distinguish between the public versus more private aspects of themselves.

CONCLUSIONS

These men and women face challenges in trying to incorporate genetic information into their lives and construct a sense of identity. They wrestle with these issues in ways that are not straightforward, but involve subjective interpretations and choices concerning categories related to genetics and disease states more generally. They seek and define these categories and terms in widely differing ways.

Issues of identity arise with other diseases as well, but can do so in unique ways concerning genetics. In many regards, genes constitute the self, and can shape one's future. Yet individuals, especially if asymptomatic, encounter challenges in gauging the extent of this predictiveness—grasping the meanings of being at risk, or having a mutation. These issues of identity in turn pose challenges for coping—how to overcome a sense of fatalism and hopelessness, given possibly deleterious genes.

Individuals who feel that their particular state of risk or illness does not fit into existing socially established categories (e.g., "predisposition," "sick," or "healthy") then try to make sense of their genetic states and decide whether they conform to a pre-existing label in any way, and if so, how and to what degree. They draw on their prior understandings of themselves and try to squeeze their genetic state into their ongoing lives, seeking narrative coherence. Whether and how they do so varies, shaped by several factors.

Though the "sick role" involves certain rights and responsibilities (e.g., to do everything possible to get better),[17] genetics can present particular challenges, involving more inchoate states. Dilemmas arise for a mutation that has not yet produced symptoms, or has been treated but may recur.

The category of being at genetic risk for a disease but being asymptomatic poses particular problems. With these disorders, identities are based on seemingly objective data that in fact vary widely, falling across a spectrum based not only on symptoms but a range of genotypes, phenotypes, and testing states. The objective correlates on which subjective identities may be based can be more fluid for genetics than for other kinds of diagnoses. Hence, while David Armstrong[14] suggested that genetic identities involve adjusting to revealed aspects of one's self, the men and women here highlight many other complexities involved—multiple processes and factors, and a range of genotypes and phenotypes that individuals interpret and apply to themselves in different ways over time. Individuals vary in what aspects of a genetic marker they focus on and how—for instance, as meaning that they are a "mutant" or not. These individuals highlight how notions of both genetic identity and illness identity are multifaceted and highly complex.

How these individuals integrate genetic information into their identities can shape decisions about testing, treatment, and disclosures of risk to family members and others. Yet these implications of genetic identities have received little attention. It is not clear, for instance, how often individuals see themselves negatively due to having a particular genetic marker, and the degree to which individuals who do so may be less likely to disclose their test results to at-risk family members who might then in turn get tested.

Between these diseases similarities and differences emerge, though overall, the similarities in themes and challenges outweigh the differences. Still, many who have a family history of breast cancer but have neither undergone genetic testing or displayed symptoms often see these states as constituting their identities less than do those similarly at risk (without symptoms or mutation) of HD or Alpha. The latter two disorders are more penetrant, and HD is untreatable and invariably fatal.

These findings shed important light, too, on possible future uses and implications of other genetic tests—including, potentially, markers associated with ancestry and various behavioral traits. Individuals may similarly interpret such genetic information in widely differing ways, relying on pre-existing personal and cultural narratives. Individuals may vary widely in what aspects of such information they focus on, and how and to what degree they do so, reflecting uncertainties of how and to what extent one is in fact shaped by genetic versus other factors. Even decisions of which *objective* elements to focus on are in the end subjective. Genetic information can disrupt prior narratives, depending in part on the strength of the narrative and the perceived penetrance, predictiveness, lethality, and severity of the genetic marker. These interviewees suggest how the complexities involved in genetics can potentially mold—and be molded by—our deepest notions of ourselves.

CHAPTER 6

"Lightening Doesn't Strike Twice":

Myths and Misunderstandings about Genetics

"I always thought that because I looked more like my mother, I was more at risk of getting the disease," said Roger, who found he had the HD mutation after he had problems driving. Misunderstandings about genetics frequently arise—for example, that genes for mutations and for physical or psychological traits sort together, and that offspring tend to resemble one parent more than the other, rather than receiving equal amounts of DNA from both. In trying to grasp the meanings and effects of genetics, these individuals struggle to understand the scientific mechanisms involved, and generally have trouble doing so. They hold many misunderstandings that then affect their other decisions. Miscomprehensions emerge party because genetics is relatively new and ever-changing. Scientists, searching for continued funding, and private companies, seeking to market tests, often tout the field's promises—and individuals yearn for information about their future.

Overall, patients, physicians, and the public have relatively little knowledge about many aspects of genetics,[1,2,3,4] but the full extent and impact of these misperceptions have been little examined.

Much of the public does not know basic aspects of genetics—for example, that genes in fact reside in chromosomes in every cell in the body,[3,5,6] and that humans have 46 chromosomes.[3] Most people view mutations negatively.[7] Members of certain groups believe that fathers contribute more genetic material than do mothers,[8] and that a child is more likely to inherit a disease mutation if he or she more physically resembles the parent with the mutation.[9] Patients also misapprehend statistics—having difficulties in quantifying, and tending to overestimate, risk.[10]

Patients may experience and construct perceptions of risk based on both their own and their family members' medical experiences. Overestimations of the likelihood of cancer[4] may impede health, and lead to inappropriate use of prevention and surveillance.[10,11] Several models have been proposed to make sense of how individuals subjectively view the nature and cause of disease and how they personalize their risk for familial disease.[2] For common chronic familial illnesses such as diabetes and heart disease, individuals may assess the salience for themselves of a relative who is newly diagnosed with a disease, which can shape coping and sense of control.

Yet questions remain of how these risks and genetics are viewed by individuals who themselves are at risk for diseases for which genetic tests exist and have been marketed. It is unclear what types of misunderstandings arise related to genes and statistics, and how these may interact and affect health decisions. Questions also persist about what kinds of misunderstandings, if any, patients have about genetics *after* undergoing genetic counseling, and why. Though not all beliefs about a disease represent misunderstandings, some may—raising questions as to when, how, and with what implications.

MISUNDERSTANDINGS ABOUT GENETIC TESTS

Men and women here reveal a wide variety of misunderstandings about genetics, shaped by various factors, and in turn having several critical implications.

Many of these individuals see genetic assays as similar to other established medical tests—viewing genetic analyses as more definitive and predictive than these assays in fact are. "My sister thought that if she got tested, she would know whether she was going to get breast cancer," said Karen, the lawyer with breast cancer and a family history but no testing. "Her gynecologist was encouraging her to get tested."

Physicians may thus contribute to these beliefs in these tests' predictiveness. Often, patients assume that a test must be worthwhile if a physician encourages it—that doctors consider a test important because it is predictive. This misunderstanding appears fairly common, especially before undergoing genetic counseling. Individuals may sense these limitations intellectually but nevertheless seek certainty, leading to conflicting perspectives or anxiety. As Karen added,

> People think the test will tell you whether you will get the disease or not, rather than it being a piece of information that says, "You're probably at higher risk for getting this disease, but it doesn't mean you're going to get

it." Intellectually, I understand that. But emotionally even *that* is hard to wrap my head around. Part of me is afraid that at some point they'll find out that if you have the gene, you will get breast and ovarian cancer . . . part of me, this Nervous Nelly in the background, says, "Someday those numbers are going to be different."

As a well-educated lawyer, she understands that scientific consensus can shift over time. But emotions can nonetheless outweigh intellectual subtlety. Individuals wish to reduce anxieties generated by uncertainty and want definitive answers, though such absolutes may not be obtainable.

This notion that a cause is simple and singular reflects both common lay beliefs and broader desires for certitude in a chaotic universe. Folk myths, media reports of genetic discoveries, and physicians' implicit or explicit attitudes all frequently bolster beliefs in the predictiveness of genes, which could potentially encourage patients to pursue testing.

Many feel that the identification of a gene implies that treatment exists, or will soon be developed—that prevention and treatment is possible, as is generally the case for other clinical tests. Yet tests for genetic markers, though increasingly available, often have less clinical utility than long-established assays. Francine, the unemployed HIV-infected woman who has not had breast cancer symptoms or testing but has seen the disease in her mother, said:

> I don't know a lot about genetic testing, but if you could tell me I'm predestined to get something, at least let me know, so I can prepare myself and my kids. This way, I'll be able to pass this information along. I'd rather know now, so I'll know what to look forward to, and not have it sprung on me. If I know ahead of time, there are things that may be done—I can't say to prevent it, but early treatment.

She imagines that tests reveal pre-destiny. Such beliefs arise in part because of views that genes reflect etiology and cause, not chance and unknown factors. Individuals often see science, more broadly, as able to produce treatments. Diane, who had an unexpected mastectomy but no mutation, said,

> Genetic testing will probably allow people to discover much more about their DNA. Certainly, research can provide treatments somewhere down the line, maybe even alterations of the DNA. One day, maybe we're going to beat death.

As a teacher, she maintains hope in the progress of science, despite her experience in surgery.

Many people see information for its own sake—that is, without it having a clear practical benefit—as conferring advantages. As suggested earlier, in this way, they suggest "diagnostic misconception," akin to "therapeutic misconception,"[12] in which patients assume that they will benefit from treatment provided in a research protocol even if they are participating in a randomly controlled clinical trial in which they may in fact be receiving a placebo.[12]

The media also fosters popular myths that behavioral genetics can uncover clear explanations for certain complex behaviors. Karl was skeptical, uncertain how much to hold HD responsible for his father's abusiveness:

> You hear a lot about predispositions for drug addiction and alcoholism, and "the gay gene"—folk information. My wife works with scientists. They know what's going on, but are the minority.

People who have studied basic biology at an advanced high school or college level may grasp basic genetic concepts more, and view claims more warily than do others. But these myths reflect, in part, wide cultural beliefs.

MISUNDERSTANDINGS ABOUT GENETIC MECHANISMS

For most of these men and women, genetics are too abstract, entailing statistical probabilities that are far from their lived experiences. A few have vague or partial understandings of aspects of genetic mechanisms, and try to grasp basic notions of dominance and recessivity. "I don't know," said Wilma, who had breast cancer along with her mother, and bipolar disorder but no testing. "Is there such a thing as genes being just *slightly* there—you have this gene in a minute, not a more dominant way? I don't know how that works."

She illustrates how individuals, especially if they have not undergone counseling, can have a very poor understanding of genetics. Most have problems comprehending the basic aspects of Mendelian patterns of inheritance described earlier. With Alpha, for example, homozygous patients often don't realize that all their offspring will be at least heterozygotes. As Dorothy, the former TV producer awaiting lung transplants, said,

> Even people who have Alpha don't understand: that their children are going to be carriers. It happens all the time on the e-lists. They say: we want our children tested. And the children turn out to be carriers. Instead, they could have had the husband tested. There's no need to test the child, and have it in his or her record.

She highlights how misunderstandings can prompt testing that can in turn lead to unnecessary discrimination, confusion, and stress.

Beliefs about Inheriting Mutations and Physical Traits Together

Even individuals with scientific training frequently think that an individual is more likely to receive a mutation if he or she physically most closely resembles the parent with the disease. Some feel they are mutation-positive because of *psychological* similarities to an affected family member. As Mary, the housewife with HD, said: "Me and my mother are like two peas in a pod."

Others grapple with these issues, drawing on their observations of their family over time, which may or may not lead to consistent conclusions. Many attempt to articulate these similarities and differences. For instance, Oliver, who continued to pursue a PhD despite having the HD mutation, feels that he looks like his father and uncle, who had the disease.

> As a man, I'm obviously physically more like my father and uncle than is my sister. But there is also a certain way I move. I've always thought that my sister is much different. Something physically in her, the way that she carries herself, was different.

His memory may be colored by his recent genetic test, but it also comforts him, providing a sense of temporal and narrative coherence in his life. Conversely, some feel that they have escaped the mutation, since they look less like their affected parent than a sibling does. Such beliefs provide a sense of both definitiveness and closeness to a beloved affected parent.

These conceptions of jointly inheriting genes for diseases and other traits extend across all three of these disorders, and reflect in part broad cultural myths. These beliefs suggest views of behavioral genetics and physiognomy—the notion that a child takes more after one parent or whole side of the family than the other. As Gilbert, the factory worker, said about Alpha,

> My oldest son is obviously his mother's child. I've always thought of him as more his mother than me. My younger son is more me than my ex-wife. It's obvious in body construction, and the problems they have—related to her lineage versus mine.

These notions that behavioral and physical traits sort together along with predispositions for disease persist strongly, and lead to assumptions about one's own and others' future test results, even in the face of contrary evidence and education. Sarah, the computer programmer without breast cancer or the mutation, said,

> When my sister came up positive, I thought I'm probably going to be positive as well. *I know it's not logical.* But I figured I probably got a good, big healthy *dose* of genes from that side. I remembered my high school biology, about what the percentages would be. But, it still struck me as probably a good chance.

She in fact wanted to have the mutation, because she thought it was associated with intelligence.

Folk beliefs and personal observations grounded in apparent common sense, rather than abstract intellectual understandings of genetic mechanisms, prove persuasive. As we shall see, despite counter-evidence and recognition of their illogicality, these beliefs can prevail in part due to desires for certainty in the face of ambiguity and anxiety. The persistence of these misunderstandings indicates their strength, and the challenges that clinicians thus face in addressing and correcting these errors.

Desires for certitude and explanation over randomness and chaos led some to search through history and photos of ancestors for answers regarding the source of disease. Before she found that she had the HD mutation, Linda, the art teacher, "sat down and looked through all these old family pictures—a box of old black and whites. I tried to trace the disease through us—like 'She's got it.'" She sought concrete visual links to other relatives, in part to feel less alone with the disease.

These men and women struggle with the possible illogicality of these beliefs. Individuals may recognize the fallacy of their assumptions but still hold them, seeking evidence of being mutation-free. Albert, the policeman who tested for HD to help his children make reproductive decisions, commented, "I look more like my father's side of the family. I think that's stupid, because I don't think it really makes a difference who you look like. But I guess I'm hoping for the best."

At times, attempts to balance acknowledgment of genetic risks with desires for hope also prompt beliefs that genetic diseases can in fact skip generations.

Getting More "Biological Material"

Individuals conceive of other genetic mechanisms in a variety of self-reinforcing ways. Sarah, as mentioned earlier, and others imagine that people receive different "doses" of genetics from each parent, as if genes were drugs. Bill, the salesman who thinks he will get HD because he resembles his father, conceptualizes "more" biological material as "cells": "I must have the most traits, or cells, or I don't know what from my father . . . [I] assume that if he has the disease, and I look like him, there's a good chance I'm going to get the disease."

Socially supported folk wisdom can fuel these beliefs that offspring receive more genetic material from one parent than the other. Outsiders may point out resemblances between a parent and a child, strengthening these notions that parents contribute unequally. As Bill continued,

> As you grow up, you start hearing, "*You're just like me when I was a kid.*" So you assume: if I look more like him or her, then I'm probably going to get what he or she has. In high school, hereditary means: two parents come together and pass on what they have. Whatever they have, you have. So, if you look like your dad, then most likely, if he has green eyes, I have green eyes. My dad's got big teeth, I got big teeth. My dad had pretty big hands, I have big hands. He was a pretty fast runner, I was a pretty fast runner. Now, [I] hear my dad has that disease, and it's hereditary, so: "I got the disease . . . I probably have more of his cells than her cells."

As a lawyer, he is highly educated and cites high school biology, but suggests the potency of these misunderstandings. These beliefs also affect and are affected by views of complex behaviors, such as athleticism—some aspects of which may to a slight degree involve genetic differences in predispositions between individuals.

To understand the nature, meanings, and implications of genetics, many therefore search for metaphors, though these can remain elusive. Individuals struggle to grasp notions of chromosomes, drawing on analogies from architecture, computers, and weapons, though the precise details can be murky.

Controllability by Metaphysics

As mentioned earlier, many of these individuals also believe that metaphysics, and the power of the mind over the body, can control the "fatedness" of a genetic disorder—that the power of positive thinking can alter disease. Many are aware of the lack of clear scientific grounding for such beliefs, but adopt them nonetheless.

These men and women also invoke metaphysics by expressing altruistic wishes that a family member would not have a mutation. Joyce, the spa employee who blamed her breast cancer on urban stresses and had a strong family history but no mutation, felt that "my siblings are never going to get it—because they're my siblings, and I don't want them to."

Similarly, notions emerge that a parent would simply not give his or her children a mutation—as if it were a conscious choice—or that an individual has the power to eliminate a mutation from the family. Individuals thus assign agency and volition to genes. Linda, the art teacher who felt overwhelmed by the "HD nightmare," felt that her father was here on earth to get rid of the disease in the family. She lacks the mutation, and believes that her father willfully, stoically, and heroically "took it on" to eliminate it. Beliefs about parental responsibility for transmitting a mutation or not can thus reflect misunderstandings of genetics.

> I had this real strong feeling that my dad had come to clean it up—to finish off this nasty, ugly business, and that my sister and I were going to be fine. He took this thing on, and was going to wrestle it down for us. I also thought that if anybody has it, it would probably be her. Three days after my dad's funeral, she was going to get her results. She sat in front of me in the car, and I put my hands on her, and thought, "Take it away. Make *me* have it, so you don't have to." My dad was the best support I ever had. I just really thought that he wouldn't have given me such a thing.

Even after genetic testing and genetic counseling, individuals may maintain these misunderstandings. As we have seen regarding causality, people may actively pursue ways of supporting such prior views.

MISUNDERSTANDINGS OF STATISTICS

Misunderstandings arise about not only genetics, but statistics as well. For instance, people do not always grasp differences between percentages and proportions. As an engineer, Benjamin said about Alpha,

> A lot of people don't understand arithmetic odds. I'll say, "There's a 3% chance that your mate is going to be a carrier." They'll say, "Well, talk to me in *real* numbers." So, I say: "There's a one in 35 chance." I try to explain it in simple terms. They don't understand percent. I've always worked with numbers. I'm kind of anal.

His professional experience and psychological and cognitive predisposition help, and distinguish him here.

Misunderstandings emerge as well concerning interpretations of absolute versus relative risks. A genetic test may triple a patient's risk from 1 in 1,000 to 3 in 1,000, though the odds of occurrence in fact remain relatively rare. Individuals may accept only one of these sets of statistics, rather than both. Beatrice, the Latina math teacher with breast cancer but no mutation, recognized how other patients may frequently confuse these two sets of figures:

> Somebody said that if I took tamoxifen, I was going to double my chances of uterine cancer. That was scary. But then I said, "Well what are my chances if I don't take it?" They said, "1 in 10,000." I said, "That means it could be 2 in 10,000?" I said fine, just give it to me. People throw numbers out, and if you don't understand or question it, it could be scary.

Thus, individuals need to look at both absolute and relative risks. Yet even clinicians may fail to do so, and use statistics incompletely and sub-optimally. Due to her advanced quantitative education, Beatrice knew to ask about absolute risks, which were still small. Yet many patients may understand these numbers only partially, if at all.

Beatrice wonders how less educated patients handle all this information. With graduate school training, she feels she was able to make an informed decision, but she is concerned for others. She continued,

> In the waiting room, there is a wide range of socioeconomic levels. How do some of these people deal with this information? How is it presented to them? A lot of information comes at you fast and furious, and you're trying to decide what applies to you.

Each Toss of the Coin as Independent

Misunderstandings of genetics and statistics often occur together. Even many well-educated people feel that the probabilities of susceptibility among siblings are not independent, but linked. Hence, some think that if two siblings are at risk for HD and one is found to have the mutation, then the other will therefore *not* have it.

Many at risk of HD, in particular, find the alternative—the fact that each toss of a coin is independent—to be counterintuitive, in part because of countervailing emotional desires and beliefs in cosmic fairness. Several individuals feel that an inherent logic of cosmic fate operates here (the notion that "you can't escape twice"). John, who had dropped out of graduate school when learning about HD in his family, said that before he learned he lacked the mutation he became frightened when his brother tested mutation-negative.

> Irrationally, I thought for sure that we couldn't *both* get away unscathed. I know they're independent events, so the fact that he tested negative does not influence my testing at all. But *emotionally*, it didn't feel that way at all.

John held this belief for a period of time, despite recognizing its illogicality.

These misunderstandings can affect *coping*, and responses to both one's own test results and those of others. John added that when he learned that his brother lacked the mutation,

> I was devastated. I couldn't talk to him. I got off the phone, and cried, thinking, "I've got it for sure." I knew it was irrational. I told him a few days later, "Look, I just can't celebrate this with you. I'm sorry. It is good news. But I'm having this irrational response, you're just going to have to enjoy this without me."

John eventually learned that he, too, was mutation-free.

Genetic counseling can help alter these beliefs, but many individuals may get tested through either physicians or direct-to-consumer marketing companies that provide little, if any, counseling. Hence, these misunderstandings can drive testing and other decisions, without counseling. Individuals may realize only later that they misunderstood, and may then feel overwhelmed. As John continued,

> One woman in my support group had a sister, and convinced herself that this sister had the gene—because she was so much like their father in personality. Then this sister got tested, and didn't have it—so this woman flips out. She had never worried about HD. She was 45, had this 8-year-old kid, and suddenly thought, "Holy shit, I got it all wrong!" She was a wreck, very agitated. I was worried.

Benjamin, the engineer, observes this misunderstanding among patients and family members with Alpha, too, and often has to correct it, telling them, "It's the same odds every time you flip the coin."

These beliefs appear widespread, tapping into ostensibly common sense notions of statistics and risks. At times, even patient support groups and advocacy organizations implicitly disseminate these notions. Before learning she lacked the mutation, Linda, who felt overwhelmed by the "HD nightmare," said,

> When my sister didn't have it, it was like, "Oh geez, it couldn't really be that we would both escape." I gather it's not that unusual. But when you tell that

to a support group, they all go, "Mm-mmm . . ." because the likelihood is not high, if you have two or three siblings in a family, that they all escaped.

Misunderstandings of statistics and genetics can in fact reinforce each other. Individuals may be aware of classic Mendelian principles, but misinterpret them. Roberta, the former nursing student who had breast cancer, as did her mother, but has not been tested, explicitly cited Mendel's law. But she misconstrued it, in explaining why her relatives, who are both sickle-cell carriers, attempted to have a child without the mutation. "We went back to old Mendel's law about four," she said. "They said you have two kids already, so you need to hit it this time, or we'll miss it altogether. So they tried it once more."

The Existence of Two Options Means the Odds Are Fifty-Fifty

As we have seen, some assume that the existence of two outcomes—having or not having a mutation—means that the odds of either outcome must be fifty-fifty, regardless of epidemiological data to the contrary. These individuals thought that the number of options predicted the odds, again reflecting misunderstandings of both statistics and the predictiveness of a particular test. Laura, the graphic designer and former environmentalist with a strong family history of breast cancer but no symptoms, said, "If you test negative, you have the same risk as the general population, so there was a 50% chance that I really didn't need to be going through all this, because I might be negative."

She appears here to confuse several phenomena. Odds of 50% apply for HD, but not for other tests such as *BRCA*. In fact, she has a higher risk than the general population because she has a family history. If she *did* have the same risk as the general population, the chance of her being mutation-negative would then be over 98%—not 50%. The risk of breast cancer in the general population is approximately 12%,[13] and the prevalence of *BRCA1/2* mutations is approximately 0.24% among non-Ashkenazi Caucasians, and 1.2% among Ashkenazi Caucasians.[14] Though Laura has already undergone genetic counseling, she nonetheless maintains these misunderstandings. Importantly, her miscomprehension led her to think she could have avoided testing. She suggests here, too, how miscomprehension of epidemiology can prompt misperception of one's own risk.

FACTORS INVOLVED

Several factors may shape the types and likelihood of individuals' misunderstandings. As suggested, education both generally and specifically in science can potentially reduce these errors. Miscomprehension can prevail, fostered by irrational beliefs (such as that desires to avoid disease can by themselves prevent illness). Individuals may realize intellectually that their beliefs are illogical, but nonetheless hold to them.

Emotional factors such as minimization, denial, and hope can bolster these misperceptions. Several of these men and women mentioned "denial," which suggests a psychodynamic defense mechanism, but has entered general parlance more widely and can perpetuate misperceptions about genetics and risks. Joyce, as mentioned earlier, "was in incredible denial." She did not think that the fact that her grandmother and aunt had breast cancer would increase her own chances of disease. People may have little desire to counter such minimization of their risk. Yet such denial, if challenged by external events, can crumble, leaving a person devastated. As Joyce said, when the diagnosis hit her it was "like a ton of bricks."

Several people believe that they received a mutation or a disease as punishment that they deserved. Questions arise about the accuracy of such metaphysical notions. As Karen, the lesbian lawyer with breast cancer but no testing, said,

> I felt I must have really fucked up. Did I fuck up because I had done immoral things? I was living an immoral life, not eating well, not exercising, not paying attention to my body. Am I being punished? I also had an affair while I was with my partner. If I hadn't had an affair, or if I lived a more morally upstanding life, I wouldn't have gotten cancer. My rabbi said, "I don't think about God as punishing in that kind of way." I'm 95% over that.

Though a well-educated professional with a family history of the disease, she has still not entirely moved past these beliefs. Some may argue that these beliefs, though unscientific, are not necessarily misunderstandings per se, and may merely reflect religious views. Nonetheless, these concepts may inadvertently impede health behaviors, and awareness of them is therefore important.

Various social contexts may abet or challenge these misunderstandings. Support groups, the media, and hearsay can all promulgate myths. A patient may feel that in certain social contexts other people may view such beliefs as irrational. But he or she may nonetheless maintain these views. Linda, the art teacher who thought that her father would eliminate the disease from the family, said about the period before she tested mutation-negative:

> I was very much a part of the New Age claptrap. A friend sent me a guru healing tape—this guru believed that some people came into the

world to extinguish a genetic disease in the family. Now, it's a little embarrassing to me. I'm from California, so you can take this with a grain of California salt.

As she suggests, friends and family members may fuel beliefs that an individual may accept or reject. But disagreements about these understandings can produce strife. Carol, who had breast cancer in her family and had her breasts and ovaries removed due to the mutation, said,

> My boyfriend is Mr. Holistic Vitamin Guru, crazy nut. He thought my breast cancer could just be treated with vitamins. He is dead against everything I've done, downright mad that all this has gone on, which has been difficult. He doesn't really understand that in every single gene in my body, this one gene is mutated. He just thought this one mutation is on one something, but not on every chromosome. I had to have the doctor tell him: this is in every single gene in my body . . . It cannot be fixed. He just thought it was just a small corruption of some sort that can be corrected in one place in my body, like my breast. So, he didn't understand why all this stuff had to happen, having my breasts and ovaries removed.

She confuses the meanings of "gene," "cell," and "chromosome," but underscores tensions that can exist about misunderstandings of mutations and their treatability.

An individual's disease can also distress a spouse who struggles with his or her own anxieties about the diagnosis, and miscomprehensions or desires not to understand. The fact that disease can result from a mutation can be both frightening and counterintuitive. Carol added about this boyfriend:

> I don't think he *wants* to understand. My breasts and ovaries had to be removed, but those genes are still lingering there . . . I could still get cancer. It could metastasize to another part of my body.

These misperceptions can impede health behaviors and coping, leading to avoidance of testing or treatment. Joyce, with a family history of breast cancer, said that before she got the disease and found she lacked the mutation:

> I thought: if I didn't have a mammogram, I wouldn't have breast cancer. So I've never had a mammogram. I always thought breast cancer was overtreated—that the whole thing was a crock. Why not get a mammogram? Foolish risk-taking—it was exciting. I also did exercise and diet. That strategy did not work.

She suggests magical thinking here—if not tested, she wouldn't develop the disease—and wariness of shifting medical science, and concluded that behavior, rather than biology, controlled her disease.

CONCLUSIONS

A variety of misunderstandings about genetic mechanisms, tests, and statistics emerge here. These tests are frequently seen as being more predictive than they actually are, and genetics are viewed as able to predict even behaviors and traits for which no markers have yet been identified. Misunderstandings arise about genetic mechanisms, carrier states, homozygosity versus heterogeneity, and the amounts of biological material one inherits from each parent. Misconceptions about statistics concern percentages versus proportions, absolute versus relative risks, and independence of odds. As we will see, these miscomprehensions shape testing, treatment, coping, and reproductive decisions.

Expanding use and direct marketing of genetic tests to both patients and providers make these issues critical. Private companies, scientists, journalists, and physicians may overly encourage genetic testing, taking advantage of and contributing to beliefs in the intrinsic value of this knowledge. Genetic testing often then becomes imbued with undeserved magical power—as potent and portent.

While earlier studies have noted that the general public misunderstands genetics, and that individuals at risk of common chronic familial diseases for which no definitive genetic markers have been identified (e.g., hypercholesteraolemia and diabetes) view these disorders in highly subjective, personal ways,[15] the men and women here confront disorders for which definitive tests exist. Frequently, they have already interacted with genetic counselors and other providers regarding these issues, but nonetheless still display numerous misconceptions.

While prior researchers have proposed possible frameworks for genetic counseling that include perceptions of risk,[16,17] the men and women here suggest how such perceptions of risk may be based on misunderstandings. Multiple factors such as views of cause, control, and family influence have been suggested, and may affect perceived risk. But the interviewees here reveal how some of these variables can in fact interact and vary, based on emotional and psychological needs that can collide with or override intellectual understandings of genetics. Broader cultural and social myths and misunderstandings can clearly affect these perceptions as well.

Several of these issues have received little if any attention among providers and researchers. For example, the notion that disease mutations are linked with physical resemblances to an affected parent has been suggested among individuals at risk for HD,[9] but arises here with other diseases as well. These men and women also elucidate other aspects of this phenomenon—how it persists despite awareness that it may be illogical, and how it supports and is supported by other misunderstandings and reflects desires for order in the face of anxiety and despair.

Misunderstandings about statistics and genetics fuel each other. Prior research has tended to separate misperceptions of statistics, genetic tests, and genetic mechanisms. But these three sets of misconceptions can in fact reinforce each other. The notion that genetic tests are more predictive than they actually are can both result from and contribute to misconceptions about statistics. Patients overestimate not only their risk, but the predictiveness of genetic tests. These overcalculations can bolster and be bolstered by beliefs about genetic mechanisms. Difficulties grasping complicated statistics (e.g., concerning relative proportions, and independence of odds) can exacerbate misunderstandings about genetics. Misperceptions of statistics and genetics may both also reflect emotional states and desires (related to hope, denial, and control). These emotions can outweigh educated understandings of how genetics and statistics actually work.

Personal experiences, education, inherent scientific uncertainties, emotional issues, and social inputs can all contribute to these miscomprehensions. When test results challenge prior assumptions (e.g., that physical resemblance among family members predicts the presence or absence of a disease mutation), some individuals conclude that these assumptions were incorrect. But others strive to maintain these beliefs, and reconcile these divergences.

At times, a sense of therapeutic misconception about testing appeared—that tests must be helpful in and of themselves in providing answers. Individuals frequently overestimate the power of genetics—for example, believing in genetic bases for behavioral traits for which no genetic markers have been found. Many think that testing is inherently beneficial in and of itself—that knowledge is invariably power—and that physicians would not offer medical tests if these were not beneficial. On the other hand, especially for HD, with its particular stigma, patients who are relatively well-educated about genetic risks (frequently due to family experiences) may value testing less for its own sake, since they are more aware of the potential discrimination that can result.

Patients seek perceived personal control,[18] and many come to believe that they can in some way affect genetic disorders (even HD). Yet these beliefs may in fact be incorrect, impeding coping. Hope, denial, and despair can shape and be shaped by these misconceptions.

Kahneman and Tversky[19,20] described difficulties in grappling with statistics, and the heuristics people then use, and suggest that humans are generally risk averse. The individuals here try to view and frame genetic information positively, seeking hope. They also respond to these challenges by seeking to reduce uncertainty, seeing genetic tests as more predictive than these in fact are.

Notions that genes are highly predictive and that metaphysics can alter health reflect widespread cultural views—disseminated in part by the media—and can enhance personal beliefs. This social reinforcement underscores needs for improving public education about genetics. At the same time, providers need to recognize that patients' misperceptions may partly stem from such widespread social attitudes, which thus need to be addressed. A patient may recognize the inaccuracy of socially disseminated notions about genetics, and reject or be swayed by these. Alternatively, patients may hold inaccurate beliefs that providers or the media can correct. Nonetheless, as we have seen, given the ambiguities of genetic information and competing emotional needs, inaccurate perceptions can persist.

Prior research has suggested that individuals who were at risk for HD, whether symptomatic or asymptomatic, generally had lower levels of distress than expected.[21] The men and women here elucidate how patients in fact manage to incorporate positive test results and symptomatology into their lives through social, cognitive, and other psychological processes. Yet these processes may at times involve miscomprehensions that can impede health behaviors.

These data illustrate how individuals conceptualize genetics within the contexts of their other beliefs. At times they have almost mystical senses of fate—of "things meant to be"—as opposed to diseases occurring through biological processes. Individuals ponder genetics not in isolation, but as part of larger cosmological beliefs and understandings, seeking order and fairness.

Earlier researchers have also suggested that patients personalize their views of genetics, yet the men and women here highlight the importance of examining not just how views of risk are subjective, but of what specific elements these beliefs actually consist (i.e., the specific *content*) as well, and how these perceptions may in fact be erroneous. Moreover, these misunderstandings are not always wholly idiosyncratic, but reveal patterns related to cultural myths and reflect underlying desires. Clearly, not all subjective impressions of genetics are inaccurate, but some are, and patients may benefit from clinicians, patients, family members, and others recognizing and trying to correct these.

With these three diseases, some possible differences emerge. Specifically, the genetics for HD is less ambiguous than for these other two disorders. *BRCA* mutations involve more uncertainties, given the reduced penetrance of the mutations and the potential effects of other, nongenetic factors in disease onset and severity. Similarly, for Alpha, confusion can result since environmental exacerbants can worsen symptoms, and heterozygotes can themselves get sick, though less severely than homozygotes. Thus, misunderstandings of absolute versus relative risks arise for breast cancer and Alpha, but not for HD. Nevertheless, many similar patterns clearly emerge across these disorders.

Correct perceptions in one domain can potentially help counterbalance misperceptions in others. While genetic counselors are trained to probe and address misunderstandings, physicians, nurses, and family members may be less aware of the breadth and prevalence of these misconceptions and the ways these may shape patients' health decisions. Yet these areas need to be addressed carefully, given the sensitive emotional issues of denial and hope. With rising amounts and murkiness of genetic testing, heightened appreciation of these issues is vital.

PART IV

Genes in the Clinic

CHAPTER 7

"What Should I Do About My Genes?":

Deciding on Treatment

These men and women struggle not only to understand their genetic risks, but to decide about possible treatments. They face dilemmas about not only testing and disclosure, but potential therapeutic options as well. The unclear predictiveness of genetic tests muddles the pros and cons of various treatments. Thus far, genetics research has uncovered causes of disease more than therapies, advancing diagnostics far more than treatments and creating uncertainties about how to respond.

As we will see, compared to other types of disease, genetics poses particular dilemmas because a person may learn that he or she is at risk or has a mutation, but never develop any symptoms or do so only years or decades later. Usually, symptoms of a disease prompt treatment. But with genetics, that is not always the case. Rather, knowledge of risk or a mutation can be far more abstract. One can lack any symptoms, yet still benefit from invasive interventions. Questions surface of how men and women navigate these tensions and figure out how to make the abstract real. They make these decisions in the contexts of complex interactions with family members, clinicians, and patient communities.

Challenges arise from the fact that these diseases have genetic bases, as well as other aspects of symptoms, therapeutic options, and treatment side effects. These features of a disease, though not explicitly genetic per se, nonetheless form the backdrop against which individuals then confront additional implications of their disorder. These diseases each raise their own difficulties, but share several common themes.

THE STRESSES OF SYMPTOMS

Both physical and mental symptoms of these diseases produce stress. Symptoms vary from minor to severe, but can all carry great psychological and symbolic weight, foreshadowing future problems. Such symptoms can be the most difficult part of a diagnosis. As Yvonne, who had lung transplants for Alpha, said, "The hardest thing is just being disabled: Not being able to do what everybody else does." If not for Alpha, many patients would have been more physically active. Dorothy, the former TV station producer reliant on an oxygen machine, added, "If I didn't have Alpha, I'd climb mountains, do a lot more with my children."

Due to its psychiatric manifestations, HD generates particular stresses. These symptoms can be the major challenges patients face, and prove more disturbing than cognitive deficits per se. But doctors may underestimate these difficulties. As Mary, the housewife with HD symptoms, said,

> I don't mind tripping, being stupid, or having memory problems. But I don't like paranoia or anxiety. I can deal with just about anything, but anxiety. That's my biggest obstacle. You can jerk around in the store, and still pick up fruit. But if you have anxiety, you're not even going to enter the store.

The difficulties of these psychiatric symptoms astonish many patients. Jim, the physician with HD, was surprised at "how debilitating *depression* was: that it can keep you from performing your duties. When I was depressed, I couldn't write down phone numbers. I just didn't remember."

As mentioned earlier, psychiatric symptoms can also impede treatment. Patients with psychosis or depression may fear and reject psychiatric care.

Confronting Mortality

Mutations trigger fears of early death. But the predictiveness of mutations, even for HD, is imprecise. Poor prognoses may prove incorrect. As Benjamin, the engineer, remarked about Alpha: "People are told they're going to die in a year or two, but are still alive 10 years later." Nonetheless, to come to terms with the threat of such limited prognoses can be hard. Dorothy, a 59-year-old, added, "It's sad that I'm not going to make it to my eighties. I hope to live for another 20 years, but I don't think that will happen."

These threats can foster fear and denial that can in turn hamper treatment. For HD, some eschew doctors and testing because of having to confront and acknowledge the disease, yet they may then delay help for treatable symptoms such as depression. Even Jim, the physician with HD, delayed such care. Though a doctor himself, he avoided addressing his depression because he feared it meant he had HD.

> My depression was getting really bad. I wouldn't even leave the house. In retrospect, I was just denying it. I was afraid of being diagnosed. That's why I ignored it for so long. And when I was depressed, it was hard to think—that was part of the problem. I liked being a doctor, and doing what I was doing. I was worried I wouldn't be able to do it anymore.

He suggests here a complex process of denial—part conscious and part unconscious. In the presence of genetic risk, early possible symptoms, even minimal or mild, can readily be feared as harbingering worse disease.

Yet despite his psychiatric problems, Jim thought it was nonetheless possible that he didn't have the mutation. "Since I had symptoms, I knew the odds were higher—more towards 100 than 50. But there was still a chance that I didn't have it." Here again, individuals altered their perceptions of their risks based on their symptoms.

Patients often have poor insight about the presence, magnitude, and impact of psychiatric symptoms. "I was working on the wards, and got pulled off," he continued. "There must have been something that happened, that I wasn't doing right." But he remains unsure of what that was.

HD symptoms can prompt rejection of help. Patty, who pushes the disease "under a rug," said about her affected mother, "She insists she's fine, but she's unstable. A couple of weeks ago somebody stole her wallet, but she insists she misplaced it. She's extremely stubborn. She's not going to get any help." Patty also tries to avoid thinking about her own risk. Yet once symptoms develop, poor judgment—a symptom of the disease—can in fact further hamper care. Patty's affected brother even canceled his health insurance, further illustrating how symptoms can hinder treatment.

PREVENTION

These individuals confront quandaries, too, of how much prevention to pursue. Alpha poses decisions of exactly *how* precautious to be, given the potential costs and benefits involved. Benjamin, the engineer, for instance, defended his visits to smoky environments despite the potential dangers.

I still go bowling, where you can still smoke. Is it good for me? No. A lot of people think I'm nuts for going in a smoky bowling alley. But what kind of bubble do you want to live in? What kind of walls? Stay away from your kids because they are a major source of infection? It depends on how much of a chance you want to take, and how much you want to shut down your life. I've got to have a little bit of a social life. I've always bowled.

He sees the dangers of smoke as possible, but not absolute, and makes tradeoffs between quality and quantity of life. Not surprisingly, family members can disagree as to whether and to what degree they should each take precautions. "My boys have respiratory problems," Dorothy, the former TV producer, said regarding Alpha. "One is involved in clay and glaze. He wears a mask, but that doesn't really help your lungs." She thinks he should stop this work immediately, but he refuses.

Given the possibility of receiving bad news, individuals may also fear and avoid medical visits, and follow-ups can fuel anxiety. Waiting for test results can be tough—even for those who know they don't have the mutation. Beatrice, the math teacher who had breast cancer along with her sister, but no mutation, understood risks very logically, but remained afraid.

The hardest thing is: every six months I go for a mammogram. During the six months, I try not to think about it. But during the last week, it plays games with my head. The worst is actually sitting in the corridor waiting. I just hope.

SPECIFIC TREATMENTS

Treatments for these disorders vary in availability, effectiveness, and expense. Each therapeutic option poses potential benefits and risks that must be weighed.

As it progresses, Alpha can be treated with Prolastin, and later, potentially lung and liver transplantations. Yet these interventions all present personal as well as broader social challenges. Undoubtedly, genetic markers will disproportionately be found for rare diseases (such as Alpha). Yet since these ailments affect relatively few people, the demand for drugs for these conditions is less than for many other disorders. Hence, pharmaceutical companies have historically invested little money into research and development for these relatively ignored or "orphaned" conditions. The U.S. Orphan Drug Act of 1983 sought to remedy this, and did so to a certain degree for a few disorders, but not others.

TREATMENTS FOR ALPHA

Prolastin

Prolastin can replace the deficient enzyme, the absence of which causes symptoms, but whether, when, how often, and to what degree it will work is not always clear. Benjamin, the engineer, said,

> There's no scientific proof that Prolastin works. Most Alpha doctors think it works, but there's been no clinical trial. In England, it's not permitted. It was approved in the United States, not because it was efficacious, but because it brought down the blood level of active Alpha-1.

Uncertainty hovers concerning the drug's effectiveness—which may vary among patients. As a former nurse, Kate is more aware of the subtleties of assessing medication effectiveness. "At best, it slows down disease progression," she said. "But in some people, it doesn't. In me, the progression continues. Who knows whether the drug is slowing the disease down or not?"

Importantly, for many years, manufacturers simply did not produce enough of the drug, leading to conflicts. As Dorothy, awaiting lung transplantation, described,

> Every year, they shut down the factory, and none of us get it. Your name goes on a wheel, and comes up in 28 to 35 days, depending on how many people. Everyone gets it for 11 months of the year.

Many patients accepted the pharmaceutical industry's claim that it could not produce more, but others were wary and frustrated. Individuals varied in whether and to what degree they accepted the profit motive of the main drug company (Bayer). Some people acknowledged the motive, or the need to triage the drug as legitimate. As Benjamin said,

> Bayer claims they're making the drug at their full production capability. But a lot of people are angry. The company improved its factory, but doctors are finding more Alphas. So the company can't keep up with demand. There may be another product. Another company is now on the horizon . . . But I've heard of possible breakthroughs too many times before. It costs a lot of money to make these drugs. The company is not in it to be altruistic, but to make a profit. I understand that. People say Bayer should be making more, and not charging as much. I kind of agree. They say Bayer cornered the market, and is ripping off the community.

Many patients thus felt that they were victims of industry interests.

As a result of drug shortages, the Alpha community took upon itself the task of helping manufacturers ration the drug.

Yet these communities then had to address several challenges. Profound questions of justice surfaced concerning how the shortage should be handled—whether all patients should be cut back equally or new ones should not get any. As Dorothy explained,

> Since there is not enough Prolastin, we've had arguments about who gets it. Doctors said it only works with moderate emphysema, so the community decided to measure people with moderate emphysema. But it was very hard to measure.

These thorny justice issues can be difficult to resolve, and communities may not be prepared to address these. As Dorothy wondered about the plan to target moderate disease, "Is that taking away from other people?"

In the end, the community helped ration the medication. Benjamin continued:

> The community asked for patient allocation, which Bayer then did. Basically, you were put on a list. When your turn came up, you'd get some shipped. Bayer tried to ship enough, but if they were running low, they would later just stop shipping, and would resume where they left off.

Yet this triaging posed tough pros and cons, and added frustrations. He added:

> At the same time, they raised the price 25%–30%. I didn't like that. Prolastin is available only in certain countries. In Canada, some people can't get it. In the U.S., anybody can enroll, but you just get put on the rotating list, and nobody gets enough. Last year, I got 10 months' worth over the 12 months.

Many concluded that, given the constraints, the system was equitable. As Benjamin said,

> It turned out fair. I think companies price-gouged, but other people disagree. Even if Prolastin doesn't do a damn thing, Bayer funnels money into the community, for research. Maybe not for us, but for our kids.

Shortages had a range of unintended effects. Uncertain supplies of Prolastin generated anxiety, which individuals tolerated to varying degrees. Betty, the designer who carries an oxygen concentrator, "learned to stretch it out, and not panic." But others worried far more.

Many patients responded to these shortages by strategically stockpiling the drug. As Benjamin observed, "One recommendation is: save it up. When you're well, skip doses." Patients were then acting in their own self-interest rather than that of the group—obtaining slightly more than they needed to cover possible later shortages.

Questions also arose about whether patient organizations, in distributing drugs, may then become too close to pharmaceutical companies. Drug companies can help fund patient advocacy organizations, but patients may be suspicious of such industry ties. Jennifer, the schoolteacher, added about Alpha,

> There's a valid criticism in the community that one Alpha organization is really a lackey for the pharmaceutical company, because that's how the organization really became effective. The organization existed before, but was sort of touch and go. The company now paid them for their services, and for taking medication orders. They became a more viable organization.

In response to these shortages, some patients even felt that physicians have begun testing less often for the disease than before. "A few years ago, there was a lot more pressure to test," said Peter, the Alpha support group leader. "Then doctors backed off, because of the shortage."

More recently, pharmaceutical companies have managed to produce ample supply of the drug, ending these shortages. But these experiences, now past, are noteworthy in revealing the potential problems that orphan diseases may pose, and that, as we will see, genetic communities may therefore confront.

PORTABLE OXYGEN

Alpha may worsen to the point that patients require portable oxygen and must carry around either an oxygen concentrator machine or heavy tanks on wheels. Such equipment poses added difficulties—immediately identifying individuals as ill. Initiation of oxygen can be hard because it represents a physical as well as psychological milestone, marking further onslaught of disease. The possible need for such oxygen thus incites deep ambivalence. As Benjamin described:

> If I have oxygen, it means I really am sick, pathetic, unable to take care of myself, or to contribute to the world. I'd have no reason to live. I'm thinking now that I could still go on, but it took me a long time to come to that. I really admire Alphas on oxygen who keep going.

Organ Transplants

Alpha can also necessitate organ transplants, which present additional dilemmas. Renée Fox and others have written about some of the complexities posed by organ transplantation for other diseases—quandaries about how the limited supply of organs should be distributed, and how recipients think about donors, whose body parts are now inside them (e.g., how indebted to feel).[1] But particular issues may arise more strongly here than with other conditions.

Though transplant may be essential when Prolastin no longer works, not everyone with Alpha is in fact eligible, raising questions of how to distribute a limited numbers of organs. Complications from transplantation can also present insurmountable barriers.

For Alpha more than for other disorders, whether to pursue the possibility of organ transplantation may be a patient's own choice. Yet weighing marginal increments of quality versus quantity of life is hard. Nonetheless, some feel they would readily accept the risks. "I would want a transplant," Gilbert, the factory worker, said, "if I can buy five good years, as opposed to 10 crappy ones. I might as well enjoy what I've got."

Still, others are less sure. Organ transplants present complex challenges, having to weigh high potential benefits against high potential risks. Charles, the accountant, said,

> The decision is going to be tough. Surgeons transplant a lot more hearts than lungs. The survival rate for lung transplants is about 70% for the first year. I'd probably die on the table. But, this winter was tough.

The waiting list for organs is long, and once transplanted, recipients' bodies can reject them. Immunosuppression medications, designed to reduce the likelihood of such rejection, induce their own side effects, making patients far more vulnerable to infection.

Unlike transplantation as a result of injury to a particular organ, in the case of Alpha the disease continues even after organ transplant. Consequently, transplanted organs, even if not rejected, may have only limited success: they can reverse past devastation from the disease, but not stop future progression. The newly transplanted organs will themselves become diseased. As Charles said,

> You're really rolling the dice. If it's successful, you're only back to where you can *dream* about being healthy. Occasionally, I have dreams about having good lungs again. But, you are indebted to antirejection drugs for the rest of your life. Even a year after a successful transplant, you can still reject it. You're changing one disease for another.

His fatalism contributes to his continuing visits to smoky bars.

In part, lung transplants are not always successful, due to recipients' prior medical histories. Yvonne, who had lung transplants, said, "For me, it worked. For others, it didn't. Another Alpha got transplanted with me. Last week, he died. He made it a year and a half."

Patients may face quandaries, too, of whether to accept one lung, if it is available for transplant, rather than waiting for two. Dorothy, the former TV producer awaiting lung transplants, said,

> You're changing one disease for another. A university offered me one lung. But you could die on the table, and people with double lung transplants do better than those with a single lung. If you only wanted three more years of life, you can go with the single lung, but the double lungs extend your life more. You really need the two lungs.

Questions also arise as to *when* to get a transplant, and how to balance the status quo against potential benefits and risks of waiting. Dorothy continued, "It's a tradeoff. I'm living, but can't do anything. Maybe if I hold off another year, I'll have an additional year to live. But a time comes when you just have to bite the bullet and say: it's time."

Still, waiting lists can take years, and promises of possible lungs are not always met. Donor lungs may seem to become available, but then not match. As Yvonne, who eventually received two lungs, said, "Mostly, you get 'dry runs.' They call you, and the lungs they have don't match, or are the wrong blood type. Chances are you go there two or three times before it happens."

Patients with Alpha, unlike those with other diseases, frequently also require more than one organ. Yet needed organs are usually not all available simultaneously. Patients then face questions of where to go for such an invasive procedure. Yvonne went out of state because a hospital there seemed better. But that decision ended up adding logistical problems.

At least in the short term, surgery can significantly reduce symptoms. After the operation she felt she was in fact "normal": "As soon as it was done, I sat up in bed, and was talking and breathing without a problem. I was a normal person."

Indeed, because of her new, transplanted lung, she felt she no longer had the disease.

> I don't think of myself as having Alpha now. I don't have to take Prolastin. They explained that I have Alpha, but I don't, because the new lungs don't have it. The new lungs will get it, but it takes 20 years to develop. I used to read the Alpha newsletter. Less recently.

She raises dilemmas of what it means to have a disease, if the diseased organ has been removed. She now has only a slow disease process, but no current symptoms, highlighting a distinction between the cause versus the effects of a disorder—what it means to continue to have the causal process but no longer the impact of the disease. The former alone, because it does not impair her function, does not trouble her.

QUESTIONS OF JUSTICE AND ORGAN DISTRIBUTION

Worldwide organ shortage creates multiple conundra of how to distribute organs fairly, and optimally, and how to decide. Questions of who should receive the limited supply involve balancing competing demands based on age, prognoses, and patients' culpability for their disease. These individuals reflected on how the larger system does and should operate. Yvonne said,

> Who's to judge? An 8-year-old got a transplant and maybe has 10 years. If I get transplanted, I get 10 years. But I've already lived 40 years. The child should have first chance, because 10 years means more to a child than to a 40-year-old. But I haven't a clue how it's divvied up.

Though she feels that the child, more than she, should receive an organ, she has already in fact received two. Hence she has few criticisms of the current system. Indeed, she feels that Alphas have an advantage: they can put themselves on the transplant waiting list before they actually need an organ. Yet she also suggests that Alphas may in fact unfairly take advantage of the system. Some try to jump the cue: since the disease is genetic, they can anticipate that they will worsen, and they can sign up for an organ before they actually need one. "The system now is kind of fair," she said. "Everybody has to wait. But with Alphas, you're way ahead of the ball game, because you know what you have."

She admonishes patients to "game" the system in this way.

> Alphas make a big mistake not getting tested and going on the transplant list. Just because you're on the list, doesn't mean you have to take the transplant. You can just keep saying, "No, I'm not ready." Then, they keep bypassing you. That is what happened with me. I went on it five years in advance. I was at the top of the list, but wasn't ready, so they just kept going by me. Which was fine. Because when I needed the transplant, I was there. If Alphas don't do that, shame on them. Other diseases don't have that time: in three months, if they don't get transplanted, they're gone.

Possible transplantation may thus also constitute an added reason to undergo genetic testing.

Yet she poses disturbing questions of distributive justice—how to determine the appropriate distribution of organs, and whether each disease should receive a quota, and if so, what. Dorothy, still awaiting lungs, added,

> It shouldn't be done by disease, but by individual medical necessity. Everyone should have equal access. One doctor believes that cystic fibrosis is not getting its share of lungs. But I don't think it was ever their share to begin with.

Given the ongoing shortage of organs, these dilemmas continue to evolve.

QUESTIONS OF RELATIONSHIPS WITH DONORS

Transplant recipients face complex psychological issues, too, regarding their real and imagined relationships with their organ donors. Recipients often want to express thanks but do not do so, wishing to keep the relationship mutually anonymous. To receive the gift of someone else's organ—to have part of someone else inside of you—challenges notions of selfhood, indebtedness, and guilt, and evokes notions of mystical connection. These relationships are odd, unique, and in many ways unprecedented. Yvonne, after her transplant, said,

> Some people with transplants think: "part of this other person's inside me," or they feel indebted, or wonder about the other person. That's very weird to talk about. You *do* have somebody else's parts inside you. Some people want to know who the donor is. They want to meet the family to say thank you. Others, like me, would love to just send an anonymous thank you card. I don't want them to know who I am, and I don't want to know who they are. Because it's not just lungs: it's a *person*. It's got a name, an identity. I've even heard stories where the family has actually said: you owe me, because my son gave you those lungs. Yes, but the guilt is uncomfortable. In other cases, the family doesn't want you anywhere near them. The donation may not have been the family's wish, but unfortunately there are not enough donors.

These emotional issues prove far more powerful than organ recipients anticipate. Dorothy, a tough, assertive businesswoman, felt that issues of donorship would not bother her. But in the end, even she recognized that her attitudes may waver over time. "Getting someone else's lungs inside of me doesn't bother me at all," she said. "It might bother me later on, but not today." Indeed, she ponders whether she will name her future lungs, and has already picked out names for them.

BREAST CANCER TREATMENTS

Breast cancer poses a different set of therapeutic dilemmas. Genetic testing for breast cancer can affect possible treatment in several ways: from type and frequency of monitoring to chemotherapy, radiation therapy, and prophylactic surgery.

Genetic testing for breast cancer can motivate more vigorous follow-up by both clinicians and patients. "Finding out that I had the gene," said Rhonda, the nurse with breast cancer and a strong family history, "my doctor recommended I be followed much more closely for ovarian cancer as well."

For those who have not already had cancer, a mutation-positive genetic test can prompt more aggressive follow-up. In fact, untested or mutation-negative individuals may feel less justified using medical resources. Thus, some women undergo testing in order to motivate themselves to monitor more. For Laura, the graphic designer, and her providers, a mutation-positive result clarifies and justifies decisions, and "makes things really black and white."

On the other hand, subsequent treatment decisions can pose more complicated and stressful choices. Chemotherapy can treat breast cancer but have painful side effects, and is not always successful. Many women thus consider or opt for prophylactic surgery instead. Carol was glad to be tested after developing cancer, but at a certain point she declined additional chemo and instead chose prophylactic mastectomy—despite her boyfriend's objection. She wanted to make her own decision, and feels in retrospect that the surgery saved her life.

> They wanted me to have more chemo, but I refused. Chemo obviously didn't do anything. So why do it again? I decided to nip everything in the bud, and have everything removed—to take matters into my own hands, and have prophylactic surgery. I had a double mastectomy, with reconstruction, and had the other ovary removed. Lo and behold, they found some microscopic foci on my removed ovary, and I wound up having Paget's disease in one of my nipples. So it saved my life. I'm thrilled I had the genetic testing, because otherwise, things would have gotten worse. Maybe they would never have caught the ovarian cancer.

Physicians' recommendations can also conflict, adding to patient confusion. Patients feel that at times, doctors are too quick to perform invasive medical interventions, and hence, in the end, that patients need to make key decisions on their own. "I don't do everything they tell me," Carol added. "But I try to do what I think is realistic. One doctor was very adamant that I do the chemo. The other doctors thought the cancer was tiny." She has not always followed her doctors' advice, but feels she carefully evaluates and weighs what they say.

Prophylactic Surgery

Women who have or are at risk for *BRCA1/2* mutations or breast cancer also face dilemmas of whether to undergo prophylactic surgeries, and if so, when. The uncertain predictiveness of *BRCA1/2* testing complicates these decisions. Women confront these choices in the contexts of complex interpersonal interactions.

Since the effectiveness of ovarian screening is relatively poor, professional groups recommend prophylactic ovarian surgery for *BRCA* mutation carriers by age 35 or by the completion of childbearing,[2] and bilateral prophylactic mastectomies for those who are willing. Prophylactic oophorectomies and mastectomies reduce cancer more than do chemo or surveillance,[3] and for mutation carriers are the most cost-effective strategies.[4]

Yet many women who might benefit from prophylactic surgery do not undergo it. Rates vary depending on country of origin and other factors. For instance, asymptomatic women with mutations opt for prophylactic surgeries much less in the United States than in the Netherlands.[5,6,7] The reasons for these differences are not clear.[8,9,10] In general, young women with children opt more for mastectomies, while older women opt more for oophorectomies.[11] Psychological factors such as perceived risks and benefits, trust in tests,[12] and being a "monitor" rather than a "blunter" of information[13] can also affect these decisions.[14,15,16] Women may choose oophorectomies based on perceptions of risk, cancer in family members, family obligations, concerns about fertility and menopause, and fears of surgical complications.[17] In general, women must balance potential benefits of anxiety reduction against potential complications of surgery.[18]

Clinical guidelines for mastectomies and oophorectomies differ, and leave much open room for questions. For oophorectomies, women have to decide exactly how long before turning 35 they can wait before undergoing surgery. Women considering prophylactic mastectomy must balance risks of disease against the risks of surgery for each type of operation (i.e., lumpectomy or mastectomy). But how women actually balance these various issues and make these disturbing tradeoffs about surgery, and when, remain unclear. Though potential factors have been suggested, the decision-making processes and the ways women view and experience these decisions remain murky.

Though the issues in contemplating each of these procedures vary in certain regards, common themes arise. Women face similar dilemmas, having to weigh conflicting psychological desires and communicate these tensions to providers and others. Differences emerge as well, but overall, the similarities appear to far outweigh these.

Women confront a series of agonizing decisions of whether to undergo each of these procedures, and if so which, when, and how. They seek input from providers, family members, friends, and breast cancer communities. Many women face these decisions either simultaneously or sequentially; and experiences confronting one procedure often shape subsequent decisions concerning other operations.

Series of Stressful Questions Faced

Women face dilemmas of whether they would develop cancer if they have the *BRCA1/2* mutation, and whether to undergo a lumpectomy or mastectomy, prophylactic mastectomies, breast reconstruction, or oophorectomies. The fact that operations had uncertain prognoses and unpredictable side effects complicates these conundra.

As we saw earlier, some women undergo genetic testing to see if they should indeed undergo prophylactic surgery. Others, who decided *not* to undergo testing, nonetheless consider surgery. Some women avoid testing because they will then have to face these quandaries. Despite her breast cancer and family history, Karen, the lawyer, viewed surgery in ways that affected her testing decision:

> So far, I have opted not to get tested. I asked my oncologist, "What difference would it make in my treatment?" She said, "At some point I would say: take out your ovaries, if there were a genetic link." So, do I want to have my ovaries taken out . . .? Or, do it prophylactically even without the testing?

She wrestles with this quandary, and has thus far not tested.

Women who decide to undergo surgery then face uncertainties of *when* to do so. They have to weigh desires to delay (in order to become comfortable psychologically with the possibility) against desires to eliminate cancer worries, and stop possible disease progression as soon as possible. Many women struggle with how long they can wait after a mastectomy before having oophorectomies. Rachel, who had breast cancer and a mutation, but not much information about her family history due to the Holocaust, concluded,

> I'm pretty much certain that I'll have my ovaries removed . . . My oncologist said I don't have to have it done now. They're suggesting: before

I'm 50. I'm 40. Could I wait 10 years? As I get older, the incidence of ovarian cancer increases . . . [After] what I've been through this year, I feel that if I were to do it now, I could at least put this chapter in my life behind me in some way, and not worry. I'm concerned about getting a cancer they can't detect. And I don't want to be under the magnifying glass the rest of my life. I have these mixed feelings about it: real confusion in my mind about what to do.

Though she had breast cancer and has the mutation, the fact that she does not know of a family history of the disease makes surgery less pressing to her.

Exquisite sensitivities concerning threats to the body and symbolic meanings of breasts and ovaries add to these complexities. Women frequently want at least to hear about possible alternatives, and to have these options addressed as sensitively as possible. But they often feel disappointed. Rachel added,

I left the first breast surgeon because he said, "O.K., here's what we do: we're going to remove your breast, and you're going to have chemotherapy and potentially radiation." My husband and I sat there saying, "We don't need it sugar-coated, but what about alternatives?" He said, "You could pursue these, but . . ." In the end, I ended up doing what that doctor said, but with a breast surgeon who worked with my integrated medicine oncologist—they had worked together before, and respected each other.

Rachel values holistic approaches and CAM, which this first doctor dismissed. As she explained,

An integrated medicine oncologist is very different than a traditional and conventional doctor. Part of my protocol, besides doing the conventional stuff, has been to integrate meditation, acupuncture, massage therapy for stress reduction, lymphatic massage, and a variety of supplements, not just vitamins, but antioxidants, Vitamin C, algae, and very large doses of dehydrated vegetables and fruits.

As we saw earlier, many women valued such alternative adjunct therapy, even if doctors denigrated it. As Rachel suggests, a physician's presentation of or openness to such alternatives may enhance patient satisfaction and trust.

The fact that these decisions arise in the context of ongoing risk and illness adds stress, since each decision is part of a much longer sequential series of choices. Hence, many seek to postpone decisions, though doing so may reflect denial. Mildred, who worked in finance and also had breast cancer, the mutation, and strong family history, is five years older than Rachel and feels closer to menopause. She wishes to wait until then.

> I don't want to think about it. I picked a number: when I hit 45. Next year. I guess I haven't decided. I mean: I've decided, but I keep on putting it off. For doctors, it's easy. They say: "take it out right away." That's fine, but for me, it's: *"Can't I just wait?* I've gone through enough." I understand it's increased my chances of getting ovarian by 40% over [my] lifetime.

She distinguishes the cavalier stances of physicians about these procedures from her own hesitation. Her past operation frames her outlook toward a future one. She understands the medical risks, but given these troubling tradeoffs, tries to delay the procedure, creating excuses. "I wanted to wait a year after surgery," she said. "Then, 'I'll wait until I go into menopause.' I'm going to constantly give an excuse."

Women face ambiguities, too, about the side effects that may result from surgery—including whether it will harm their physical attractiveness, relationships and sex, and views of their bodies and selves. To answer these questions definitively is hard. Arlene, the asymptomatic nurse who studied religion, has a sister and aunt with breast cancer. She debates whether to undergo genetic testing, based on the possible implications for prophylactic surgery.

> I've been looking at other women's breasts, thinking, "Is it really that big a deal?", wondering what some of the sensations [would] be like. Arousal in your nipples is not going to be there. But how much does that interfere with having a loving and caring intimate relationship?

She is uncertain about both sexual experiences, and the potential effects of these on romance.

Communication about Stresses

Given these quandaries, women generally seek and receive input from several sets of others, and various factors in turn shape how assistance is both offered and received.

Clinicians offer input, but it often proves complicated. Many women want clear, unambiguous medical opinions. But the subjectiveness of decisions about prophylactic surgery leads many physicians and others to feel uncomfortable giving such unequivocal recommendations. Beatrice, the math teacher who had breast cancer along with her sister, but no mutation, was unsure whether to have a lumpectomy or a mastectomy. She understood the risks logically, but still sought advice: "I called my internist, because she's a good friend, to help me make that decision. But she just felt she really couldn't." Physicians may feel torn—wanting to help, but recognizing that simple definitive opinions may not be best.

Patients may acknowledge the elusiveness of such firm input, but nonetheless feel frustrated. Beatrice continued:

Sometimes we want to hear that there is one answer, but there is none. Sometimes I wished somebody said, "This is how you do it . . . this is the pill. That's it. End of story." Whereas with this, you have to make a judgment call. A lot of information comes at you fast and furious. Sometimes it's a lot easier just being a little kid: Your mother says this is what you're having for dinner.

She highlights the difficulties of having to confront these quandaries and assess relatively large amounts of information without sufficient guidance, while at the same time desiring certainty. Surgeons may have less difficulty treating women newly diagnosed with cancer (where direct approaches may be well-suited) than women contemplating prophylactic operations (where nondirective discussions may be more appropriate). Yet Beatrice suggests that ambiguities arise in decisions involving both therapeutic and prophylactic considerations.

As we saw, doctors may vary not only in how directly they make recommendations but in whether they present other treatment options. Physicians range widely in the degrees to which they provide input versus leave decisions up to the patient. Due to the ambiguities and subjectivities involved, physicians may not say definitively what to do; instead, they may leave much of the decision making up to the woman herself. Yet selecting between these surgical options can be overwhelming. Carmen, the Latina former clerical aide who had breast and thyroid cancer and a *BRCA* mutation, but no family history, said, "It was my choice whether to have the breast removed or leave it. I decided to have it removed. It was very hard—like the world was coming down on me."

At the other extreme, given these uncertainties and sensitivities, some physicians may provide input *too* readily or forcefully. Particularly for oophorectomies, given their reproductive and psychological implications, doctors can appear somewhat callous regarding the stresses involved, not seeing these issues from patients' points of view. Doctors vary not only in the content and directiveness of their input, but their tone and sensitivity. Bonnie, whose mother and sister had breast cancer, said,

When my sister was getting the mass removed from her ovary, the doctor said, "We'll go in, scoop it out. We'll be out in a minute." Scoop it out? It drove me insane. He was "one of the best," but I feel so bad for any woman who goes to him. I've seen other doctors like that, too—male and female, it didn't matter. For doctors, it's just another day at the office.

Doctors may appear callous in both the information they present and the context in which they present it. Susie, having worked for an HIV organization, was acutely aware of these issues, and said about an ultrasound that found ovarian cysts,

> This doctor tried to discuss the results of the sonogram over the phone. I said, "Hi, Doctor," and suddenly I'm being told about this stuff. I didn't want to hear it over the phone. I don't think she was a good doctor. I don't see her anymore. My experience was bad.

The information this doctor provided may have been scientifically accurate, but Susie did not like the manner in which he conveyed it—without emotionally sensitive framing or any introduction to contextualize the information to try to lessen the trauma. From a relatively young female physician, such perceived harshness can be unexpected and surprising. Such patient reactions, though subjective, can nonetheless shape patient trust and treatment adherence—and thereby therapeutic outcomes. Physician gender does not seem to matter much.

Given these vagaries, doctors' time frames also differ in both raising the topic of surgeries and recommending these procedures. Physicians range in the degrees to which they push patients in these choices. Some patients feel urgency from doctors to undergo surgery, and perceive insensitivities in timing.

Clinicians may face conflicts in deciding when initially to raise options of surgery, to allow patients to prepare psychologically. The possibility of prophylactic surgery emerges not only after a mutation has been found, but before, when considering testing as a hypothetical possibility. However, women often saw providers as presenting options either too early (e.g., before genetic testing) or too late. Providers may want to prepare patients for the possibility of surgery by broaching the topic before genetic test or biopsy results are available. Yet women may then feel that these conversations are premature. Susie continued:

> Before I got my test results, the doctor jumped ahead to tell me: if you're positive, you should just take out your ovaries. I wasn't sure. I said I didn't think I wanted kids. She said, "Then it's easy. You'll just take the ovaries out." She seemed very confident. I thought, "What?! *You don't even know what I have! Why are you telling me that?*"

She ended up not having the mutation. Yet patients may feel uncomfortable expressing these objections to providers, thus impeding feedback to doctors.

Mildred, with breast cancer, a mutation, and a family history, also feels conflicted about prophylactic oophorectomies, and is thus waiting until menopause to undergo them. She continued, "My gynecologist and oncologist are O.K. with me waiting. My breast doctor is the only one *pressuring* me." Mildred highlights tensions between autonomy and paternalism—doctors encouraging what they think is best as opposed to what the patient may want.

Patients sense that institutional factors may also hamper provider communication. Some women feel, for example, that providers may defer from being more directive in these decisions because of legal liabilities or insurance concerns. "If they say, 'This is what you do,'" said Beatrice, the math teacher, "and things backfire, somebody's going to turn around and sue. No doctor wants to take that legal risk." Hence, patients at times feel that doctors may not discuss certain options unless patients specifically ask about these. Ori, the Israeli woman with breast cancer but no mutation or family history, said,

> The doctor recommended a mastectomy only on the sick breast. I asked, "How about this other one? Do I run the risk of developing something there?" The doctor said, "Yes, it's a good idea. I'm glad you asked: I'm not allowed to raise it by myself." She couldn't recommend it without my asking for it.

Lacking the *BRCA1/2* mutations or a family history, the need for such surgery was not clear, but Ori, at age 55, did not want to take any chances, in part due to the possibility of other genetic factors. At her age, she was also less bothered by losing both breasts than were many younger women. She suspected that in her case, insurance or other constraints limited the doctor's options, though the precise nature of these constraints was not wholly clear. Nonetheless, Ori highlights how patients feel that the larger health care system can at times restrain physicians.

Implications

As a result of some doctors' low levels of input, finding the "right" physician can be hard. Women may shop around for a provider, though not all patients have flexible insurance plans or out-of-pocket funds. Difficult tradeoffs arise. Even with a lumpectomy, questions emerge as to how extensive an operation to have.

As Karen, the lawyer with breast cancer and a family history but no testing, said,

> I went to four different surgeons. The first one seemed too busy. Another was too paternalistic. A third one wanted to take out a bunch of nodes, rather than do a sentinel node biopsy, so I eliminated her, though I liked her a lot.

Women have to consider *what* a doctor recommends, as well as *how*, and when. Karen balanced one physician's bedside manner against treatment recommendation, and weighed the former over the latter. Physicians can vary considerably in styles, timing, and recommendations. Women, in turn, range widely in weighing these factors, making it difficult for providers to know how best to approach these issues with any one patient.

Communication with Family and Friends

Given these stresses and often disappointing provider interactions, women frequently turn to family members and friends. Yet these additional interactions also differ considerably. Family members and friends can be either too aggressive and opinionated, or, on the other hand, too removed. Isabelle, the social worker with breast cancer and a mutation but no family history, feels pressured by her employer to undergo a prophylactic mastectomy:

> My boss always pushes me to get the surgery. She has multiple sclerosis. Living with her situation, unable to do anything about it, she thinks, "Are you crazy? You can do something! Do the surgery. And don't have the reconstruction—do it the simple way." But I just don't think I can deal with a double mastectomy, seeing what it looks like.

These highly personal issues can lead women to clash with their friends and family. Isabelle has thus far undergone an oophorectomy, but not a mastectomy.

When a woman's main social supports disagree with her or one other, she then has to balance these conflicting views. As Vera, the Asian executive, said about a possible oophorectomy, "My siblings are leaning towards 'no': why have surgery when you might not need it? My friends are leaning towards 'yes: cancer is bad.'" This opposition arises in part because no one in her family has had breast cancer. Still, she and others must then negotiate between such clashing arguments, and may remain undecided.

Ultimately, families and close friends generally uphold, rather than oppose, the patient's preference. Spouses, in particular, usually see their own opinions as secondary to the patient's. Family and friends may voice strong opposition, but in the end usually respect—perhaps more than do physicians—a "feminist" position that ultimately, a women's decisions about her body are her own. Carol, whose boyfriend opposed her prophylactic surgery, said, "In the end, despite the fact that he was so against it, and people said, 'Oh my God, it's so drastic,' it was *my* decision. It's *my* life." The risk worried her far more than him. She had both breasts and both ovaries removed.

Communication with the Breast Cancer Community

Given these stresses and frequently unsatisfying inputs from clinicians and others, many women turn to patient communities. These groups—both formal and informal—can fill gaps left by providers and families. Yet complications arise here as well. Within breast cancer communities, women vary in terms of what information they share and how. Debates about these surgeries fill much communication, and information from websites and patient advocacy organizations (either online or through support groups or meetings). Isabelle, for example, the social worker with cancer and the mutation, had undergone an oophorectomy but has had difficulty facing the prospect of additional surgery (a mastectomy). She finds it helpful hearing about others' decisions, though she sees women as varying widely in their tolerance and acceptance of risk. The degrees to which some patients take strong positions surprise her. She feels unable to do so herself.

> Online, the biggest issues are: whether to be tested or not, and have surgery, once you know you have this gene. Some women are really pro-surgery . . . Others feel they don't need to go to such extremes. Women who haven't had cancer, but have mothers or sisters who have, go to extremes and have preventive surgeries. I give them a lot of credit; that's very brave. I haven't been able to come to terms with surgery.

In these communities members can clash, and potentially sway each other. When initially considering testing and its implications, Susie, with no symptoms but an extensive family history, spoke to other women. She contemplated the possibility of prophylactic surgery as a reason to undergo testing.

> Other women have had double mastectomies—because their mothers died early—and feel it saved their lives. For them, it made sense. So I did hear some positive stories to counter this insane invasive surgery.

She then decided to pursue testing, and turned out to be mutation-negative.

The specific venue can affect these discussions. For example, the Internet offers certain advantages over direct face-to-face interactions, providing large amounts of information (including, importantly, photographs of surgical results), and permitting anonymity. Within these communities, members can share intimate experiences and even photos of breasts after surgery. Generally, group norms value such sharing, altruism, and communitarianism over protection of confidentiality. This communality forges and in turn further strengthens social connections. Women may not even see an alternative to such sharing. Carol, who dismissed her boyfriend's opposition to prophylactic surgeries, said, "if someone asks me, I'd probably show her my breasts: how great they look . . . I show everybody who wants to look. I'm not shy. How can you be?" With breast cancer, a strong family history, and the mutation, she had undergone both sets of prophylactic surgeries. The breast cancer community had assisted her, and she wished to help other members.

This camaraderie provides key information that physicians, family, and other friends often do not. Patients frequently seek as much advice as possible, and hence value the vast amount of data and experience, both visual and verbal, available online. A strong sense of community exists on the Internet, encouraging and facilitating mutual assistance. Nevertheless, patients range in the degrees to which they are willing to forego confidentiality in exchange for additional social support.

Women also differ in the amounts and kinds of information they pursue. Some women are highly proactive, looking at outcomes even before receiving their own genetic test results in order to help decide what prophylactic or other surgeries to undergo. Patients may even shop online for surgeons before receiving their genetic test results. Even before testing, Sarah, the computer programmer who is asymptomatic but has an extensive family history, including her sister, said she

> went to some of the big plastic surgery sites. You can go through lists of hundreds of surgeons, and look at their patients' pictures before and after. I looked at the pictures of people who had had prophylactic work done versus mastectomies only after developing cancer. The prophylactic ones looked a hell of a lot better. I even looked at the different techniques.

She wanted to see other women's results herself—highlighting the importance of *visual*, not only verbal, information in confronting these uncertainties and anxieties. She continued, "Someone might say, 'Why not ask your doctors for recommendations?' But I wanted to *see* what kind of work they do."

As suggested earlier, women have to assess the content and validity of information they receive, which can be difficult. Within these disease communities patients have to judge each others' views carefully given possible biases, personal preferences, and personalities. Patients vary in how much to accept versus how much to question information received—especially online from anonymous sources.

CONCLUSIONS

Genetic markers offer diagnostic—but not necessarily therapeutic—advances, and patients thus confront stresses concerning treatment. These challenges can vary due to the differing treatability of each condition. While HD has no effective treatment, Alpha does, though these therapies have posed obstacles.

Women with BRCA1/2 mutations face particularly difficult decisions regarding prophylactic surgeries. They confront questions of whether to undergo surgery, which operations to undergo (prophylactic mastectomy, reconstruction, prophylactic oophorectomy), when to do so, and how to decide (whether to accept or reject input from others). These issues even shape decisions of whether or not to undergo testing.

Choosing surgery or no surgery both pose ambiguous risks. Limitations of the health care system related to insurance or liability concerns may also constrain providers. While some women feel disappointed that a physician is not more directive, others reject doctors' input as too callous and forceful.

Providers, friends, and family may feel frustrated, caught in a double bind, wanting to offer more definitive advice but feeling unable to do so. Physicians and family members often need to be more sensitive to these issues, and prepared to broach these topics related to sexual functioning, reproductive plans, and physical attractiveness, and to help patients with these decisions, acknowledging these subjective and taboo concerns as legitimate. These others may also need to be more aware that they may view the form and content of communication far differently than do these patients.

Prophylactic surgery raises particular anxieties because the risks of both having surgery and not having it are considerable, yet abstract and hypothetical, and involve stigmatized issues concerning sexual organs, sexuality, and physical attractiveness.

These issues highlight several additional complexities and paradoxes of genetic testing, which can yield incomplete information that these murky treatment options make even more difficult. To face a mutation without any symptoms is a unique scenario in medicine. The fact that thus far genetics has yielded diagnostic far more than therapeutic knowledge presents dilemmas that will no doubt arise as well with many other genetic markers identified in the future.

CHAPTER 8

"Passing it On?":

Reproductive Choices

"Should I have kids, adopt, or abort?" these men and women repeatedly asked. They wrestle with difficult medical decisions about not only treatment, but reproduction as well—whether to have children "naturally," or by screening embryos or testing fetuses. Diseases associated with a genetic marker differ from other disorders in posing stark reproductive choices: the possibility of eliminating the mutation from one's descendants. But such removal, while offering potential benefits, also poses moral quandaries and the prospect of eugenics. How then do individuals face these conundra? How much responsibility do they feel to eliminate these mutations from future generations versus avoiding interference with embryos and fetuses, and what social, moral, and other factors are involved? As we will see, these reproductive choices can be shaped by prior decisions about testing and disclosure, and understandings of genetics, fate, and identity.

For several decades, prenatal testing has been possible for certain genetic markers of disease, using amniocentesis or chorionic villus sampling (CVS) of a fetus, followed by the option of terminating the pregnancy. More recently, preimplantation genetic diagnosis (PGD) has also been developed,[1,2] in which mutation-negative embryos are implanted in the uterus (either with or without parents' knowledge of their own genetic status). Patients who do not wish to know their own gene status are thus able to assure that they have a mutation-negative pregnancy,[3] while not learning if they themselves have the mutation. Yet the medical treatments involved with PGD can be stressful.[4]

Reproductive issues have received some attention with regard to HD, but much less with regard to other disorders. For HD, individuals not at risk have thought that at-risk individuals should prevent transmitting the mutation to offspring. For example, 94% of Swiss law and medical students support the systematic proposal of prenatal testing for at-risk pregnant individuals.[5]

Of Mexican neurologists, psychiatrists, and psychologists, 38% thought that mutation positive individuals should not have offspring[6] (though this study did not consider PGD). A study in three European countries found that most geneticists, obstetricians, lay individuals, and pregnant women would hypothetically undergo an abortion of a fetus with the HD mutation.[7]

However, in the past decade, rates of prenatal testing among at-risk populations have been found to be relatively low: 5%–25% in the United Kingdom[8] and Australia,[9] and approximately 18% in Canada.[10] In a French study of couples pregnant at the time of presymptomatic testing, 73% opted to continue the pregnancy, and only 9% opted for prenatal testing.[11] Women more than men have been found to undergo predictive testing for themselves and to request prenatal testing.[9,10]

For HD, many at-risk individuals have decided to have children despite possibly carrying the mutation. In the Netherlands, for example, only 19% of at-risk individuals have had genetic testing done. Of these, 44% already had children.[12] HD carriers, compared to noncarriers, may have fewer subsequent pregnancies.[13,14] In Europe, for instance, one study found that 14% of HD carriers versus 28% of noncarriers had additional pregnancies.[15] Among carriers, prenatal diagnosis did not occur in one-third of pregnancies. Among those who were motivated by family planning to get predictive testing, 39% of carriers versus 69% of noncarriers had subsequent pregnancies.[15] Thus, test results may predict pregnancy decisions, although differences may arise between countries.

Possible reasons suggested for low uptake of prenatal testing include objections to abortion, hope that a cure will be found, avoidance or minimization of the issue, and desires to first seek predictive testing for the parent.[9,16] Of note, Australian and Canadian reports above did not mention *expense* as a potential barrier. Indeed, such testing may cost much less there than in the United States.

Major ethical questions surface as to which genetic markers should be screened for using PGD or other prenatal procedures to avoid defacto eugenics.[17] Controversies arise about embryo selection based on sex or inheritable deafness.[18] Nondisclosing PGD presents additional ethical challenges, given that egg extraction is not entirely benign, and a large team of health care providers is involved in PGD, potentially challenging maintenance of confidentiality. Due to these concerns, at least one HD clinic has not offered PGD without disclosure.[19] Yet the ways in which at-risk individuals actually view these issues have not been examined. In the future, individuals may seek "designer babies," using IVF and testing embryos to select for intelligent, tall, or attractive progeny—though as of now, no markers have definitively or clearly been identified with these so-called desired traits.

In one of the only prior studies to look at reproductive issues among people with mutations, Claudia Downing,[20] a psychologist, emphasized the importance of *responsibility* toward others as a factor in reproductive decision making about HD. But other concerns may emerge as well. Indeed, her data involved testing through linkage analyses that necessitated families acting together to arrange for prenatal testing.[20] However, technology has since advanced to allow direct testing for the gene. Moreover, Downing presents three cases, but additional scenarios and conflicts may arise among other individuals.

With regard to individuals' decisions about testing themselves for HD, "stages-of-change" models have also been suggested (e.g., that individuals enter a series of phases from precontemplation to contemplation to action).[21,22] With regard to reproductive decisions, individuals confronting mutations may undergo such a process, yet what exactly occurs during these stages remains unclear. Individuals may face conflicts and have to balance desires to act altruistically and responsibly toward others against wishes to follow their own needs.

Several critical questions thus remain: in making reproductive decisions, do at-risk individuals in fact balance responsibility toward others against alternative considerations and concerns, and if so, what, and how?

REPRODUCTIVE OPTIONS

The men and women here encounter a series of reproductive options, and usually make these decisions not unilaterally, by themselves, but dyadically, as part of a couple. Additionally, couples often make these reproductive decisions not in isolation, but with input from family members, friends, and clinicians. They feel responsibility toward others but differ in who these others are—parents, spouses, or future generations. Moreover, in each of these interactions, conflicts ensue. Even within the domain of "responsibility toward others," multiple considerations exist and can compete.

These reproductive choices often prove to be among the most difficult that these individuals face. Tensions can emerge between individual desires and perceived responsibilities toward spouses, families of origin, current offspring, future offspring, and broader society. One's own symptoms, family history, personal and religious views, and mutation status can strongly shape one's attitudes. But these factors can also conflict.

For many, the key characteristic that distinguishes a disease associated with a genetic marker from another diagnosis is that the former can be transmitted to offspring at conception. As Beatrice, the math teacher with breast cancer along with her sister, but no mutation, said, "If it's genetic, I'm more concerned, because I could pass it on to my two children. It's not going to die with me. If you get hit by a bus, your disease stops there." She therefore underwent testing.

Some differentiate between genetics and familial history, seeing the former as connoting a higher likelihood of transmission. "Before testing, I had a strong family history," said Rhonda, the 31-year-old nurse with breast cancer who at age six had seen her mother die from the disease. "Now, I definitely have it, and can pass it on." Individuals like Rhonda then confront stressful reproductive dilemmas.

HAVING CHILDREN

Most of these men and women have seriously considered having children, and have then had to decide how to proceed. Rhonda's gene status changed how she viewed the prospect of offspring. She still struggles with this dilemma.

> I think: fifty-fifty chance I pass this on. My mom was in her thirties, I was in my twenties. It occurs younger in every generation. Now patients are in their teens. The mutation is not enough to make me not have children in the future. But the future is far away. I can't say for sure.

Others already had children before knowing about the risk of a disease. But many remain uncertain whether to avoid spreading the disease to other generations. Once they have developed serious symptoms, parents often choose not to have additional offspring. According to Benjamin, the engineer with Alpha and two young children,

> Younger couples who already had a kid don't know what to do about having *other* kids. Some of them just do. Sometimes they're lucky, sometimes not. I don't know anybody who had a liver transplant, and then a second kid — although I could see it happening.

HD, because it lacks any treatment, poses these issues most starkly. On the one hand, notions of responsibility toward others lead many at-risk individuals to oppose having children without first eliminating the possibility that these offspring may have the mutation. These patients feel they could—and should— help stop the spread of HD. Moreover, the parent may become sick, and not live long enough to be able to help offspring fully develop. At times, these concerns about dying and being unable to raise the child outweigh fears about transmitting the gene. As Evelyn, who had seen a psychic after her husband opposed her testing, said about her HD risk, "My biggest fear then was not, 'What if I pass this gene to my child,' but 'What if I get sick before he's old enough to take care of himself?'"

Still, others at risk for HD proceed to have children because of their own desires for offspring, or lack of knowledge about HD. At times, children are born at risk for HD because the infant's grandparents had not disclosed the risk of HD to the parents. As Georgia, who has HD, said, "It was only three or four years ago that my mother first mentioned it to my brother and I. My brother already had a son."

Individuals may also know that HD is in the family, but not think about the risks to future generations. Patty, who pushes her HD risk "under a rug," said, "I never thought in terms of the disease being hereditary, and my children having the disease." In part, she was single, 43, asymptomatic, and untested, and not considering children in the future or the potential impact of her risk on them. But the fact that the risk did not occur to her is revealing of the psychological disconnect that can exist.

Decisions to have children can be divorced from concerns about mutations. Some have children after being aware that HD is a risk, but before fully acknowledging it. Denial may operate here, in part because of desires to avoid confronting the potential burdens of the disease to oneself or others. Chloe, the 28-year-old asymptomatic and untested secretary who was terrified that she was turning into her affected father, said about her brother, "He didn't know it was genetic. I don't know *how* he didn't know. How wouldn't you know it's genetic? He says, 'If I had known that, I wouldn't have had any kids.'"

At times, an unplanned pregnancy forces decisions of whether to give birth or undergo an abortion. As John, who dropped out of grad school, and later learned that he lacked the HD mutation, said:

My brother's first child was a mistake. It was their anniversary, and they celebrated, had dinner, and had sex, and the condom broke. So they spent the whole night talking about what the hell they should do. They decided to take a day-after pill. Three months later, she's pregnant — the pill didn't work. They have the kid.

But they worry that the child may have the mutation.

After weighing the possibilities, Others have children, and consciously take the gamble that the child will be mutation-free. Children can bring joy and continue life, and hence be seen as helping the extended family, partly by compensating for deaths from HD. "We decided to have another baby," said Evelyn, untested and asymptomatic. "It's the best decision we ever made. He's just brought a lot of happiness into my family since my dad died."

The possibility that a cure may eventually be developed can further justify childbirth. "I want to have children," said Tina, who told her future husband about HD on their first date and had no symptoms or testing. "If I do have the disease, hopefully by then there will be treatment." Yet therapy may or may not be developed, prompting others to feel perplexed, anxious, and cautious.

Adoption

Those opposed to the possibility of giving birth to a mutation-positive child face several options, including adoption. Rather than hazard transmitting the gene, many try to adopt, though they then have to weigh varying options. Adoption might result from a sense of responsibility toward others (i.e., unwanted infants). In general, given large numbers of unwanted children in the world, to produce offspring oneself—regardless of genetic disease—may be seen as selfish. As Laura, the graphic designer with past depression, said, "there are babies in the world who need homes."

With HD, too, many consider adoption. "If I test positive, I probably will adopt," said Bill, the married salesman who fears he will develop HD because he resembles his dad, but who has no symptoms. "I would try and 'make' a baby's life that someone else couldn't take care of."

The fact that parents with HD could die before their child reaches maturity also shapes these considerations of what is morally "better." Adoption raises ethical questions of exactly *how* responsible to be to others: whether the benefits of giving an uncared-for baby a home for several years outweighs the possible moral objection that the parent may eventually become incapacitated and die from HD. Due to the threat of a parent's eventual incapacity, Ron, whose brother committed suicide, said, "in certain states they won't even let you adopt."

Amniocentesis or CVS, and Abortion

Some individuals had, or would choose, amniocentesis followed by abortion of a fetus with a mutation. HD often presents these dilemmas most boldly. Walter, symptomatic but untested for HD, and on disability from his government job, said that his niece underwent such a procedure and "had an abortion. I go along with her on it: it's her baby and her life."

Though desires for an abortion can reflect responsibility toward a future child (ensuring that he or she does not have the mutation), many of these individuals nonetheless see termination of a pregnancy for this reason as morally problematic. Many draw lines as to what genetic markers justify abortion or not. Some judge that such termination was permissible for a very serious disease such as HD but not for many other disorders. "I wouldn't recommend it for just any illness," Walter added. "It has to be something as devastating as HD."

Ori, the Israeli with breast cancer but no mutation or family history, would not abort a fetus for her disease but would do so for certain other conditions, such as Tay-Sachs, which has an increased prevalence among Ashkenazi Jews.

> I don't think I would kill for cancer, because it's survivable. But if the child will die anyway, like in Tay-Sachs, then I believe that abortion is good. A rabbi I know insists on testing people for Tay-Sachs. He allows abortions when the child would die anyway.

As she suggests, clergy may also provide input, and at times mandate decisions. Moreover, the fact that her disease does not appear to have a genetic component shapes her view that abortion should not be performed for it. But patients with the mutation at times see these issues differently.

Family and friends can disagree as to what is morally permissible. For example, if both parents are sickle-cell carriers, dilemmas emerge of whether to try assaying the fetus. Roberta, the African American former nursing student who had breast cancer along with her mother, but has not been tested, faced this scenario in her family. Given the severity of the disorder, she would abort a fetus if it had full sickle-cell disease, but not if it only had the trait. She would want "to have a kid that comes out as much on top as possible. If it was just the sickle-cell trait, we'd work with it." She would not abort for breast cancer, despite her family history, because she feels that treatment for that disorder is improving.

Regardless of their own moral qualms, many feel that the potential parents' preferences are paramount. Yet these preferences can encounter complications. For a child with severe illness, not only the patient but the parents may face obstacles. Carmen, with breast and thyroid cancer and a mutation, said, "If I knew I'm going to bring a baby into this world and she's going to suffer, I'd rather not have it. Because *you* suffer, too." Though Catholic, her medical history leads her to support abortion in such cases.

Despite the disease's severity, high penetrance, and lack of treatment, a right-to-life stance leads other people to oppose aborting a fetus even with the HD mutation. Concerns arise that permitting abortion for certain mutations would prompt abortions for other traits that individuals feel are undesirable—raising the specter of eugenics and, ultimately, Nazi Germany. As Tim, the Catholic lawyer with the HD mutation, but no symptoms, said,

You could test embryos and opt for a selective abortion, but I'm really Catholic. It just offends my sense of morality to decide which embryo lives or dies. It has the *potential* to become a human life. I just don't think I could live with making those kinds of moral distinctions. I don't feel it's up to me.

Of note, he lumps together moral objections to selection of both fetus and embryo—seeing them both as steps toward eugenics.

Resistance to abortion because of HD also emerges because individuals with HD can still lead full lives before becoming ill. "My brother has HD, but is a beautiful human being," said Bill, the salesman. "I'm taking care of him. He's not draining society." Yet Bill implies that the fact that his brother does not "drain" societal resources may affect this determination, suggesting that if his brother did use such resources, the moral equation might then shift in favor of abortion.

Even if pro-choice, some feel they would not undergo amniocentesis and abortion, due to wariness of eugenics. Many oppose the possibility of so-called designer babies, arguing that rejection of potential infants on genetic grounds violates something sacred. A sense of responsibility to the optimal health of one's future children can also clash with broader moral qualms about the specter of eugenics, which may reflect responsibility to broader social equality. In deciding to have a child, many feel that a parent must be willing to accept the child no matter what. Childbirth should not be akin to ordering and returning commercial goods. As Bill added:

I disagree with: "Oh, this person's going to have leukemia. Throw him out." You were willing to take that risk by having a baby. You could die having a baby. If that baby is sick, you have it. That's the decision you have to make up front. It's not like ordering a meal: if you don't like it, send it back to the kitchen. It's not like buying a pair of pants: send it back and get something else. You have to accept what's given to you, and make the best of it.

People can thus differ widely in perceiving responsibilities toward others—as mandating termination versus protection of a pregnancy.

In considering abortion, many of these individuals tend to draw on visceral moral feelings more than principles. They do not follow rigid dictates but consider the specific circumstances, implicitly or explicitly weighing various competing factors. Bill added,

Abortion for HD just doesn't sit right with me. Not because the Church says abortion is wrong. It's just not right. I'm not against abortion.

A woman has a choice. But the choice is made based on her ability to provide for the child.

Opposition to abortion arises, too, due to the argument that one could potentially have been aborted oneself. "Just because I'm at risk for HD doesn't mean I shouldn't have been born," said Evelyn, untested and asymptomatic. "What if my parents had detected it before they had kids?"

At-risk individuals justify decisions to have children who might have a mutation, responding to possible objections of not acting dutifully toward others. Despite being at risk of HD, they argued, one can still have a good life. "I've had a great life and wouldn't change anything," Jim, the physician with HD, added. "Even with HD. I don't regret being alive."

Others disagree, and believe in eliminating a serious mutation through abortion, though they have difficulty reconciling this stance with the fact that, following this logic, they themselves would not have been born. They cannot always reconcile these two opposing viewpoints. Jennifer, the 65-year-old schoolteacher who learned she had Alpha after her son was tested, said,

> People shouldn't have kids unless there's a cure for Alpha. They could just test the fetus, and if it is positive, abort. Would people actually do that? I would, because for years I worked with handicapped kids. Someone could say that *I* would have aborted. How do I put those two together? I don't. There is no right answer. It doesn't make sense.

Of note, she does not appear aware of PGD as an option.

Principles of autonomy (the right to make one's own reproductive choices) can also conflict with notions of beneficence (responsibility toward others). Many people distinguish between their own reluctance to undergo an abortion and a legal prohibition against anyone being able to do so. These individuals would choose not to have an abortion themselves, but think that others should be allowed to make their own choices, except for purposes of eugenics. This opposition to abortion often clashes with a pro-choice stance otherwise.

The possibility of amniocentesis followed by abortion arises for breast cancer as well, but is generally viewed less favorably, than for HD in part because the mutation is less penetrant and the disease far more treatable. Yet here, too, moral or religious objections could preclude abortion and thus amniocentesis. As a staunch Catholic, Beatrice, the Latina math teacher with breast cancer but no mutation, opposes abortion. When she had her two children, she even refused amniocentesis, though at the times of these pregnancies she was 36 and 38 years old—ages at which amniocentesis for Down's syndrome may have been warranted.

Both times, I declined amniocentesis because I would not have acted on it. I do not believe in abortion. The second time freaked me out more than the first — thinking I got away with it once. My Ob/Gyn said, "Being 38, you're at a higher risk. But if you're not going to act on that information, don't have it."

She weighed the risks, but followed her moral beliefs, though anxious about the outcome.

Others remain unsure of what they would do if faced with this dilemma. Not everyone who would undergo amniocentesis assumes they would abort a fetus if it had a mutation. Presumably, physicians only recommend amniocentesis or CVS if a patient is willing to have an abortion. Yet at-risk individuals ponder and wrestle with hypothetical questions of whether, if pregnant, they would undergo amniocentesis and, depending on the result, abortion. People also recognize that over time their views might change. Chloe, the asymptomatic and untested 28-year-old secretary, who fears she is turning into her HD-affected father, said,

I think when I get pregnant, I'm going to test the fetus. *I would just feel better if I knew.* So our child, if he showed symptoms, wouldn't have to think he was crazy, because we would know. But I don't know if I would want to get an abortion. I don't know if I'll be able to do it.

Yet a child could be tested after, rather than before birth. She remains conflicted, in part because she does not know her mutation status. She wants amniocentesis because of her desires for information, but has moral concerns.

I'm pro-choice, but don't know how I'd deal with it. Why would God give me a baby that had HD? Am I supposed to just abort it? At the same time, the only way we can stop the disease is not to pass it along.

She remains undecided as to how she would resolve this dilemma, balancing innate desire for knowledge and feelings that the knowledge could help her child against public health concerns that reflect broad social responsibilities toward others.

A few individuals would want amniocentesis not in order to abort the fetus, but only to prepare themselves psychologically for the child's problems. Clinicians appeared to oppose use of the procedure for this reason, but patients at times remained undeterred.

Knowledge, even if murky, is presumed to confer power. As mentioned earlier, marketers of genetic tests may take advantage of this widely held assumption. Such testing is presumed to have benefits that it may not have. Through the course of evolution the quest for knowledge has offered selective advantages—but can now clearly pose disadvantages, too.

PGD

Given the moral difficulties posed by amnio followed by abortion, many consider PGD. Several interviewees screened embryos in this way—or knew those who had—and saw the procedure as advantageous. Others pondered it, or said they would potentially do so. Roger, tested for HD after having problems driving, said that his sister underwent nondisclosing PGD.

> They take out and test 10 of her eggs, and find eight that don't have the disease, in case she has it. But if she has it, they don't tell her. Then they put the eggs back in, and don't tell her if she has it or not. So she knows her kids don't have it now, which is great.

The advantages of this procedure are clear: allowing couples to have children without the HD mutation, and without informing a parent if he or she has it.

Many individuals oppose abortion of a fetus because of a mutation, but would support PGD since it involves embryos before implantation. "I'm definitely pro-choice," said John, who dropped out of graduate school and lacks the HD mutation. "But I *personally* would have trouble with abortion for HD. It would feel immoral. But with IVF, there is none of that." He is pro-choice for others, but feels that to abort a fetus himself is wrong. Hence, as an alternative, PGD proves appealing. Not surprisingly, several people would consider PGD if they knew they were mutation-positive.

With Alpha, too, a few would use PGD. Yvonne, who had lung transplants and now wants to move south, feels that individuals should have the right to undergo PGD and abort a fetus because of this disease. She and others feel that PGD can ultimately help eradicate the illness. "They should get rid of this disease so no one ever has it again," she said. Her own experiences as a caregiver for her severely ill grandmother helped mold her perspective.

Several African American women support the use of PGD for sickle-cell disease as well. Francine, for example, who saw breast cancer in her mother and has HIV, supported PGD to eliminate the disease: "They should be allowed to say: we want the egg that doesn't have it."

For breast cancer, too, several women would opt for PGD. Still, individuals drew careful moral distinctions: supporting PGD for diseases, but not for nonhealth preferences such as gender. Vera, the Asian executive with breast cancer and the mutation, said,

> I would have my own embryos tested, but wouldn't pick the sex. You shouldn't be able to choose the sex. That sounds like so Nazi, so "concentration camp." Then, you start discriminating against people who are mentally ill. I would have embryos tested just to make sure they're healthy.

Many recognize the moral dilemmas involved, but feel that for medical problems the benefits of PGD outweigh these concerns. Still, logical paradoxes exist if one has the disease for which one would thus reject an embryo.

Given potential misuses of PGD that might border on eugenics, some try to differentiate further among disorders, but doing so is not always easy. Dorothy, the former TV producer on oxygen, sees PGD for Alpha as more subject to a patient's discretion. "We should screen out things that cut your life short," she said. "It's a personal choice, but I wouldn't wish Alpha on my worst enemy. You can't lead a full, normal life."

Given these competing moral, social, and psychological issues, others remain conflicted. As a lesbian lawyer, Karen is deeply concerned about discrimination and struggles with several competing issues regarding PGD for breast cancer.

> All kids are going to have genetic frailties that interfere with the so-called perfect life — whatever that is. So the intellectual part of me says, "There's no way I would test them when it doesn't matter." Who knows what treatment is going to be available in 15, 20, or 40 years? Then, part of me projects into being a parent, with a daughter who would get breast cancer, and I think, "How could I do this to her?" She's going to be treated as being at higher risk for cancer. She'll probably have an earlier baseline mammogram, and would need to be more careful, and aware at an earlier age than most of her peers.

Karen is thus torn.

Others remain more wary, not seeing PGD as a panacea or even a realistic possibility for them due to moral qualms as well as economic, psychological, and physical costs, particularly if more than one IVF cycle is needed. As John, himself without the HD mutation, said,

> I have seen just how tough the in vitro process is — physically and psychologically—all the hormones you take . . .My sister's boss tried three times and failed. My sister has witnessed very close-up how emotionally draining that can be.

The financial costs of PGD can be prohibitive, since insurance usually does not cover it. Patients, once they are aware of their genetic risk, may also be too old to realistically consider the procedure. Benjamin, the engineer with two children, said about a woman who wanted PGD for Alpha:

The insurance would not cover it. She was upset: $300,000 for a liver transplant, and $50,000 for IVF and screening. It's available, but I don't see it used too much. Most people who are sick are also not in the childbearing years.

High costs of PGD can combine with moral scruples to help make childbirth seem as if it is not meant to be. This sense of destiny and cosmic fairness in the universe suggests how metaphysical beliefs may lurk beneath these decisions. Laura, the graphic designer and environmentalist with no breast cancer but a strong family history and a mutation, said,

If no cost was involved, I still would not screen to make sure the breast cancer gene is not passed, partly because it seems *unnatural*. Even if I had that much money, I would have a problem with IVF. I don't judge anybody who's done it. But it's forcing something that wasn't meant to be. Children already out there need a home. If you have to try *that* hard to have your own offspring, maybe it's a sign that it's better to adopt. It's not that I believe in destiny. But if you have to try too hard, you can jinx it.

She sees the "natural" as morally and medically better. If she had had the disease herself, perhaps she may have sought to prevent its spread—though that is not wholly clear.

For breast cancer, some are wary of PGD, too, because of the chance that endocrine treatments involved in IVF might increase risks of disease. "The hormones may put you at higher risk for developing new cancer," Rhonda, the 31-year-old nurse with breast cancer and the mutation, warned. "They tell you to wait five years after you're diagnosed to begin IVF."

Many women who already had children would not want either to risk doing so again, or to have to consider PGD. Rhonda has met many fellow patients who were glad to have had a child, but who did not want to chance having another: "Knowing they're *BRCA1*, or have had cancer, women say, 'I'm lucky to have had one. I don't think I'd risk passing it on now.'"

Still, despite the limitations, PGD can reduce anxieties—even if the technological details are not fully understood and instill moral concerns. As Simone, the 29-year-old bookkeeper, said, "it is all like *Star Wars* to us. But . . . the peace of mind is huge."

Yet while some people are aware of PGD from film and articles in the media, not everyone knows of its existence. Many, particularly those at risk of diseases other than HD, are less cognizant of it. In response to a question about PGD, Laura, the graphic designer with a breast cancer mutation, asked me more about it.

Of note, people confronting the diseases here all supported the notion of PGD, but only those confronting HD had known of anyone who had in fact undergone the procedure for their disease.

NO CHILDREN

Given these complex moral quandaries, some are grateful, in retrospect, not to have had children. Yvonne, who underwent lung transplants, said,

> I thank God all the time that I never had any kids. If I had kids, they'd most likely have this disease. I see people in my support group: the husband and two or three of their children have it. They already know the children are going to go through it.

ABSTINENCE FROM REPRODUCTION OR MARRIAGE

As we saw earlier, in discussing dating, the fact that marriage is linked to having children may contribute to some individuals with the HD mutation eschewing serious relationships altogether in order to avoid having children or confronting these reproductive choices. They feel they should not burden a spouse with potential limitations in abilities to have or raise offspring. As a result, some individuals with the mutation refrain from long-term commitments. Genetic risks of other diseases can also lead to avoidance of marriage and children. As Gilbert, the electronics factory worker with Alpha who had his children tested, confessed,

> Had I known my wife's history when I was dating her in college, I might not have gotten myself in as deep. Her father had manic depression. Her older sister committed suicide, and another one was hospitalized. My older son got my wife's family genes. My younger son got *my* family genes, which were fortunately free of those problems. Everyone has something genetic. But you assess *how dangerous* you think it may be, what percentage chance your children will be afflicted. If somebody knows that I've got Alpha, and that having children is going to result in a carrier, they have to assess that—what the disease is likely to do over time, whether they want to be involved in that. There is no cure for Alpha-1.

Similarly, he would not have married a fellow Alpha carrier.

ROLES OF OTHERS

As suggested earlier, patients feel moral responsibility to a range of other people, and these obligations and inputs can collide. For instance, a spouse's preference can conflict with an individual's own sense of the best interests of a future child. Preferences of other family members (e.g., a sibling) or input from a physician (that a cure might be developed) can counter a spouse's views. As we will see below, the outcome may depend on the nature and strength of each factor.

Members of a couple can disagree about these issues, clashing in their sense of responsibilities toward future generations and others. For instance, members of a couple can disagree about undergoing genetic testing before having a child. Evelyn, asymptomatic for HD, whose spouse opposed her testing, said,

> I went back and forth with my husband. I kept telling myself: "I can't have another baby." We both wanted another child. But he said: we will not have another baby *if* you're going to get tested first.

Her husband's refusal to permit her to undergo genetic testing suggests the degree to which a couple can quarrel about these issues. Spouses can view these issues very differently from each other.

In a couple, power relationships may operate such that one member may overrule the other, who in turn may be forced to yield, or consider responding surreptitiously. Evelyn said about her husband's desire to have another child without her testing:

> He was so adamant! I was going to have myself tested, and if I came out positive, I was just going to say: No, we're not having another one. I don't know if I was going to admit I had the test. I never told my husband this, but I called [my OB]: "Can I come in for a blood test?"

While she felt compunctions about potentially passing on the mutation, he did not. Unable to reach consensus, she explored testing clandestinely.

At-risk individuals may believe that scientists will eventually develop treatment. As Evelyn said, "They swear that my children are not going to have to worry about it—that there's going to be a cure." Providers may not actually make such explicit assertions, but express optimism about the prospect of future treatment that individuals may then misinterpret.

Disagreements in a couple may reflect differences in not only desires for other children, but views of fate, morality, and the cosmos. Linda, the art teacher who abhorred the "HD nightmare" and tested mutation-negative, said that her husband wanted to risk having another child and felt they should not be too concerned about potential moral qualms.

> While I was getting the testing, he was still saying he would be willing to have another baby without me going through with it. He thinks . . . you have to run a little rough shod over those kinds of things.

Doctors could impact these reproductive decisions in several additional ways as well, and could disagree with patients' decisions. Linda said about her having a child before having tested for HD,

> There was that awful moment when the doctor put two and two together: that we had had our son without having that test. I saw the look on her face. In a flash, I felt the full weight of her judgment: That I had done such a thing. That was excruciating.

In part, Linda felt rebuked because of her low self-esteem, and feelings of having deserved HD. Such perceived criticism engenders anger and, possibly, future secrecy. "Finally, I didn't tell doctors the truth," she added. "I wised up."

For breast cancer as well, because of increased rates of recurrence, providers may implicitly or explicitly oppose desires to have children. Carol, who disregarded her boyfriend's opposition to prophylactic surgery, said,

> I would have loved to have had children, but it just wasn't going to work for me. I was diagnosed at 30. The doctor said, because I had breast cancer, "You shouldn't get pregnant." Four years after the chemo, I actually did get pregnant. My doctor freaked that it would bring back the breast cancer. I had an abortion because everyone said I shouldn't have a baby. There went my only chance.

She understood the doctor's logic, but remained rueful and frustrated, given her strong desire for a child.

GUILT AND BLAME

Stresses arise concerning not only *future* reproductive decisions, but *past* ones as well. However, since what has already happened is too late to change, parents can end up feeling guilt and blame. As suggested earlier with regard to views of disease causality, occasionally, affected offspring do indeed blame their parents. Bonnie's sister, who has breast cancer, faults their mother for the disease. As Bonnie explained:

> They have a very complex relationship. "If Daddy didn't marry Mommy, I wouldn't have to deal with this." I don't feel that way. If Dad didn't marry Mom, we wouldn't be who we are. She thinks it's solely genetic: that because my mom had cancer, my sister will. I don't agree.

Bonnie's sister needs to assign blame far more than does Bonnie, who has been disease-free. Causal understandings of a disease can thus also shape emotional responses to it, such as regret and culpability.

Parents may indeed feel very badly about having passed on a mutation. Chloe, the 28-year-old secretary who feared she was turning into her father, said,

> My sister has three boys, and got HD, but says that if she knew then what she knows now, she would have gotten the test, and had an abortion . . . She feels *guilty* — like she passed it on to one of the boys. But there's nothing she can do.

Those who have had children without testing may later feel regret about having done so, even though their children remain of unknown genetic status. Linda feels this way because she had a child before learning that she lacked the HD mutation.

> I could not believe that I put my little boy at such a risk. I wanted to have another baby, and knew I could never ever do that again in the same way I had. It seems like the most irresponsible thing. At this point, since I had a child, I was determined to make sure I dotted every "i," crossed every "t," to make sure he was taken care of. I was no longer going to play so fast and loose. It was fine to do it with myself, but suddenly to have done it with him was *unacceptable*.

Yet outsiders, including members of the same family, may feel that such guilt is unwarranted, since the parents did not know of the danger.

Regrets may be stronger for HD, given its higher penetrance and lack of treatment, than for breast cancer or Alpha. Yet regret may nonetheless arise for these other diseases, too, in part because of the threat of a parent's relatively earlier death. As Isabelle, the social worker with breast cancer and the mutation but no family history, said,

> When I had cancer, it was the first time in my life that I said, "I wish I didn't have kids." Now, I don't feel that way. But when I was in the throes of having cancer and not knowing, "Am I going to be fine?", it was very scary . . .I thought, if I didn't have kids, this would be a whole different experience.

The fear of possible guilt in the future *if* they had kids led some to avoid having children at all.

The guilt of having unwittingly transmitted the disease to one's offspring can be overwhelming. Simone, the 29-year-old bookkeeper, said about her father, "When they told him HD was genetic, he couldn't live with that. He lost all interest in living."

Questions arise of whether one *should* feel guilt about passing the mutation on to one's children. As we saw earlier, regarding blame, such guilt can persist even when it is seen as irrational.

Yet others feel that such genetic transmission is not culpable, since the tests are still new, and have only recently become available. Gilbert, the factory worker who might not have married his wife if he had known her family's psychiatric history, nonetheless said about Alpha,

> I don't fault anybody for this. My parents couldn't have known, because they didn't discover it until '63. So they didn't have any informed basis on which to decide whether they should have children. So, I don't wish that my father or mother had married somebody else.

The absence of knowledge confers innocence: he might have avoided marriage if he had known, but would not blame parents who had unwittingly passed on the disease.

Still, uncertainty hovers as to how future generations would view present decisions—the fact that tests now exist, but might not be used. Potentially in the future, children could blame parents for not having prevented transmission of a mutation—which further deters some interviewees from having children.

To blame parents was felt to be absurd, since disease is inevitable and parents transmit many genes—good *and* bad. Chloe, the 28-year-old secretary without HD symptoms or testing who feared she was becoming like her father, felt that he had nonetheless given her "a lot of other good stuff . . . Even though my life's been a little rough, I still like my life—who I am."

In addition, some avoid blaming parents because the latter experienced their own struggles and difficulties, and blame would thus be unfair. Perhaps disease transmission could have been prevented, but these parents faced other exonerating problems. Carol, with breast cancer and a mutation, was not angry with her mother or grandmother for transmitting their mutation because "they had really horrible lives."

Others do not, in the end, fault parents, but the lack of a scapegoat can make a disease with strong genetic components harder to deal with. As Gilbert added about his Alpha,

> I don't blame my parents, but find this disease much more difficult to live with than something I caused myself. I would much rather have something that was my fault—because I'm willing to take the consequences of my actions. This is not my fault.

RELIGIOUS AND POLITICAL ISSUES

These dilemmas clearly relate to much broader religious and political views as well. Facing the terrible potential costs of these gambles, some seek spiritual consultation. Several simply decided that whether or not they got pregnant and had a child was God's will—not theirs. Chloe said,

> I don't think God gives you anything you can't handle. That's why I don't know if I could deal with an abortion—because why would He give me a baby that has HD if I can't handle it? It's just too much to think about.

Given the complexity of these issues, the feeling that what happens is "all in God's hands" can offer sustenance. In part, for God to give Chloe a problem she could not handle would suggest that she was being punished—an idea that was anathema to her.

One's own moral intuition can also mutually support or compete with one's larger political beliefs. A sense of broader social responsibility can lead one to oppose having a mutation-positive child because of the eventual costs to society. "It seems unfair to ask people to forgo childbearing," said Karl, who lacked the mutation. "But at the same time, you're burdening society with people who are going to get sick." Still, these men and women, despite or because of their varied and often confusing experiences, generally feel ill-equipped to comment adequately on these larger political issues. Karl concluded that those questions were "a little too big."

CONCLUSIONS

These individuals face a range of reproductive dilemmas, balancing personal and moral factors. They confront quandaries of whether to get pregnant and deliver, have fetal testing and abort if the fetus is positive, screen embryos, adopt, or have no children. In confronting these decisions they weigh numerous colliding desires and concerns. A sense of responsibility can embody conflicting notions that have to be weighed against both each other and additional competing factors, posing one's own needs and desires against those of spouses and larger moral concerns. Broader ethical issues and perceptions of the best interests of current or future offspring can clash. Thus, quandaries arise of *how much* and *to whom* to feel responsible, and whether one should end the spread of the disease or follow particular religious or moral dictates (e.g., about abortion). A schematic "model of responsibility" has been suggested in which, in part, one establishes oneself as a "responsible decision-maker."[20] Yet the men and women here highlight complex tensions that can be involved. Moral decisions are frequently disputed and murky. The perceptions of others may conflict with an individual's own moral views.

Not surprisingly, over time, with each pregnancy, some individuals were uncertain or changed their perspectives—they may have taken a gamble with a first pregnancy, but subsequently became more cautious, using PGD or avoiding additional pregnancies altogether. Family members also frequently voice preferences and pressure individuals about these choices. Though the interviewees here are mostly pro-choice, many say they would not undergo abortions themselves, and have qualms about aborting a fetus because of a mutation. Thus, varying notions of social and moral responsibility lead to different pro-choice stances that are not always unequivocally pro-choice but depend on the specific situations involved. Many interviewees here are *pro-choice but anti-eugenics*, suggesting that social concerns about eugenics could outweigh feelings about autonomy and individual rights. Indeed, women undergoing abortions have been found to experience complex emotions related to socioeconomic status, self-efficacy, guilt, blame, and beliefs about the fetus.[23]

Individuals weigh pros and cons concerning their decisions, but moral values about eugenics and current and future children also influence these choices. While rational decision models have been put forth, the individuals here highlight key emotional, moral, unconscious, and imagined factors as well. A range of other social and psychological factors also affect whether these interviewees either seek or eschew information about their future children. A person's earlier reproductive decisions may affect later ones, but sexual behavior is not always planned and reproductive decisions are generally dyadic, not unilateral. These men and women thus underscore the limitations of theoretical models in this area, and the need for developing appropriately nuanced understandings of these complex, multifaceted issues.

Decisions about conflicting ethical dilemmas are rarely a simple choice between good and evil, but more often involve weighing competing ethical goods.[24] People have to balance responsibilities toward others against their own needs. The men and women here frequently have difficulty knowing *how* to resolve these conundra. Given the complexities of these issues, these choices may not always be consciously determined. Rather, some pregnancies occurred without planning, or before genetic risks were fully known or acknowledged. Unconscious psychological defenses such as denial can affect these outcomes. When couples disagree decisions may be deferred, one party may prevail, or a compromise may be reached. Notions of responsibility toward others are in part *subjective,* involving interpretations and applications of moral principles that can vary. Thus, though individuals may present themselves as acting responsibly,[20] more complex and nuanced questions emerge here as well.

Several specific issues arise concerning PGD—the use of which appears limited by cost, and knowledge of its existence. The fact that not all at-risk individuals know about this procedure highlights the need for more education about it. Yet understanding such reproductive technologies can be difficult. PGD also remains controversial, and along with the use of other reproductive technologies—abortion and stem cell research, for example—has fueled intense political debate due to fears, religious beliefs, and moral objections. PGD has been outlawed or strictly regulated in several European countries,[25] and is debated in the United States.[26] If use of PGD increases in the future, concerns arise that norms may change to the extent that its use may become expected. Some parents wonder if they will be blamed for not using this procedure and then having mutation-positive children. Individuals born with mutations for particular diseases may therefore encounter increased stigma.

In upcoming years, as more tests become available, patterns of and reasons for abortions may also change. Among multiple reasons for seeking abortion, women commonly mention wanting to postpone or stop childbearing, and socioeconomic factors. Only 13% of women in the United States in 1987, and 7% in Australia in 1992 cited the possibility of a fetal defect.[27,28] Yet with the spread of genetic testing, that proportion may increase.

Awareness needs to increase of how reproductive decisions are made within the complex dynamics of couples. Most doctors would like to be involved in post-test counseling and support,[29] but may not have the training or expertise to do so. Providers need to be able to raise and address these topics with patients and couples as part of medical care, and learn how to do so. Currently, doctors may work closely with only the one at-risk individual, yet spouses may disagree about these reproductive choices, posing dilemmas of how providers should address and mediate spousal conflicts. If a husband insists that an at-risk spouse *not* get assayed before becoming pregnant, should providers intervene and support the at-risk individual's insistence on getting tested? If the disagreement persists, does the woman or the at-risk individual have more decision-making power, or should the decision be entirely mutual within the couple? Though the principle of autonomy can dictate that these choices be left wholly up to the individual, questions arise of whether providers have—or feel they have—ethical obligations in these decision-making processes, and if so, what. Dilemmas emerge of whether, when, how, and to what degree clinicians should inform at-risk individuals or encourage them to consider these various reproductive options. Arguably, genetic counselors and other providers should ensure that at-risk individuals are as aware as possible of the existence and availability of PGD.

More psychosocial services may help at-risk individuals confront these quandaries. The fact that these dilemmas can hamper at-risk individuals in entering or maintaining committed relationships further underscores the need for psychotherapeutic services to help in confronting these issues. Indeed, couples therapy may be helpful in decisions about not only genetic testing,[30] but reproduction as well. Providers may focus on whether to undergo genetic testing—not how to make reproductive decisions. The Huntington's Disease Society of America advocates a team approach, but it is not clear how these issues in fact get addressed: by whom, when, how well, and to what degree.

The fact that those with genetic disease may face obstacles in being able to adopt children poses important policy concerns. The 1994 Federal Uniform Adoption Act provided some general guiding principles,[31] but gray areas exist in how agencies evaluate the physical and mental health of prospective parents. Anecdotally, at least some adoption agency application forms inquire about genetic disease in the family.

As whole genome testing becomes more prevalent, infertile individuals, without known genetic risks, who seek IVF, may be offered PGD as well. More genetic tests will surely become available—including those for incompletely penetrant diseases and genetic modifiers (which are normal variants but might influence treatment response or disease progress). Hence, these issues are becoming increasingly important, and these men and women underscore challenges that increasing numbers of others will no doubt one day face as well.

CHAPTER 9

"There's Only Privacy If You Make It":

Problems with Privacy and Insurance

"I lied to my doctor," John, who dropped out of graduate school when learning about HD in his family, told me. "I said that I hadn't seen a doctor in so long, I couldn't remember his name, and didn't know where this new doctor was going to be able to get my old records. I was trying to kill the paper trail that stated that I was at risk for HD."

But, I wondered, what if his old record contained information that a new physician would find valuable in John's care?

These men and women face dilemmas concerning not only which medical procedures to pursue, but how to pay for them, and specifically whether to use insurance—thereby divulging their genetic risk to others. Genetic information can prompt treatment, but also discrimination. These individuals struggle to pursue medical help while avoiding stigma. But these dual goals often prove hard to achieve. Patients with other medical problems face these frustrations, too, but genetic tests pose added challenges—since one may lack symptoms, and information about one's own genetic risk also implicates one's family, potentially revealing information about *their* chance of disease as well.

Awareness of one's own genetic risk also forces one to confront larger political and economic issues about health care financing and delivery. While in the United States concerns about health insurance discrimination loom large, in the United Kingdom, which has national health insurance, discrimination arises related to life insurance more than health insurance. There, banks maintain the right to obtain results of certain genetic tests in determining mortgages.

In May of 2008, the Genetic Information Non-Discrimination Act (GINA) became law in the United States, and some patients, family members, and even providers feel that potential problems have thus now been resolved. Yet debates continue as to how much actual genetic discrimination exists. Indeed, in April of 2010 a woman sued an employer, stating that she was fired as a result of her genetic background after she underwent prophylactic double mastectomies.[1]

Critics have asserted that complaints of discrimination have been exaggerated,[2,3,4] and based on subjective, anecdotal impressions, rather than objective facts. Some have insisted that objective data are needed to assess whether alleged instances of discrimination have indeed occurred, and if so, whether they have been legal or illegal.[5,6,7]

Given the need for data, the Australian Genetic Discrimination Project recently surveyed 951 genetic clients in that country. Of these, 10% reported discrimination, citing several domains: life insurance (42%), employment (5%), family (22%), social (11%), and health (20%).[8,9] Yet questions remain concerning the degrees and circumstances of such bias. Experiences may also differ between countries based on whether national health insurance exists (as in Australia and the United Kingdom) or not (as in the United States), and the nature and scope of implementation and enforcement of antidiscrimination legislation.

GINA intended to prevent genetic discrimination—generally defined as discrimination faced by an asymptomatic individual who has a genetic mutation. Bias faced by a symptomatic individual would presumably be based on a disability, and hence be covered, in the United States, by the Americans with Disabilities Act (ADA). GINA stipulates that employers and insurance companies cannot discriminate against individuals on the basis of potential genetic conditions, punishable with fines of up to $300,000.

Yet surprisingly, little data have been published concerning how patients who have or are at risk of genetic disorders actually view these issues, and when, how, and to what degree they have experienced discrimination.

These interviewees express many concerns about discrimination, which they see as taking a wide range of forms from explicit and overt, to implicit and subtle—and therefore being hard to prove. Laws may be limited in their protections and effectiveness. Several factors may be involved, including the visibility and disease-specificity of symptoms and the nature and age of employees, and these concerns can hinder testing, disclosure, treatment, and major career and life decisions. Many individuals are concerned that they may fall between the cracks; they are either uncovered by GINA or ADA or uncertain as to whether they are covered.

INSURANCE CONCERNS

For patients with other diseases as well, insurance can be precarious. But genetic information may provide a degree of knowledge about the future, heightening worries. Most Americans have limitations in their insurance that can severely restrict choices in choosing doctors, obtaining second opinions, having genetic testing, and accessing reproductive technologies. Insurance—for those lucky enough to have it—can be confusing. What services are covered, and to what degree, can be unclear. A patient may decide to use insurance depending in part on how much exactly it reimburses. When genetic risks are involved, these issues can become even more perplexing. "We weren't sure exactly what was covered where," Karen, the lawyer, said. "And if you test before you get sick, there can be problems."

Obstacles arise concerning not only health insurance, but life, disability, and long-term care insurance as well. Before Linda, the art teacher, learned that she lacked the HD mutation, she was anxious about coverage and felt she had to proceed as if she might indeed get the disease.

> With life insurance, if after two years you don't die, and they don't find anything bad, then the insurance remains. I think I found out that it was the same for long-term care insurance, but I wasn't sure. I hope the clauses in the long-term care insurance policy said that if they *did* take it away, I would get all my premiums refunded.

People grapple to understand the intricacies of each type of coverage. Disability insurance, for instance, can also be bewildering, and insurers may not provide full or accurate information. Jennifer, the schoolteacher with Alpha, said,

> The insurance representative should have told me that I could have kept Blue Cross, and Medicare could have been my *secondary* coverage. I didn't ask. I just assumed. I didn't research it sufficiently on my own.

As she suggests, even fairly well-educated patients struggle and have to teach themselves.

Insurance companies can also be vague. For instance, they may provide coverage for only limited periods of time. "My insurance says, 'We're taking you on for one year. Then, we will review,'" reported Diane, the Spanish teacher who had had an unanticipated mastectomy. "At least that's what I think I understood in that letter." She remains uncertain. Insurance can be fleeting and fluid; one can have it, but it can be taken away.

With HD, many feel that it is important to arrange for disability insurance coverage before undergoing testing. As suggested earlier, genetic counselors and patient advocacy groups often recommended doing so. "My father gets a pretty good chunk of money from his disability policy," Karl said, "because he had it in place beforehand."

Many worry that insurance company policies or laws can shift, or that one's own or one's spouse's job could change, jeopardizing coverage. "I don't know if my husband's going to change jobs, or not work, or if I have to go to work," said Rachel, whose family died in the Holocaust and who now has breast cancer and a mutation. "Everything could change."

Similarly, a patient or his or her spouse could be laid off, jeopardizing insurance. In the US, the continuation of insurance coverage mandated by the Consolidated Budget Reconciliation Act of 1985 (so-called COBRA insurance) lasts only 18 months. Companies can also change insurance companies, each of which can have different policies. Uncertainty hovers as well since current or past employers that had arranged for insurance can eventually become insolvent. Gilbert, the factory worker with Alpha, said that his company

> . . . declared bankruptcy. It's a virtual certainty that retirees will be losing their health care coverage. I may have eligibility for an 18-month COBRA extension. I don't know whether I can be turned down in this state or not, but I'd just as soon not even find out.

Many with insurance coverage worry about threats to it in the future due to government alterations in policies. Peter, the former businessman who now runs an Alpha support group, said,

> I'm now on Medicare, and my wife is a retired teacher, so we have the state health benefits plan, and a very high percentage of my costs, about $60,000 a year, are covered. But who knows what will be coming?

Patients fear that possible health care reforms can impose additional changes and restrictions. Insurance companies can also change their regulations and practices in the future or increase their rates, heightening apprehension.

Not surprisingly, these individuals tend to fear that the presence of a mutation could threaten insurance more than jobs. Rhonda, the nurse with breast cancer and the mutation, said, "I've never heard someone say, 'I tested positive and am worried about getting fired.' But I have heard concern about being able to maintain insurance, and switching jobs, because of insurance."

PROBLEMS WITH PRIVACY

Insurance companies induce anxiety about not only coverage, but threats to privacy as well. The possession by insurance companies of highly personal health information generates visceral discomfort. Many interviewees feel these corporations know more than they should. Bonnie, the saleswoman whose mother and sister had breast cancer, felt personally exposed—that her private information could be purloined.

> It's like a thief coming in your house, and looking through your underwear drawers. You don't know who it is, but you know someone's been there, and you feel violated, even if they're faceless. You go to a therapist to share something you can't share with the world. Some executive looking over your records is just not fair—even if you don't know who they are.

A few rare interviewees felt that privacy was adequately protected, and that concerns of violations of confidentiality were overblown. Individuals may have little concern since they have not seen or experienced discrimination or possible harms, and hence may not appreciate these potential dangers. These views vary in the degree to which they acknowledge the possible complexities involved. Benjamin, the engineer with Alpha, lost his job because his employer realized that Benjamin could go on disability. Nonetheless, Benjamin felt that privacy was well-protected, and that concerns can be exaggerated.

> We get a little overzealous. I don't see where it's of that much interest to anybody. People are afraid that if the Alpha registry is not protected properly, Mr. Evil can get in there. But what would anybody want to do with this information? I don't think insurance companies are going to go break laws to get it. I don't know too much about it, but the government is sure throwing up all sorts of regulations. You've got to go through all sorts of hoops. A lot of people believe we're not protected enough. I'm saying: there's got to be a happy medium. I don't know where.

Though he is wary of the need for regulations, he remains unsure. Some individuals thus have faith in confidentiality, though at times this trust may be naïve.

A company's large size can itself alleviate fears of such personal discrimination. Karen, the lawyer, feels confident that her employer is "such a huge bureaucracy that the information wouldn't go anywhere."

But most others are far more wary. Often, they do not know much about privacy laws that might protect them, but remain suspicious and cautious. As Laura, the graphic designer with no breast cancer but a mutation and family history, explained, "I'm worried, but don't feel I have much information. I don't even know how much I'm protected. Genetic counselors told me you can't be turned away." But the risks of losing insurance were too high for her—in part as a freelance artist—to feel wholly comfortable.

Others know of at least some of these laws—for example, the Health Insurance Portability and Accountability Act (HIPAA)—but remain wary of the ability of such legislation to safeguard confidentiality. Karen added,

I do not believe in the power of HIPPA to protect privacy. With HIV, I've seen confidentiality broken too many times. In theory, we have this patient protection law. But I'm not sure it's going to work.

She and others assume that information will leak: "You have to expect that your genetic results are going to be told to people whom you would not necessarily want to know."

Most patients are also wary because they have been regularly asked to sign away their rights to privacy in order to receive treatment. Many people just authorize such forms without reading them. Technically, patients have the right not to sign. But they generally feel that they have little choice. "On the one hand, you are told that you are entitled to privacy," said Diane, the teacher who had an unexpected mastectomy. "But instantly, everyone makes you sign all these release forms, so it's totally meaningless." Hence, in the end, options appear illusory. "If you refuse to sign, and want a job, you are free not to apply. That's your only choice." In part due to her surgery, she remained somewhat fatalistic about her options.

Refusal to authorize release of information could in itself raise suspicions. To decline to sign may suggest that one has something to hide. Faced with this double bind, some dissemble or lie.

Even with recent legal protections, ultimate privacy can thus remain elusive. A patient's medical information is not disseminated unless he or she gives permission. But if one does not agree, one will not have coverage. "If you want life insurance, you have to sign your life away," said Ginger, who as a medical secretary, is savvier than many. "I never knew a life insurance company that didn't ask you to give all your medical records."

Some had in fact seen violations of privacy occur, leading to discrimination. Ginger, for instance, had seen physicians provide information to insurance companies that should not have been sent. Due to such a lapse, her brother had been denied insurance.

People with Alpha should probably tell their family doctor, but then, life insurance companies can obtain those records. In the office, we often got forms in the mail from insurance companies, wanting information on patients. But some doctors I know just copy the whole chart, and mail it. One doctor did that to my brother. An older doctor in her seventies sent the whole chart. He was denied insurance. He blamed the internist. But it was the secretary, not the internist, who sent the records to the insurance company.

INSURANCE DISCRIMINATION: WARINESS OF PRIVACY LAWS

More overt forms of discrimination occur as well. Oliver, who decided to pursue a PhD after learning of his HD mutation, said that his sister was once refused one kind of insurance as a result of their family history: "The form asked, 'Do you or anyone in your family have one of these diseases?' It didn't ask which. She said yes, and was denied because of that." Such discrimination is particularly unwarranted since family history is, of course, no guarantee of having the disease. For breast cancer, a positive genetic test alone may never lead to symptoms.

Disagreement exists about the degree to which laws can ensure the protection of privacy and information. Numerous advocates hope that GINA will prevent such discrimination, but this law does not cover life, disability, or long-term care insurance. Many people remain wary. Laws may be inherently limited in practical scope or effectiveness, and such discrimination may inevitably result because of human nature—tendencies toward selfishness and greed. Joan, the psychiatrist whose daughter had breast cancer, was pessimistic because industry can profit from information and will thus continue to seek it.

> I'm basically fatalistic: You may prevent certain people from getting information, but drug companies and people who have something at stake financially are going to find ways to get what they want to know.

Laws may inevitably be limited, because human greed will invariably overcome patients' rights. Consequently, Peter, the retired businessman who now leads an Alpha support group, feels that legal efforts must continually be made to protect privacy "because mankind, for social and economic reasons, will discriminate—misuse their knowledge of someone else's condition."

Others worry about the possibility of future discrimination in as yet *unforeseen* ways. Discrimination due to illness may be illegal, but it does happen and can be hard to prove. Before he tested negative for HD, John felt such apprehension and dropped out of graduate school:

> I worried that if I were positive, a corporate chief who doesn't know me, just sitting in the back room crunching numbers, might be worried about the liability. A woman who is young and probably going to have kids isn't

discriminated against. But society knows: if you hire this person, you might be stuck with a huge maternity leave bill. That does influence people, even good people, indirectly. It would be illegal. But I'm sure a little bit of that goes on.

Privacy of genetic information is also important because it could affect one's children—though uncertainty enshrouds this possibility. As Rachel, whose family died in the Holocaust and who had breast cancer and the mutation, said, "This is going to follow my kids—any health insurance company will note a genetic disposition, and communicate about it in ways I'm not aware of. It's a big black hole to me." Confusion, ignorance, and doubt persist about current laws and their implementation.

Given economic pressures, some patients distrust not only insurance companies but also policy makers, economists, and providers. The high costs of treatment can determine what companies and the government do.

At Ginger's office, patients do not even own their medical records. As she explained, "Patients ask, 'Can't you just give me my records? They're my records?' 'No, the records belong to the corporation. The information is yours. But we have to copy it. We can't give away the originals.'"

Patients are keenly aware, too, of recent antiterrorism laws that can further erode privacy. Diane, the Spanish teacher, added, "Privacy is not sacred. It's being withdrawn." The degree to which privacy is an inalienable right is now increasingly contested.

Current privacy laws, especially HIPAA, can also be cumbersome and have unintended consequences, impeding the transmission of information between doctors. As Beatrice, the math teacher with breast cancer, commented,

A doctor calls for information, and has to jump through hoops. It's a good policy, but when my internist wanted my information, my [oncologist] knew he was my internist, not some random person. But I still had to get releases.

Problems thus arise in *how* physicians each carry out the policy in daily practice. Even people who support the policy at times feel frustrated.

Others think that HIPAA has important symbolic value, and hence some effect—sending the message that privacy is significant—even if not always adhered to. Karen, the lesbian attorney, said, "These laws need to be there. They help create a standard, even if not followed all the time. But it's unrealistic to think that a law is going to be followed, *just* because it's there."

Several factors can affect these attitudes. Personal experiences may be involved—the vulnerability of one's economic position and future. Persons who are younger, and middle or upper-middle class, may have more to lose, and thus be more concerned. "If I were trying to move up the corporate ladder, or were younger, I might feel differently," Beatrice, the 56-year-old math teacher with breast cancer, continued. "But given where I am, I just deal with it."

A few others are relatively less pessimistic because of professional or personal experiences. Based on his job as a policeman, Albert has faith in law enforcement. But he could afford to trust that his HD risk would not jeopardize his job, partly since he is a member of a strong labor union, and his supervisor is a friend. "I'm close with my boss, who actually hired me, so he knows," he explained. "He's a friend. You probably could get discriminated against, but I [am] in a little different position."

As suggested earlier, threats to confidentiality related to insurance companies occur against a backdrop of threats to privacy from other sources—the Internet and increasing electronic storage of financial and other records. Some believe that privacy simply no longer exists. Rachel, with breast cancer and a mutation, invoked Orwellian notions of *1984*: "We're living in a whole other world as far as privacy: The Internet and exchange of information, and the whole Big Brother theory, credit card fraud, people taking social security numbers . . ." For many, these threats blend together. Several think these threats are even worse than in Orwell's novel, since information now takes on a life of its own—known by not only government, but vast corporations as well.

Clearly, threats to privacy concern not only health but finances. Yet threats to financial privacy are ultimately more remediable than those to health. Usually, one can merely cancel a credit card, and get a new one. Violations of medical privacy are not always as readily and permanently reversed.

RESPONSES

Resignation

Many just accept these inherent limitations to privacy. They feel that their genetic risk forces them to sacrifice confidentiality. "There's only so much I can do," said Laura, a freelance graphic designer with no breast cancer but a family history and a mutation. "I can keep information about my genes private, but not if insurance is going to pay for treatment."

With Alpha, too, loss of privacy often seems inevitable, given the choices involved. "My medical supplies are delivered," said Betty, the designer who carries an oxygen concentrator. "Neighbors can potentially see these." The machine, too, reveals her status as a patient.

Against these larger social forces infringing on privacy, patients may feel powerless. As Ginger, the medical secretary, said,

> I once worked for a doctor who said, "Give me 24 hours and I can find out everything there is to know about you: your medical history, financial history, anything." I guess you have to accept it. What can you do? That's the way the world is.

These tensions have broader implications for ongoing policy. These individuals recognize inherent cost-benefit calculations involved in determining how much privacy is optimal, realistic, or desired. Ginger added, "I don't want people discriminating against my children, but you can't afford to increase insurance rates too much. People are going to have to give up some of their privacy and some of their rights in order to keep costs normal."

Others are willing to trade off privacy protection in return for advances in research. Scientific studies can endanger privacy, but they can also potentially yield vital benefits. "I don't care if anybody knows, if it's going to help someone," Mary, the housewife, said. "I trust people, because I'm at a really good place in my life. I'm very private, but research is important—finding a cure." In addition, she is unemployed, and hence in relatively less financial jeopardy since she cannot be fired.

Concerns about privacy could also potentially go too far, hindering treatment access. "My father is so anal about privacy, he won't get any help," Mary continued, "You really hurt yourself with all this privacy stuff."

Feeling Stuck

Worry about insurance and privacy can shape other life decisions about relationships and work. Laura decided to wed because of health coverage. "My health insurance would be more protected," she said. She has had no breast cancer, but a mutation and family history.

Alternatively, regulations and requirements can impede marriage. As Yvonne, who wants to move south, said about her Alpha,

> It's been rough on my boyfriend: Insurance issues have actually caused us *never* to get married. If I marry him, my insurance would cancel, or I would have to go on his. He's on disability also. If we get married, it cuts our disability insurance in half.

She feels that insurance prevents her, too, from being able to move out of state.

I can't move out of state, because my insurance is a [company in this state]. It doesn't go with you. They can't cut me off, but I can never move out of the city. I want to move to the South, because the winters are warm. . . But I'm stuck.

Patients may also stay in jobs they dislike because of anxieties about losing insurance if they switch. Fears of forfeiting disability or health insurance from a new employer impel some to feel trapped in positions they would otherwise leave. They may feel sick, but force themselves to keep working. "In the middle of chemo, I was feeling horrible," Joyce, the spa employee with breast cancer, but no mutation, said. "But I didn't want to lose my health insurance. So I stayed in the job, and pushed myself."

Striving to Maintain Privacy

Others try to protect their privacy proactively in varying ways. They are often unsure how worried to be about privacy threats, and range from unconcerned to feeling paranoid, uncertain whether they should or could do anything to limit this threat. In attempting to protect their confidentiality, they fall across a spectrum from more to less aggressive.

At one extreme, some at risk for HD or breast cancer decide not to use their insurance to pay for testing, not wanting to take the risk. Others seek to hide even their *risk* of a disease. Therefore, some restrict the information they not only provide, but obtain. For instance, in searching for online information, some do not use their name, and instead rely only on paper. Yet in so doing, they may avoid patient groups and services, thereby incurring potential personal costs.

Others visit disease websites but remain anonymous. As Benjamin, the engineer, said about the Alpha community, "One person wouldn't tell me their identity, but wanted to get the organization newsletter. I don't know how the organization found *me*, either." A few attempted to preserve their privacy by shredding all disease-related documents. But those who are overtly symptomatic or undergoing treatment for a disease may simply not have the luxury of protecting privacy to the same degree. Dorothy, who wheels an oxygen canister, said, "Privacy doesn't matter to me, because I have the disease. It's not going to go away." As we will see, others proceed very carefully at work, trying to avoid revelations about their risk.

Whether to Use Insurance

Given these threats, these individuals face a series of Catch-22 situations related to whether to use health or disability insurance. As suggested earlier, high costs can deter testing. Some individuals decline or defer a genetic assay since they would have to either use their insurance (and hence face possible discrimination), or pay out-of-pocket, which they cannot afford to do.

Patients may also face stark tradeoffs about seeking treatment. Insurance companies might pay for a procedure if it is medically indicated, but could then nonetheless discriminate—for example, raising premiums. At times, individuals are utterly unsure how an insurance company will respond if they have testing and then surgery. For those confronting breast cancer, discrimination might occur because statistically, the recurrence of a second cancer is higher. Bonnie, who has not had breast cancer or testing though her mother and sister had the disease, said:

> If I couldn't afford treatment, and had to release the information for the insurance company to pay, I would do it. It's twisting your arm, bullying. If they obtain information that one of their employees has cancer, they're going to raise the rates. They're punishing you for being sick.

Yet using health insurance could then affect whether, how much, and when one can obtain life and disability insurance. As Mildred, with breast cancer and the mutation, reported,

> I used to sell life insurance and disability insurance. Everything in your medical records is in some database. Life insurance companies say, "You have to sign a form to release information." So if I get tested only for disability insurance, I can get it, but if I become disabled because of ovarian disease, it would be excluded because I carry the breast cancer gene.

Individuals must also decide whether to apply for Social Security disability, and thus have information about their mutation further disseminated, potentially impeding their own or their offspring's future health or other insurance. Some feel they simply had to forego privacy to access disability benefits. Mary, the housewife with HD, said,

> That was a big decision: money or insurance. We didn't know which was going to outweigh the other. Once you tell Social Security, it's out there. There's no turning back. Are a few extra bucks worth jeopardizing my insurance? I don't know but I'm sure that somewhere down the line, I'm going to be screwed. The insurance company's probably not going to pay for something I'm going to need, because I'm going to have known about it, before I switched to them.

Not Telling Insurers

Many of these individuals confront quandaries of whether to disclose genetic information to insurers. Some would simply not tell insurance companies about genetic test results. Harriet, an African American schoolteacher with a family history of breast cancer but no symptoms and an indeterminate test result, is wary of discrimination and said she would feel justified in withholding all genetic information, because the insurance company would interfere with her doctors' decisions. "If the test was positive, I wouldn't tell the insurance company," she said, "because I don't want them making decisions about my health."

Several anticipate that they will simply leave questions blank on insurance forms, though this strategy might be impossible or backfire. Ron, the motorcyclist, said,

> For disability insurance, I could have passed the physical exam. But, if I do come down with HD, they're going to know that I knew about HD or had reason to believe, because my brother and father died of it.

Some feel that the major privacy concern they face is their children being denied health insurance in the future. As a result, these patients admonish their adult offspring to avoid volunteering any information unless absolutely necessary. Ginger said,

> Privacy is a concern not for me, but for my children. I told them, "When you apply for life insurance or a job, don't tell them anything that they don't ask about." No one's going to ask, "Do you carry the gene for breast cancer or Alpha?" I don't volunteer any information. If they say, "Do you have any diabetes in the family?" you have to tell the truth. If they ask, "Any breathing problems in your family?" tell them your mother has emphysema, but don't mention that it's genetic. You're not lying.

Many feel few qualms, since insurance companies compel patients to dissemble. "These companies put people in a bad position," Peter, the retired businessman who now leads an Alpha support group, added. "So, I say: tough on these companies, because *they* are the ones who have caused this problem."

Nonetheless, others do not feel that lying is a viable option. In fact, some who dissembled to insurance companies have been caught. Simone, the bookkeeper who only learned of HD when getting engaged, said,

> After my dad was diagnosed with HD, my mother tried to get life insurance. She paid into it for 10 years. When he died, she tried to collect. They

reneged, because she had known he had HD. They wouldn't pay out. They gave her back all the premiums she paid.

Hence, some patients advise at-risk individuals to test anonymously through a research study, and if one has the mutation, to buy insurance. Nevertheless, others defer from doing so. They fear trying to get insurance after testing—even in a study—because that would be dishonest and potentially punishable.

Because of these perceived needs for secrecy, Peter is not even sure whether his two daughters have been tested for Alpha, and if so, what the results are. "I think they got themselves tested, but it wasn't broadcast. Nothing said is better."

Still, within the complex dynamics of families, such preferences for ignorance may not be followed. Secondary disclosure may occur. Laura, the freelance graphic designer who has a breast cancer mutation and a family history, but no symptoms, said,

> I assumed that if my mom didn't tell me she was negative, she probably was positive. I didn't want to officially know, because if anyone asked me, I wanted to be honest and say I didn't know. I got mad at my sister because she told me. I said, "I didn't want to know!"

Lying to Doctors

Patients also face dilemmas of whether to divulge genetic risks or test results directly to medical providers, and if so, to whom, when, and what to disclose. Though many readily disclose, others are far more apprehensive and make difficult risk-benefit calculations.

Some will tell a doctor only if they judge the information to be directly relevant. For Alpha, for instance, Ginger averred that patients should not always give physicians information. "If you have no breathing or liver problems, I wouldn't mention it, unless your doctor says, 'Your liver enzymes are elevated.' Then," she said, "you almost have to, or they may not find out the truth.'

Individuals may not disclose to *all* their doctors, and instead assess *which* particular physicians to tell. Even patients with apparent symptoms might inform providers only partially. One criterion is the degree to which patients see disclosure to a specific doctor as possibly leading to insurance or employment discrimination. Some choose *which physicians* to tell based on insurance—for instance, not telling those who are covered by an employer's insurance company. Tim, as a lawyer, defended his decision to suppress information because of the risks involved.

I just don't think that it's really relevant, or that doctors need to know. They might tell the HMO or my employer, or the HMO might try to increase how much my employer pays for insurance. I don't like the risk.

Others must make more nuanced distinctions between their doctors, based, for example, on whether the physician seems trustworthy, and how he or she treats other family members. Evelyn, who consulted a psychic when her husband opposed HD testing, said, "I don't know if my family doctor knows. I told my pediatrician, because when you trust your kids to a doctor, you almost put their doctor above your own doctor."

Patients may tell only if they sense that clear benefits can be gained. But as a result, GPs may not be informed. However, assessments of these benefits versus these risks can be subjective, as patients try to gauge whether knowledge of a mutation will unduly bias physicians' assessments. In the process, rationalizations may arise. Simone, who only learned of HD in her family when getting engaged, said,

I don't tell anybody unless there is something that can be obtained or achieved. If our GP can't do anything, which we know he can't, why tell him? If I see him, and he doesn't know, he's going to treat me for whatever ailments I have. He won't start blaming everything on HD.

She continued her secrecy, though not to the degree that her mother had.

Some simply don't trust practitioners with the information. GPs may also be perceived as unreliable (e.g., because of not keeping track of all past medical details).

But patients' assessments of providers may not be entirely accurate, and bad medical practice can result. Physicians may work in the dark, unaware of a patient's actual diagnosis. Simone continued,

A gynecologist sent me to a specialist. I just said I had a physically handicapped brother and MS in my family. This went on almost a year, going to these different specialists, and *making up stories* about the family history. It wasn't until one of them suggested that I go to an HD specialist. I kept saying that I didn't know it was HD. I was trying to get them to suggest it, rather than me saying it. I was buying insurance, so really didn't want to know, until I had that sorted out. I never told my GP. I was afraid that he might write it down.

Excluding Genetic Information from the Medical Chart?

Patients wonder, too, whether to request that genetic information be excluded from their medical record. Such information can potentially help future physicians make decisions, but can also pose dangers. Others remain unsure of how to even broach the topic with physicians. On the one hand, some feel that the inclusion of genetic information in the medical chart is inevitable. "The genetic test has to be in my medical record," said Diane, the Spanish teacher with cancer but no mutation. She cannot conceive of an alternative, and feels that the data could be beneficial.

Yet genetic counselors and patient advocacy groups may encourage patients to request exclusion of such information. Still, to do that can be hard. Patients have to assess when to try to stop doctors from including it. Isabelle, the social worker with breast cancer and a mutation, said, "When they told me I had the gene, they said: make sure doctors don't put it in your record. In the beginning, I used to be on top of it: 'Oh, you're not writing it down . . .?' Since then, I don't." Even for her, as a social worker familiar with medical records, such protective efforts can take too much effort. Over time, individuals' concerns and gumption can also vary.

Health care professionals differ as well in their sensitivity and approaches concerning the storage of genetic information. Patients and their providers may agree or disagree on how the information should be handled. At times, physicians themselves may volunteer to exclude genetic information from a patient's medical file—without patients even asking. Karl said, "My doctor didn't put in my record that HD was in the family, at her suggestion. She volunteered to exclude it—I didn't ask."

For breast cancer, too, health care workers may simply leave genetic information off the record. Rhonda, the nurse with breast cancer and a mutation, reported, "The genetic counselor or oncologist said, 'Oh, that really shouldn't be in the chart, because you don't want to worry about insurance.'"

Alternately, physicians may obfuscate and hide genetic information. As Carol, with breast and ovarian cancer, explained, "It's cryptic on my chart that I'm *BRCA1* positive." Practitioners may use a broad generic term rather than a specific diagnostic label. Brian, whose wife pushed him to test for HD after a distant relative called him, and who now has symptoms and the mutation, said, "In his records, my doctor is not using the *word* 'Huntington's,' but a *generic term* that covers lots of things."

Some GPs keep genetic information *separately*, but such precautions are not always foolproof. Staff may not appreciate the potential problem, and patients may thus remain wary. Ron, with the HD mutation, said,

> A note is in my file on a loose piece of paper that the doctor can pull out if he has to send anything to insurance companies. He tells me that's what he does. But he sees 1,500 people. Is he going to remember? What if he is away, and his secretary sends it in, or he forgets? I don't have any great trust.

Physicians employed other strategies as well—for instance, giving test results to family members, but not to patients themselves. Jennifer, the schoolteacher with Alpha, said,

> One doctor I know tests people for Alpha for free, and doesn't write it down anywhere. He will never tell you the results, but will tell a family member, because employers may ask, "Have you ever been told you have a genetic disease?" You can then say no.

Patients often need to arrange and negotiate for such nondocumentation themselves, but these requests can be easy or hard, and be followed or rejected. Evelyn encountered little resistance: "I told the pediatrician, 'I need you to know something, but I don't want it in the chart.' He said, 'Absolutely. I'm glad you told me.'"

But this secrecy can prompt difficult or awkward situations. A physician may care for other family members, necessitating firewalls that may or may not be fully safe. Evelyn continued, "My doctor also treats my nieces and nephews. He assured me he's not writing it their charts, but knows they're at risk." Evelyn in fact mentioned her nieces' and nephews' risk to her children's pediatrician before her siblings agreed for her to do so.

But doctors may not all be as sensitive, or cooperative with patients' requests to separate genetic information from other medical records. Providers may simply refuse. Mildred, who used to sell insurance and now has breast cancer and a mutation, reported, "I asked my doctor not to put the genetic testing results in my file. She said, 'Why?' I said maybe I can't get a health insurance or something. She said, 'Well, that's not going to happen.'" Mildred did not feel able to push her point further. John, too, who dropped out of graduate school and later found he lacked the HD mutation, tried to push the same request, but to no avail.

> I had a fight with my primary care doctor. When I tried to get some insurance I said, "Don't tell them about HD." He gave me some legal jargon about, "Well, if they ask me, I'm legally obliged to." So I just stopped seeing him, and decided never to mention HD to a general practitioner again.

He changed providers, and lied about his prior physician to his next doctor.

To block transmission of already documented information can be virtually impossible. Once data has entered the medical records, it appears irremovable. Often, when patients inquired about deleting information from the chart, neither providers nor insurers knew how to respond. Rachel, with breast cancer and a mutation, tried to expurgate such information. Her hospital's patient services office was not helpful. But luckily, a specialized medical privacy officer eventually aided her. In the end, she proceeded even further, and attempted to "clean up" her records herself. She illustrates the need to enhance education about these issues among patients, providers, and others.

> I had my genetic testing done, and was advised by the counselors, "Tell doctors you talk to not to write this down, or put it in any medical records." My husband is an insurance investigator, so he knows that if you need copies of somebody's medical records, you get them. I had no problem insisting to my doctors that they not write it down—except for one doctor, about whom my oncologist said, "He's a little rough around the edges, but is a good doctor." In trying to get an appointment to see him, his staff didn't want to put me on his schedule until they knew the exact reason. I said, "Well, I don't want to tell you." So, I had my oncologist call him directly. I told her, "Just make sure you mention that he should not write this down." I went to see him, and said, "I have this particular mutation." He wrote everything down. I said, "Please don't write that down." He said, "You have complete control over what anybody sees in your medical records. All you have to do is exclude certain parts of what you give access to." I thought, "O.K., he's a doctor. He knows everything. Though this goes against everything I have been told, I guess I'll go along with it." When I walked in his office, I had not had enough time to sign in. The reception- ist had said, "When you come out, we'll do your paperwork." So, when I walked out, there was a sheet to give the doctor's office authorization to bill my insurance company. The last sheet is about privacy. I said, "Shit." Now, what am I supposed to say? ". . . Except that part that says *BRCA2* mutation"? My husband later said, "You shouldn't have signed it!" But could I have made the doctor stop writing? I don't think he understood the potential problem. Would a health insurance company raise my rates? Could it affect my children? I walked out, feeling like a fool: "Dammit. Now I've got a lot of work to do." I told patient services: I'd like that stricken from my records. Blacked out. She said, "Well, what do you want me to do?" I said, "I don't know, talk to the doctor." The representative said it really wasn't completely under her jurisdiction. She later said, "We have spoken to the doctor's office." I didn't feel very comforted. I called the privacy officer, whose name was on the back of the privacy sheet. He had me send a note to the doctor's office, saying, "Please strike these particular references in my record." Now, I have to ask for copies of my records, which is going to cost me money, to see how they photocopy it. It's caused me a lot of work. People were trying to help, but there wasn't a lot they could do.

Linda, the art teacher who eventually tested mutation-negative for HD, went even further, and actually stole part of her record.

My whole "at risk" status didn't really sink in until after my son was born, when I suddenly needed to get life, disability, and long term care insurance. Suddenly, I had a horrifying realization that I had just gone around spouting off the HD information to any doctor who would listen. When they had asked me about my parents, I told them. So I tried to clean up my paper trail. I had all the records sent to me from my primary care doctor. On every page was: "HD risk," "father had HD." It was my fault. I wasn't educated about it. No one sat me down and said, "You are allowed to lie to a doctor, to not tell the truth." I was determined to clean it up, and get insurance, no matter what. My doctor couldn't delete the records, but put a cover letter on the file—a big post-it to her staff— "Don't fax these to anyone, if anyone calls." We had a back-up plan, where she would write a letter stating my decent health to any insurance company that asked.

I also went to the birthing center where I had had my son. They wouldn't fax me the file because it was huge. They wanted me to pay for them to copy and send it to me. I said, "I'll come down and look at it." So I found myself sitting in a little cubbyhole with this huge fat file that said "HD risk" on every other page. My heart was pounding for 45 minutes, looking through it. Then I just decimated the file. I went through and took out every page that had HD on it. I tucked them in my pocket, and returned the file. I'm generally not such a thief. But they weren't my physicians anymore. I thought "What the hell? *This is mine!* It belongs to me. I'm the one who coughed it up." It would get in the way of me getting life insurance. After that, I left my primary care doctor, and saw a new doctor. I started a new file there.

But lying to doctors is hard to learn—going to these new doctors and not telling the truth. It gave me a sense that the universe was falling apart, and there was no stability. To have a nice gentle professional person who is supposed to take care of you, look you in the eye and ask you a very serious question about your health, and *you're not able to tell them the truth!* I felt there is no safety. I can't tell someone who is supposed to be looking after my body the truth about what might be going on with it. I don't like stealing, lying. But what is the most ethical thing to do? Make sure I get insurance for my kids! I felt exhilarated because I had done something proactive to take it back into my own hands, not just be terrified that information out there was going to screw my kid.

"There's only privacy," she concluded, "if you make it." But she also empha-sizes the need for providers to discuss these issues with patients in advance. She believes that the information belongs to her. But as Ginger pointed out earlier, it is not clear that this argument is in fact correct. Morally, the informa-tion is easily seen as hers; legally, however, the records may be said to belong to the clinic. Competing legal claims related to professional responsibility and accountability may undermine her moral intuitions.

In either case, even for Linda, it is hard to lie, since to do so erodes the trust and sanctity of the doctor-patient relationship. She added,

> A support group advised me that I could just play dumb. When doctors ask, "What did your father die of?" just say, "Oh, I don't know. Pneumonia? We weren't that close." I felt I was betraying my father. I knew what he died of. If you can't tell the doctor the truth about that, how are you supposed to trust them?

Importantly, insurance companies thus undermine doctor-patient relationships and trust.

Patients face quandaries of how far to go in trying to protect their privacy—whether to alter death certificates, too. She continued,

> Someone suggested I could have embarked on a long red-tape journey to change the death certificate. But at that point, I was just going to apply for the insurance, and hope they don't investigate. I had strung my emotional rope out for as long as it could go—six months. I couldn't go any further.

Such efforts require energy, while one simultaneously faces other testing and treatment decisions. The actual physical and psychological costs entailed could outweigh the risk of future discrimination.

CONCLUSIONS

The dual goals of obtaining health care and avoiding discrimination can clash. These men and women fear threats to both their insurance and privacy, and respond in varied ways, from resignation to refusing to reveal their genetic risks to insurers or physicians.

Discrimination can be indirect, implicit, and subtle, making it hard to prove, which in turn can have several critical implications. Many remain wary of laws meant to protect them. Fears of discrimination can impede not only genetic testing and research but disclosures, treatment, and major career and life decisions, causing stress that could potentially exacerbate illness. These fears can even trump desires for testing and treatment. Privacy concerns can hamper relationships with family, friends, and others. While some hoped for the development and implementation of stronger policies, others thought that they had to manage these issues on their own. They could not trust providers or policy makers—only themselves.

Yet wide and profound confusion about health insurance persists—for example, what insurance companies are required to offer. Misunderstandings, uncertainty, and fear regarding the law, exacerbated by mistrust of insurance companies, can trigger fears of possible discrimination that may or may not be realistic but nevertheless prevail, and potentially impede individuals in pursuing testing and treatment. Such wariness and unsurety can lead individuals to take unnecessary precautions that heighten stress.

Privacy may be more of a concern to those who feel they have more to lose, because of precarious insurance or jobs. Yet almost all here fear these possible dangers to some degree.

Many feel that no one has prepared them to handle these issues. Education on privacy has been suboptimal—but hopefully will increase.

These interviewees highlight, too, the critical need for laws to cover long-term care, life, and disability insurance. Policy makers may distinguish between discrimination faced by asymptomatic and symptomatic individuals, and define genetic discrimination as referring only to that faced by the former, but the individuals here suggest several complications. Importantly, these interviewees tend not to see this differentiation as distinctly or sharply. In part, these disorders have intermediate gray areas—possible (but not definitive) or nonspecific symptoms. For instance, those at risk for HD but untested may be difficult to get along with, which may, only in retrospect, be seen as an early, nonspecific symptom of the disease. Yet these interpersonal difficulties may nonetheless prompt discrimination.

Similarly, exposures to environmental irritants may precipitate symptoms in otherwise asymptomatic individuals at-risk for Alpha. Thus, the distinction between symptomatic and asymptomatic may not be wholly clear, and individuals may face discrimination due to symptoms that are not yet recognized as resulting from a genetic disorder. Moreover, symptomatic and asymptomatic individuals are frequently members of the same families and patient communities. Fear of discrimination against symptomatic individuals may heighten anxieties among their asymptomatic family members, affecting the latter's decisions. Fears also arise here among individuals who have not been to genetic counselors.

These results mirror efforts historically to eliminate other kinds of discrimination—for example, to address civil rights in the 1960s, and discrimination based on gender and sexual orientation. These prior endeavors illustrate how discrimination has not disappeared after any single piece of legislation but rather has required decades of battles regarding implementation, and additional laws to rectify problems and alter attitudes. In each of these past examples bias has nonetheless continued, despite initial legislation.

I conducted these interviews before GINA came into effect, and while that law represents an important advance, these data suggest several concerns. Subtle discrimination, for instance, may make it too early for patients to risk discrimination by disclosing fully and widely. To assess GINA's full eventual effects, benefits, and limitations is premature. But it is crucial that this legislation does not inadvertently promote a false sense of security. In upcoming years the amount of discrimination could potentially *increase* because of GINA, as patients may now feel it is safer to begin to disclose more. Employers may feel it is permissible to engage in more discrimination because it is not necessarily detected or detectable, and thereby punishable. Indeed, the fine for violation of GINA is only $300,000, which may cost some employers less than a patient's ongoing treatment. Therefore, some companies may feel that it is cheaper to discriminate and merely pay the fine if caught.

Just as the ADA has been found over the years to generate numerous ambiguities, GINA, too, will no doubt pose uncertainties that need to be closely monitored and addressed. Discrimination depends on the presence of unjust or prejudicial treatment. Yet definitions of justice and of being "pre-judged" vary widely,[10] and are inherently open to differing interpretations and individual perceptions.

These issues become increasingly important as genetic information expands and, despite its ambiguous meanings, is sought, and potentially used by insurers as bases for discrimination. Many of us may soon have to confront these concerns regarding ourselves, our family, or others we know.

PART V

Genes in the Wider World

CHAPTER 10

"Keep it in the Family?":

Other Disclosures Beyond Kin

"My genetics is private," Tim, the lawyer, said. "It's no one else's business, unless they're my family or very close friends." These men and women face conundra about disclosing in not only familial and medical contexts, but other social worlds—with bosses, coworkers, neighbors, and friends. In seeking to obtain social support, but elude discrimination, they confront quandaries about exactly *how private* to keep this information. Outside one's family, social and therefore moral bonds and obligations to divulge may decrease. In part, non-kin to whom a patient discloses are not ordinarily at risk themselves, and thus don't need to be warned. Medically, revelations here about genetics are not directly important. Rejection may also be more likely and costly. At the same time, norms about divulging illness in these settings are far fuzzier than in families.

These men and women inhabit multiple complex social worlds in which they have to decide whether, whom, what, when, and how to tell. People vary in the degrees to which they want to share intimate details of their lives and feel comfortable doing so, and welcome the support and advice that they may receive as a result. They tend to be more or less open as opposed to private. However, with potentially taboo or stigmatizing information, they may feel or fear rejection or discrimination. How then do they navigate between these goals?

While within families disclosures can inform members of their own risk and, depending on the disease, of possible screening, treatment, and reproductive options, outside of families disclosure has far different functions, benefits, and costs. In nonfamilial settings, some people may reveal their genetic risks because to do so could advance public education, or because the information is an important part of their identity. Yet other patients remain far more circumspect. In these situations, secrecy and divulgence concerning genetic risks is generally not an all-or-nothing proposition, but rather varied and nuanced. One may share certain information with some friends but not others.

Outside the family, social norms about sharing personal information may be more implicit, murky and unspoken. Quandaries thus arise of how exactly to decide what is "private" and what is not. Bill, the salesman who doesn't discuss HD with his siblings, described such unvoiced rules: "You know what's going on, but don't talk about it."

FROM CLOSE FRIENDS TO "GOING PUBLIC"

Patients face these questions in a wide range of relationships—from close friends to acquaintances to the broader public. Regarding revelations about genetic risks, these worlds vary widely in comfort, appropriateness, and acceptance.

Implicitly or explicitly, with different individuals patients range in the degrees to which they see genetic information as private, prompting disclosures selectively to some people but not others. Across these social spheres, secrets vary in their acceptability, and size, depth, and darkness.

Some have told only their immediate family and no one else, not even physicians. Yet as we will see, in social settings "keeping up appearances" in these ways can carry costs.

In these diverse social worlds, other individuals disclose for public and personal reasons. Several rationales cut across settings, while others appear more specific to particular situations. In general, individuals divulge because they want support, feel their genetic risk is an important part of their identity, and want to use their experiences to teach others. In certain social worlds, disclosure can also occur as a way to justify time spent on medical appointments. As Laura, the graphic designer who had been an environmentalist, said about her breast cancer,

> I want people to know, because it increases awareness, and it's a part of who I am. It makes me. I want people to understand: when I say I have to go to all these doctors, I'm not just a hypochondriac.

The information can specifically instill in others the need for disease prevention. Many women discuss breast cancer with each other to encourage self-exams. Ori, the Israeli, said,

> I'm extremely open about it, telling everybody to check their nipples, because my particular inflammatory cancer started with a tiny little nipple discoloration. No one knows to look for it. It's not an embarrassment.

She divulges not because her disease is genetic per se, but because she feels it is preventable.

Still, to disclose in these worlds, patients often have to overcome feelings of shame and embarrassment. At the same time, to keep wholly private an experience that has transformed one both physically and psychologically is difficult. Laura has worked to accept her *BRCA* mutation, compelling her to talk about it further. She feels marked as "special," though this was clearly a mixed blessing. "People like to show off their scars," she said. "It makes me tougher. I feel sort of marked, like in *The Scarlet Letter*, with a 'C'—for cancer."

As suggested earlier, others feel that because of visible evidence of the disease or treatment, they do not have a choice whether to tell or not. Physical symptoms or treatment effects can reveal disease. For Alpha, having a permanent IV line or carrying oxygen can be obvious and potentially stigmatizing. Here, disclosures may not always be planned. Jennifer, the schoolteacher, said,

> I have an infusion port for IV Prolastin. I swim, and people in the dressing room walk around with just a towel on. Over the years, a couple of people have asked me what it is. I say, "Well, I get weekly infusions." They then think I have cancer. They usually don't ask, "What do you have?" At one time, it was embarrassing. But I forget about it now, until I see somebody looking.

Genetic diagnoses may arise in conversation because of the effects of the disease in one's family, not oneself. Ordinary, casual social discourse may include information about one's family. As Ron explained, "My twin brother died, and my older brother's dying, so it's going to come up. But I don't feel a need to tell everybody. If it doesn't come up, I don't talk about it."

Others hesitate to tell friends out of concern about burdening them. One's claim on friends is often less than that on kin. "I haven't told a lot of good friends," Tim said about his HD. "It wouldn't make me feel any better, and would make them feel worse."

Yet disclosure can make friends closer; conversely, closer friendships may allow or even mandate more disclosure. One's genetics are integral to oneself, but whether one should therefore share it with others can be very unclear. To do so can feel akin to sharing one's nakedness—full, unguarded exposure. Individuals may grapple with the exact degree to which genetics *is* part of them—whether the "specialness" of this information necessitates more secrecy or more sharing. Bill, who feared getting HD, was highly concerned as a salesman about outward appearance:

> Your genetic makeup is your makeup, and it shouldn't be shared with other people. Why do we walk around with clothes on? Should we just walk around *naked*? Certain things should be left to yourself or only intimate people around you.

Information can feel shameful, or worse—incriminating. Bill added, "There are things you don't tell the world: my drunk dad, my financial status, if I broke any laws. It's private, embarrassing."

Others simply avoid talking about a diagnosis in order to avoid thinking about it, reflecting possible elements of magical thinking. As Jennifer explained about Alpha,

> I thought, "If I don't talk about it, I won't get sick." I wanted to deny I had it. If I didn't talk about it, it wasn't real. I wouldn't get ill. Only since I became more symptomatic have I talked about it.

Breast cancer, and the removal of breasts and ovaries, adds potential embarrassment related to taboos about sex and sexual organs. "I have not really mentioned to anyone that I had cancer or mastectomies," Diane said. "I feel very touchy about it." She was upset partly about her unexpected mastectomy. Shame can be irrational, but powerful.

Yet in public spaces, such self-imposed restriction can limit one's life— even if one is anonymous. "Some people are very open about it," Diane added, "bare-breasted on the beach. I don't feel that way. I loved the beach. But I had to stop."

GOSSIP

In diffuse social worlds without relatively clear boundaries, information can unfortunately spread through gossip. Third party disclosures can readily occur. Patients may want to keep certain information private, while others are eager to obtain and spread it. Only in retrospect may such leaks become apparent. Given these fuzzy social boundaries, individuals may also avoid disclosing to certain friends for fear that the information will disseminate more widely. Once information is out, one no longer possesses it. It cannot be untold.

Such private information, including knowledge of others' risks, can be seen by others as valuable social capital and sought for social and psychological, if not financial, gain. People seek and transmit gossip to advance their own standing. As Bill observed,

> People like to hear things that others don't know. They *get something on you*. It's a little competition: I heard his girlfriend's going to leave him. It makes you feel better about yourself a little bit. It makes them feel more powerful. It's sad. Everyone does it.

Yet in social situations, many people may be surprised that information about them, too, is spread. Bill added,

> We think no one talks about us. So, if you talk about somebody, it's hush-hush. If you feel someone is talking about you, you can't believe it. Yet, you talk about everyone else. That's just the way it works—it's washwoman stuff, but almost everyone does it.

Despite one's best efforts at privacy, information may flow through rumors in varying and unpredictable ways, with uncertain effects.

Some are acutely aware of these dangers and hesitate to disclose their risk, since to do so can be painful and jeopardize one's confidentiality in additional contexts. Giving information involves bestowing trust on others, allotting them power that they could then potentially use against you. Linda, the art teacher, said, "If you tell someone how you feel, you give them *a gift*: trusting them to respond to your feelings in a helpful way. It's been very useful to me to hide some things." Knowledge is a "gift" in part because it has power, and affirms closeness and trust.

At the same time, norms operate that can deem the transmission of some information to be inappropriate, illicit, and taboo. Still, people may publically disavow their desire for information, while privately still seeking it. Paradoxically, needs for privacy stem in part from the fact that people *assume* that it is elusive.

Given these complexities, a few patients confront such secondary disclosure when they learn of it, but to do so is rare. Jennifer added,

> If somebody says something to me about my illness, and I didn't tell them about it, I'll say, "If you want to talk about illness, talk about *your* illness, not mine." I don't want people to view me as sick.

Her reluctance to be perceived as sick may flow in part from her own difficulties in seeing herself as "flawed."

A few people accept secondary disclosure among a group of friends, highlighting how complex relationships may be within a social network. Yet within such a group it is not always easy to rigidly differentiate close friends from more casual acquaintances. Information may still circulate more than is desired or assumed.

Disclosures can also strengthen relationships, with listeners offering support. Yet such responses can be hard to predict.

Moreover, not wanting to disclose differs from not wanting others to know. Some patients do not want to have to tell a third party (to avoid having to manage immediate psychological reactions), but do not mind if someone else gives that person the information. At times a patient may even *want* a friend to tell mutual friends.

But friends who are told then have to decide whether or not to share the information with others. Consequently, patients often attempt to assess the trustworthiness of others—the likelihood that these friends will not spread rumors. Patients vary widely in the degrees to which they tend to trust others, and are open or private. While within families, one may feel obligated to disclose because of moral bonds, among friends, one generally has more latitude.

WHAT TO TELL IN SOCIAL SETTINGS

In these fluid and diverse social situations, quandaries also arise about what exactly to tell. Again, these issues resemble—but also differ from—those with family members, since here the social and moral bonds, expectations, and obligations are generally far less. Casual and ill-defined social worlds pose challenges of how to talk about one's genetic make-up and mutations. Particularly with acquaintances or relative strangers, some speak indirectly or in code. "If somebody is smoking, I'll say, 'Oh I have a lung problem,'" reported Barbara, the part-time professor with Alpha. "They don't need to know the whole story. I think I *pass* very well."

People may ask about one's health, but want to hear that essentially everything is now fine. Individuals may each prefer to maintain a certain safe distance and not want to get closer; disclosure of illness can threaten to narrow the separation. The two parties may or may not agree on this distance. Yet as Betty, the designer, said about her Alpha,

> Usually, people just react with, "Oh, well, you're O.K. now, aren't you?" People want to hear that everything is O.K. So, when anyone says, "How are you feeling? Better?" they usually don't really want to know any gory details.

But partial explanations may not always be accepted. Therefore, people may simply disclose as little as possible, in order to avoid having to elaborate later. Betty continued, "If I say 'Alpha,' I have to be ready for further explanation, which remains difficult for *me* to understand, so I wouldn't tell anyone in passing."

Patients may give only partial, coded information. The fact that the disease is rare can itself exacerbate social difficulties, necessitating additional explanations. For Alpha, patients may say simply "genetic emphysema"—since people have generally heard of emphysema—but not chronic obstructive pulmonary disease (COPD) or Alpha. As Gilbert, the factory worker, said,

> Typically, I explain that I have a genetic disorder that leads to emphysema or COPD. Everybody understands emphysema. They don't all understand COPD. I explain to them what it is, and what Alpha-1 is, and how the enzyme works—as much as they're interested in learning.

Recipients of information can vary widely in how much detail they want or comprehend.

Other patients will claim that they have a better-known, less stigmatized disorder. At times, Roger, tested for HD only after having problems driving, claims he has Parkinson's disease.

> People think I have Parkinson's. They'll say "Oh Parkinson's?" And I'll just say "Yes," because that's what they think. To explain what I have takes so long. No one understands Huntington's.

Yet he has trouble accepting his diagnosis himself.

The degree of closeness may also determine the extent of detail. The broad category of "neurological disease" may suffice with friends, but not with family members who may themselves be at risk.

Given the complicated pros and cons of divulgence in these amorphous social worlds, many wait to disclose until they are less vulnerable to possible adverse consequences. Karl, who eventually learned he lacked the HD mutation, said, "I didn't share the result *before* I tested. I was concerned about insurance. But, afterwards, I felt pretty comfortable telling people." Still, he reveals his risk, but not the traumatic effects of the disease on his family.

Patients also face quandaries about *how* to tell—for example, whether to do so in person, through email, regular mail, or phone. Ever widening circles of friends exist, and the logistics of telling a *group* can be difficult. Email offers advantages, but can lead to misunderstandings as well. Vera, the Asian executive, felt that emailing her *BRCA* mutation-positive test results to friends would be emotionally easiest. But problems arise.

> I emailed the information the day after I got tested. I thought it was better than telling in person. I was still a little shaken up, and thought I would start crying on the phone. Most were very supportive. One was totally in shock, and couldn't deal with it. I confronted her. Supposedly, I misunderstood her email.

DISCLOSURES AT WORK

Given blurry social boundaries and possibilities of gossip, disclosures at work can pose particularly thorny dilemmas. Closeness to bosses and coworkers has to be balanced against fears of discrimination. At one extreme, some keep their diagnoses completely secret at work. Still, they may speculate whether colleagues nonetheless know. "I've never told anybody at work," said Diane, the Spanish teacher who felt damaged from an unexpected unilateral mastectomy. "I feel very self-conscious about people looking at my chest. I always wonder if they notice."

Many fear possible discrimination, even though it would be illegal. As we saw earlier, many are wary of how laws get implemented and enforced. "While it would be morally incorrect to let me go," said Chloe, the young secretary asymptomatic and untested for HD, "things like that happen."

But silence and secrecy at work can pose burdens, and carry costs. Many find it hard to hide their diagnosis at their job. Joyce, the spa employee who was in denial, had trouble concealing her breast cancer and finding an adequate wig.

Before the chemo, I got a haircut, and a wig that was very similar in color. But the texture was different, and it was short. Everybody thought it was adorable. They just thought I had straightened it. But I was afraid the wig would fall off. I was so nervous. I had no eyelashes or eyebrows. When I put on makeup, it just slid right off. My face was puffy from steroids. I just tried to duck in and out of work, and hope for the best.

Such concealment can impede accessing disease information that could aid coping. For instance, some defer from using the Internet at work for any disease-related activities—even simply seeking information. Tim, the lawyer with the HD mutation, but no symptoms, said,

At first, I printed out some things, and an associate said, what's that? I said, "Nothing . . ." I then decided not to look at work. I don't know if they track my email. Why take the risk? But I don't have Internet access at home, so I don't know that much about HD.

At his office, he also does not talk about HD on the phone.

Between the extremes of openness and secrecy, many make more finely grained decisions, trying to temper threats to privacy as much as they realistically and comfortably can without causing too much harm—for instance by limiting their Internet use while at their job. John, who turned out not to have the HD mutation, said,

> I was concerned not about going to HD sites, but receiving HD emails at work—though I did. So I started to transition HD stuff to a private AOL account. I didn't worry too much about it, but when I saw Huntington's disease in the subject line, I thought: that probably isn't good.

Even searching for information about HD on the Internet can instill caution. Simone, the bookkeeper with the mutation though no symptoms, is more concerned—in part because she is only 29, and hopes to have a whole career ahead of her. At her office she tries to restrict her HD-related web use in other ways. Such precautions may seem extreme, but she feels that her very life and death are at stake.

> I'm kind of paranoid. I look up *other* diseases from work—MS and other neurological disorders. So it looks as if I'm just looking at WebMD in general. But I can't sign in to the HD Society site. I would be afraid somebody is watching me . . . I would hope that they would say, "Well, she's just hitting everything"—not specifically HD.

At the other extreme, depending on the nature of the organization—specifically the degree of closeness to colleagues, and fear of discrimination—people may be fairly open about their genetic risk. Anxieties about discrimination may depend in part on length of time and amount of trust with an employer. Patty, the fashion designer untested and asymptomatic for HD, said about her risk,

> Now, everybody at work knows. I've been there eight years, and *they're like my family*. I work for a small design studio. When my mother does things that really upset me, I go to work and cry. I never thought, "I shouldn't tell people."

Employers' questions about family members can reveal one's *own* risk, too. A relative's diagnosis could thus arise when being interviewed or hired for a job, or having to fill out forms for new insurance. Consequently, worries about bias can lead patients to prevaricate about their risk. Yvonne, with lung transplants, assumes that her siblings either dissemble about their risk of Alpha, or are not asked about it.

> I'm sure they lie about it, or just say no. Employers don't ask you if *any* family member has a genetic disease—just whether you or your *immediate*

family have it. My siblings wouldn't think that sister or brother would be immediate.

Needs for treatment can also prompt disclosure. Consequently, some may disclose at a prior job—when ill, and needing time off for hospitalizations and treatments—but not at a new position, when no longer acutely ill. At a new workplace, disclosures may in fact be rare—occurring only if the topic comes up, and seems appropriate. As Rhonda, the nurse with breast cancer and a mutation, said,

> At my last job, I told some people I became friendly with. Not just in a general conversation: "Hi. How are you? My name's X and I had breast cancer." But *if I felt it fit into the conversation.* Girls talk about bra sizes. Now, at my *new* job, I work with different types of nurses. Some know, some don't. If it comes up, I don't have a problem telling someone. I facilitate breast cancer support groups. So if I hear someone has been diagnosed, I'll pass the contact number along.

Thus, she tells if she thinks the knowledge will help someone. As a health care provider, she may also encounter less discrimination than do employees in other fields.

Severe symptoms and needs for disability can force disclosures as well. "Everybody knew," Benjamin, the engineer, said about his Alpha. "I thought I was going to die, and need disability." Jennifer told no one about her Alpha for 12 years—until she required time off from her job as a teacher. Exhaustion and desire for a sabbatical necessitated revelation.

One may tell because of family needs that result from a disease for which one is also at risk. Bill, the salesman, asymptomatic and untested for HD, told coworkers about his risk because he experienced stresses caring for his brother. Only later did he become concerned about the information spreading. Therefore, in work settings, as in other social networks, individuals have to carefully weigh their wishes to tell and gain support against their fears of gossip and stigma. To negotiate between these conflicting goals poses shifting problems.

Telling Bosses

With supervisors, too, patients face particularly tricky questions of whether, what, when, and how to divulge information. Bosses may have an inkling about a person's condition, yet feel constrained from asking, not wanting to be in a position of knowing too much. They may have to separate their personal and professional roles and knowledge. Patty, the fashion designer, said, "One of the partners knew that my mom had something, but never asked about it." Occasionally, bosses might be surprisingly supportive because of their own illness experiences. Employers vary widely in whether they talk about their own problems, and if so, how much. Susie, who worked at an HIV organization and had a family history of breast cancer but no symptoms or mutation, found her boss to be very open about medical problems. Susie suggests how the ethos of different organizations can range widely from for-profit to nonprofit, and from health-related to not. Still, individual personal differences and idiosyncrasies can play major roles as well. She reported,

> I told my boss I had a cyst. In the past, he had told me what was going on with him and his wife—from trying to stop smoking, to thinking he had lupus. So it wasn't out of context.

She underscores how employees may take their cues from employers in defining the boundaries and scope of these relationships.

Especially for breast cancer, female bosses may possibly be easier to tell—but not always. For Vera, having a woman as a boss facilitated disclosure:

> She knows what I've been going through. I went for the genetic test results at lunch, because I thought I was just picking them up and coming back. I ended up staying out. By four, I called her and told her what was going on. I wouldn't say she's my *friend*, but I felt comfortable telling her. I feel secure enough in what she thinks of me and my abilities. If my boss was male, it probably would not have been as easy to tell him.

She distinguishes here between the roles of employer and friend. The two roles may share some features but not others, and may be fluid but at times also constrained.

Tensions can emerge between an employer's official and unofficial knowledge—between what a boss feels is appropriate to ask or know and what is not. Complicated choreographies can result. Patients may want support and some flexibility—which can be difficult, if not impossible, to obtain. Linda, the art teacher who eventually found she lacked the HD mutation, said,

> I wanted my boss to know that *something* was up, and that he should be extra nice. I would say cryptically, "I have *a medical thing* I have to take care of," and kind of hope or convey that I wasn't really O.K., and that it would be good if he asked after me. A couple of times he did: "Are you . . .? Is everything . . .?" *I wanted a little bit of support without revealing*

anything. He felt it was private. He gave me some leeway. I didn't want to get any slack, like I was doing something irresponsible by missing a meeting.

This intricate dance—revealing the existence, but not the nature or extent of a problem—can involve much back-and-forth and indirect communication.

Patients who are themselves physicians can face additional problems, as colleagues may be surprisingly distant. Jim, the doctor with HD, got little if any support from colleagues. "No one ever says anything to me about having Huntington's," he said. "They have a hard time dealing with illness. They don't really know how to react." Doctors often feel that they must sharply separate themselves from illness, and that they wear "magic white coats," and are supposed to be healthy. They may feel that becoming ill themselves threatens this fragile veil between patient and healer.[1]

Telling Coworkers

Coworkers also occupy peculiar in-between roles—as "work friends." They may be close, but potentially convey personal information to others who could in turn tell bosses, precipitating discrimination. Still, fellow coworkers can be easier to tell than supervisors, who have the power to hire and fire. But many individuals find that their social and work worlds overlap or collide. Friends may be (or know) coworkers or employers, muddying clear and definitive boundaries. Hence, some divulge to coworkers very cautiously. Particularly in a small community, disclosure of genetic information at work can implicate one's relatives as well. Chloe, untested for HD, is a secretary at the same company as her sister and sister-in-laws. Her sister "hasn't told her in-laws yet. I definitely can't tell *anybody!*" Chloe did not mention her risk at work—largely because she didn't want to call attention to her sister's early evidence of disease.

The risk of gossip spurs efforts to gauge the trustworthiness of coworkers. But doing so can be difficult. Some struggle to assess whether coworkers maintain others' confidentiality. As Vera said, "If someone says, 'This person told me this, and told me don't tell anyone, but I can tell you'—that's a red flag." Yet concealment can carry costs as well. Secrecy can necessitate obfuscating the truth, complicating even innocuous conversations. To hide the presence of a disease in one's self or one's family can be difficult, if not impossible. Evelyn, whose husband forbade her to test and whose father had hidden a relative's letter about HD, said,

My sisters tell no one. But when my grandmother, who's 94, dies, a lot of work people are going to show up at the wake. "How do we keep Mommy home?" My sister said, "Slip her Ex-lax or a diuretic. She'll have diarrhea, and won't be able to come." We can't do that. We're just going to *lie*, and say she has MS.

Secrecy can thus span several generations, because of fears.

Concealment also entails foregoing support, and risking the possibility of getting caught. Barbara, the part-time professor and former smoker, keeps her Alpha secret but pays enormous psychological costs, as she fears being discovered.

> I have to put up a false front, and live a double life. My Prolastin comes to my house and I refrigerate it. What if someone from work comes over, looks in the fridge, and says, "What is this?" I'm constantly at the point of potentially being caught.

The fact that she used to smoke makes her feel potentially culpable for her illness, exacerbating her sense of shame.

Divulgences to colleagues may also occur unintentionally and unplanned. One cannot always suppress sudden strong emotions about one's disease. Laura, the graphic designer with a family history of breast cancer and the mutation but no symptoms, said,

> I spilled my guts to my coworker. We were having a meeting, and I just had the genetic counseling appointment, and couldn't help saying something because I knew I seemed negative.

Revelations can also become mutual. These reciprocities highlight the intricate implicit rules involved in work disclosures. Often one does not know about another's illness until disclosing one's own. Laura added,

> Everybody has something. You don't know until you talk. My coworker has been more open. He gives himself shots five times a day at work, and has to regulate his blood sugar. What a pain. But he's so discreet. I wanted to ask him more, but didn't know if he was comfortable. Maybe there's a reason he didn't talk about it before. All he needed was someone to ask.

She highlights the implicit norms of divulging only if asked, and otherwise maintaining silence. Yet it is also possible that a graphic design studio may be more open and less discriminatory than certain other kinds of workplaces.

Still, others who felt compelled to disclose because of an emotional upset later regret doing so. Secrecy can be hard to maintain at a job. An office-mate may be told—but that person then knows forever. The eventual effects of a disclosure can not always be predicted. Linda, the art teacher who found she lacked the HD mutation, said,

> I told a woman I share a little office with. Somehow, it came out. Then I felt, "Oh shit." I swore her to secrecy. I was probably on the phone, really upset, or just said, "Yeah, geez—my dad had blah blah blah." But after I told her, I had to share with her what I'm going through. I felt she's watching me, listening to my phone calls, wondering if I'm O.K. When the whole Huntington's nightmare starts—"Oh shit . . . now she's going to know." I felt exposed, and wished I had kept it to myself. Although during this very hard year, having one person out there who knew was not the worst thing in the world.

Linda highlights the conflicts involved. Disclosure can offer both advantages and disadvantages, generating social support but also worries about gossip. In retrospect, a few feel they have been too trusting—especially concerning HD. "I'm very naïve," said Patty, the fashion designer. Luckily, she turned out to lack the HD mutation.

Coworkers can respond to these divulgences in various ways. To disclose is to enter the "sick role," raising quandaries about when to enter and exit that role. Coworkers can become jealous of an employee who goes on disability without seeming to be severely ill. Even fellow teachers, for instance, thought that Jennifer, with Alpha, was "pulling a fast one over them: 'You look pretty good.'"

Consequently, individuals must assess coworkers' implicit attitudes and indirect comments. People are generally able to select their friends, but not their coworkers. At work one usually spends large amounts of time with individuals whom one has not chosen, and who may or may not be supportive. "I just get the vibe," Jan, with breast cancer, but no mutation, said about the need to be circumspect in her office. "They make little rude comments."

Telling Clients

In business, those who have worked closely with customers over several years face additional disclosure decisions. Generally, one is much less close to clients, and somewhat financially dependent on them. Carol, the saleswoman with breast cancer, a mutation, and prophylactic surgery, told only a few customers about her illness. Yet after finishing chemotherapy, she removed her wig.

I was bald, and wearing a wig, and 90% of my customers didn't even know. They'd say, "Oh, your hair looks really great. Did you change your style?" People are so oblivious. I told a couple of customers, but not others. Then I finished my chemo and took my wig off. My hair was short, and people said, "Are you Hare Krishna now?" They didn't get it. It was bizarre. The first time, with breast cancer, I might have told 5% of customers. With ovarian, maybe 20%. I tell close customers, but don't feel that comfort level with customers who I don't really have a relationship with, or don't see on an ongoing basis.

She suggests wide variations based on the individual client, rather than their social role alone.

Telling Neighbors

Patients also face questions concerning disclosures to neighbors who may see medication deliveries or symptoms. Ginger, the medical secretary, goes so far as to scrape the labels off empty prescription bottles that she puts in the trash.

When I throw any medicine bottle away, I pull the labels off with my fingernail. I don't want people picking up prescription bottles, "She takes Xanax, or antibiotics, or Theodore, or inhalers." Kids once picked up a big bag of trash from the alley behind our house and threw it on somebody's lawn. The next thing I know, the police are knocking on my door, "What's this? You're littering somebody's lawn up the street!"

Telling Schools

Dilemmas arise, too, concerning telling schools and other institutions. To inform schools about a parent's genetic risk can create problems for his or her children. Mary fears that if her children's school know her HD diagnosis, they may take her children away.

My son and daughter are speech delayed, because I can't help them. They'll say a word wrong, and I don't correct it. I don't know why. I want to tell the school, because I'm having a hard time getting my oldest son's homework done, and reading books with him. They probably think I'm a terrible mother. But I'm not telling them, because I'm afraid it will backfire, and they'll watch me, and find more wrong than I want them to. I don't want any outside agencies involved. I don't know why I don't read—why I can't get it done. I say, "Oh, we'll do it later." I'm always putting it off, and then it never gets done. I feel bad.

CONCLUSIONS

Across these varied social domains—from friendships to jobs to schools—individuals struggle with dilemmas of whether, when, what, and to whom to reveal their genetic risk. These questions require careful balancing of competing concerns. Individuals often feel they should tell others with whom they are close. Such revelations can also serve to increase awareness and education about a disease. But discrimination can ensue. Disclosures may occur in families, because of social bonds and moral obligations that can be explicitly discussed and reinforced, and physicians and insurers may explicitly ask patients for genetic information. But in other social worlds, such norms and expectations are far more implicit, fluid, and complicated, begetting confusion and conflict.

The experiences here illustrate important aspects of work and social networks—their plasticity and lack of clear or strong boundaries. Definitive boundaries generally exist in families, separating kin from non-kin, but not in these other social worlds. Outside the family, trustworthiness can be hard to gauge, confounding disclosures of genetic information and thus patients' support and experiences.

In these other social worlds people frequently try to guide and monitor the dissemination of information about their genetic risk, but they do not always succeed. The fact that one's genetic data reveals information about not only oneself but one's family makes these issues even trickier. Coworkers may meet or know family members whose illness can then suggest the employee's risk, and vice versa.

These challenges should prompt rethinking of these social norms. Increasingly, many of us will face quandaries about whether to share our own or others' genetic information. We will confront secondary or third-party disclosures, and have to weigh trust against possible gossip, and perceived benefits against potential dangers of revelation. We may try to erect social boundaries between who does and who does not know, but with mixed success. As we will see, genetic information can also fundamentally alter our social worlds.

CHAPTER 11

"Crossing Over":

Entering Genetic Communities

"A year ago, I crossed over to 'the other side,'" Joyce, the spa employee, told me, "from the people who haven't had cancer, to the people who have." She changed in critical psychological, social, and economic ways: she now had a disease, and needed government support. "When I was first diagnosed, people who had cancer were disgusting and strange. Then, one day, I realized a lot of the people I know have cancer, and I'm on Medicaid."

These men and women face decisions concerning not only their prior social worlds but new realms as well—genetic communities. Eventually, these individuals discover a wide range of organizations, both formal and informal. These groups can prove helpful, but also pose challenges. Stigma, rejection, and low knowledge of genetics in the outside world impel people to join groups of fellow patients. But fears of having to confront one's disease further and see sicker patients as a result can mitigate against such involvements. Patient communities provide both advantages and disadvantages. How then do these individuals decide whether to participate in these genetic worlds, and how to do so?

Prior studies have suggested that psychosocial support groups can help patients with a wide variety of diseases, enhancing quality of life, social support, information, and hope.[1,2,3] Yet many patients who might benefit from such support groups do not always use them, often because of being unaware of them.[1,4,5] Support group participants tend to be female, young, and better educated.[1,4,5,6] A few studies have suggested that compared to nonparticipants, participants have more anxiety,[1,5] but less stress and depression.[7,8]

Recently, online communities have mushroomed, offering advantages and disadvantages.[9] Websites can provide informational and emotional support,[10] and be empowering.[11] For good or bad, websites may also decrease physicians' "information monopoly,"[12] and challenge doctors' expertise.[13]

But many questions remain as to how individuals decide whether and how involved to be in disease communities, how they experience these entities, and what difficulties, if any, they encounter.

I soon found that communities confronting genetic risks resemble those facing other kinds of illness, but also differ, due to several unique issues. As we have seen, people facing genetic risks may be completely healthy, and their disease may be exceedingly rare, and hence virtually unknown. Genetics may thus foster particular confusion, and these patient communities can thus play especially vital roles but also present several challenges.

ENTERING COMMUNITIES

Many individuals are surprised to learn that vast genetic communities exist. Unlike participants in many other types of social organizations—based on characteristics such as gender, ethnicity, or religion, of which one is aware since early childhood—interviewees have generally learned only recently that they are potential members of genetic groups. "You have no idea that the breast cancer community is there," Joyce, the spa employee, said, "until you have a reason to find out." Joining such a genetic community can then involve surprising and unplanned social transformations. One may feel distance from prior social worlds, but suddenly welcome into others.

Individuals may first learn of the existence of disease organizations when referred by a provider, but they then enter these communities to varying extents. Some find the disease—and hence these communities—too threatening. They may shun these associations, and not even wish to hear about them. As Benjamin, the engineer with Alpha, reported, "A subset *don't want to know anything* about the disease: 'Take me off the list. I don't want to know about it.' People are afraid they will get too depressed, angry, or afraid." These groups can present tradeoffs between gaining useful knowledge and confronting emotional stress. Still, most individuals make more fine-grained decisions rather than being wholly in or out.

Given these obstacles, joining such communities may be gradual, facilitated by a guide. Occasionally, after diagnosis, patients may be contacted by a friend who has heard the news and then provides information about such communities. As Ori, the Israeli with breast cancer but no family history or mutation, said,

> Other friends had cancer before me, and arranged for this phone call that
> I got. I wasn't even looking for it. I didn't want to hear from other people

about it, or go to meetings. But it was very helpful. I would not have called them on my own.

She would not have looked for a disease community, but benefited once it contacted her.

A few patients asked a health care provider about such groups, and were then referred to them. "When the doctor first diagnosed me," Ginger said about her Alpha, "I asked him, 'Where can I find some information about Alpha?' He said, 'The Internet.'"

But overall, such physician referrals were uncommon. Instead, individuals generally had to find out about these communities on their own (e.g., though Google searches), or chance interactions, with little systematic input from anyone. Diagnoses may, after all, be new and secret, and patients may share the information with only a handful of providers and immediate kin.

THE FUNCTIONS OF GENETIC COMMUNITIES: WHAT THEY OFFER

These communities can offer a wide range of benefits—emotional, cognitive, social, and political. Patient groups provide valuable information, helping individuals and their families understand aspects of genetics from disease mechanisms to broader implications, addressing uncertainties and confusion.

Communities can offer input concerning testing, treatment, and finding medical experts. Especially for relatively rare diseases, these groups can assist in locating specialized or nearby physicians. Gilbert, the factory worker, commented,

At an Alpha conference, I discovered there was a group much closer to my home. Through them, I found another doctor. My previous doctor was great, but going to his city was . . . a hassle.

Patient organizations can also facilitate and encourage research, disseminating recruitment information and even cosponsoring studies, helping to establish disease registries or data banks.

These organizations can assist, too, in providing helpful information that doctors may in fact not know. Physicians have limited time, and may forget, undervalue, or feel embarrassed or uncomfortable discussing certain topics. Especially for rare diseases, patient organizations can fill in the gaps. Doctors may be particularly uncomfortable discussing diseases such as breast cancer and HD that involve taboo matters concerning breasts, ovaries, psychosis, sexuality, and death. The anonymity of online communities can facilitate discussion of such difficult areas.

Many of the topics discussed less by doctors than by disease communities concern side effects of treatment, about which physicians may feel embarrassed or guilty. Ori, the Israeli with breast cancer, said, "The staff simply didn't tell me what to expect in terms of my hair falling out."

These communities can facilitate discussions about taboo topics concerning the body, about which both patients and providers may feel uncomfortable. Denise, the banker, said about her breast cancer treatment:

> In chemo, anal fissures are surprisingly common, but doctors don't tell you that. People generally don't talk about constipation. There is nothing like the constipation you get with chemo. I get a lot of private online messages, because I decided that women can ask me anything, since *I never want anybody to have to go through what I did.*

Discourse about these future problems can help prepare patients. As she suggests, mutual sharing and altruism can play key roles here.

These communities can provide information, too, about how to *cope* with the vagaries of these diseases—for example, of being at risk but untested or asymptomatic.

Large amounts of information may be available online, yet recently diagnosed individuals may still feel either uninformed or overwhelmed. "There's so much confusion about genetics," Linda, the art teacher, said. "I know information is somewhere out there for these smaller diseases, but you have to do the research yourself."

Distributing and Arranging Treatment

As mentioned earlier, disease organizations may face decisions about what roles to adopt with regard to treatment access, and to what degree. In part because overall, genetic disorders are disproportionately rare—so-called orphan diseases—drug companies and researchers may devote relatively few resources to them. Thus, for example, Alpha organizations became actively involved in distributing Prolastin, though tensions ensued.

Treatment shortages raised other ethical and policy questions as well—for example, whether to advocate for widespread screening. If broader population screening for Alpha were instituted, the demand for Prolastin would have further increased without necessarily increasing the drug supply, forcing dilemmas of how to balance public health against individual treatment needs. These organizations faced challenges in confronting these decisions.

Psychosocial Support

Genetic communities can also provide vital psychological and social benefits—from informal to formal, and direct to indirect. Usually, communities institute formal mechanisms that then also have informal benefits. For instance, peer-to-peer counseling can ultimately aid individuals involved on both sides of the interaction. Communities can foster altruism that can itself abet coping. As Jennifer added, "I'm a peer guide: I have to desensitize myself to the possibility that I may be on oxygen, so I talk to other Alphas about it."

These groups can be particularly useful in reducing isolation. Especially for diseases associated with mutations that have low prevalence, individuals can feel alone and stigmatized. Joining a community of others who are similarly affected can thus counter these painful feelings. For Peter, the retired business-man leading an Alpha support group,

> A benefit of the national meetings is: You get together, and see that people are concerned about Alpha. Doctors are working on it, and there is psychological support: *You're not the only one* facing this.

Particularly for rare diseases that are less well-understood by the general public, such communities can be vital. Fellow patients comprehend the disease, while outsiders usually do not. In these communities patients do not need to explain and justify the illness. "People understand," Dorothy said. Generally, outsiders don't know that Alpha is genetic, and is not self-induced through smoking.

This support may be especially crucial for genetic diseases since affected patients share common experiences as well as intrinsic biological parts of themselves. In fact, they may all share a common ancestor. "We are literally all related," Jennifer said about fellow Alphas. "It came from the Vikings. There is that feeling of common ethnic background: Northern Europeans."

The journey from isolation to "belonging" can be incredibly powerful, producing a kind of high. Jennifer continued about her first meeting:

> Until that morning, I had never met another Alpha. It was an electric excitement, mountain-top experience. A sense of belonging—camarade-rie. I wasn't alone. There were lots of people. Many of us feel like islands: I'm the only person in the world paddling this canoe.

Patients can guide and inspire each other, promulgating hope. Given possible bad prognoses, such optimism can be vital. Carol, who ignored her boyfriend's opposition to prophylactic surgery, said, "I tell people, 'My life is O.K. I've been there.' *That's what I'm there for: to be an inspiration,* so people will see me and say, '*She* looks O.K.'"

Inspiring other patients gives her an important sense of purpose.

Contact with others who have been sicker can also reduce despair and instill hope. These communities can uniquely fill these functions. Ori, with breast cancer, added,

It was helpful that I heard from someone who had 40 positive lymph nodes and survived. I only had nine. So, to her, my case was Mickey Mouse. I drew strength from her. It was a lifesaver.

THE STRUCTURES OF GENETIC COMMUNITIES

Genetic communities are not fixed entities, but vary and evolve over time. To perform the functions above, new groups and subgroups form, defined not only by diagnosis but age, race, ethnicity, socioeconomic status, and stage and presentation of disease.

Between the two extremes of only online and only in-person communication are many combinations. Interactions range from formal to informal, simultaneous to delayed, and small to large. These differences emerge in part due to type, prevalence, and stigma of disease, and tradeoffs between facilitating social interactions versus protecting privacy.

Some communities establish one-on-one buddy systems or hotlines to assist new members in person, on the telephone, or over the Internet. In response to fears of potential discrimination, anonymous support systems can let members communicate one-on-one without divulging any identifying information.

Yet the social dynamics can become complex. As Ori described,

I have a friend, but don't know her personally. She's part of an organization, and was hooked up with me as a peer. She, too, has gone through breast cancer and is Jewish, with eight children. She had genetic testing, but I didn't ask her the results. In her Hasidic neighborhood, nobody knows that she even had breast cancer. They walk around in wigs anyway, and she was able to hide her illness from future mates—they arrange marriages. So I asked her, regarding Jewish values, how you go about not being up front with that issue. She said that if asked, you have to say; but if not asked, you don't. People in the community ask a lot about Alzheimer's, mental retardation, and cancer. So far, no one has asked her, because her children are not of marriage age. Now, one is 19, so it should come up soon.

Genetic communities can thus serve as a refuge from stigma. Subgroups can also form—based, for instance, on religion. Ori suggests as well the novel amorphous social category of a "friend" whom one doesn't "know personally"— highlighting the complex definitions, responsibilities, and boundaries of such relationships.

Given primary concerns, communication on websites can require special registration and passwords. Isabelle, the social worker with breast cancer and a mutation, trying to decide about prophylactic mastectomies, said, "One section, for which you need a special password, is just for women who have had mastectomies: It's photographs of reconstruction."

In-person support groups are common, and can be very helpful, extending for years. Formal support groups often spawn ongoing informal friendships.

National or regional conferences further enable patients to meet, learn from, and interact with each other and researchers. These larger venues further strengthen senses of a broader community, including scientists as well.

Virtual Electronic Communities

Increasingly, however, genetic communities are becoming electronic and virtual, with online mechanisms varying from informational websites and posting boards, to live chat rooms. These formats are not mutually exclusive, but can interconnect. In-person interactions can also become virtual, and vice versa.

Particularly for rare diseases, online fora may be vital, since such disorders are uncommon in any one locale but accumulate nationally or internationally. For relatively more common but stigmatized conditions such as breast cancer, online communities can serve unique functions as well.

Web communication can also offer logistical benefits—for example, saving time. Yet the anonymity of online communication can erode trust in the quality of postings. The Internet can reach many, but web information can be unvetted and incorrect.

The relative newness of the web, the rapid evolution of science and treatment, and the fact that information can be posted anonymously all make the accuracy of material offered difficult to judge. "Early on, you don't know anything, and are getting information," observed Denise, the banker with breast cancer and a family history. "But you have no idea who is giving it to you, and how accurate it is." To address this problem, these communities have frequently evolved informal self-corrective mechanisms to monitor quality. "If somebody posts bad information," she continued, "other women write, 'This is not the case. My doctors, in fact, say: don't do that.'"

Online communities also require computer and Internet access and skills that, though increasing, are not universal. Limitations still exist related to age, education, sex, race, and ethnicity. Carol, the 43-year-old saleswoman with breast cancer, surgery, and a mutation, has "never done chat rooms. I don't even know how." Some seek to acquire these skills, though doing so is not always easy. "I'm just not a computer person," said Wilma, the 54-year-old with breast cancer and bipolar disorder. "I'm just learning."

HOW TO BE INVOLVED

Individuals face decisions of not only whether but *how* and *to what degree* to be involved. Patients choose activities based on varying needs and interests, intertwining their lives with these organizations in different ways.

Volunteerism

As suggested earlier, individuals not only receive support but provide it to others, which itself can be rewarding and helpful. These communities often explicitly facilitate such volunteerism, which can potentially benefit one's relatives, future descendants, and others.

Some volunteer to help manage these organizations. Patients who legally can't work because they are on disability can nonetheless volunteer their services. Beatrice's sister took early retirement, and offered to administer such an organization for free. These efforts provide valuable indirect economic support to these communities. "She retired early, and embarked on a part-time second career, doing a lot of volunteer stuff. She thought it was fate."

Ethical claims can further fuel such reciprocity. "I profited a lot from what people had done," Jennifer said about the Alpha community. "So I wanted to give something back."

People may get involved in a disease organization because they have important skills to contribute, perceiving deficiencies that they can help remedy. Dorothy, the former TV producer, worked to help improve physician and public education about Alpha. "The organization had no PR," she said. "I used to work for TV, and knew people. I thought: maybe I could do something. That's how I got involved."

Initially, after diagnosis, individuals may try out different activities to see which prove most helpful, wholly rejecting certain engagements and choosing others. Gilbert, the factory worker, tried holistic healing for Alpha and concluded that it did not help him. "They were sitting there meditating with this holistic healer," he said. "That's just not my bag."

Participating in Research

Genetic communities also sponsor and promote research, helping to recruit participants. Once informed of these studies, individuals may decide to participate for altruistic reasons—to help other patients. Yet engagement in genetics research may differ from that in other disorders in stemming, potentially, not merely from abstract altruism. The results could benefit not only oneself and strangers, but one's own direct kin—present and future. "What if one of my sister's kids ends up having HD?" Chloe, the untested and asymptomatic 28-year-old secretary, wondered. "Maybe doing research will help them."

A version of therapeutic misconception may extend to one's relatives. While therapeutic misconception suggests that individuals often feel that they themselves will benefit from research when that is not the case,[14] with genetics many patients assume that research participation may not help them at all but will aid the next generation. This sense of gain to others may represent hope, rather than misconception, but can shift the risk-benefit calculus for a study, with individuals, as a result, at times accepting more risk than they otherwise would. These individuals may thus view research participation differently than do institutional review boards (or IRBs) that oversee research and are often more protectionist. Bill, the salesman without the HD mutation who cares for his affected brother, added,

> My brother says: "I'll be a guinea pig. Inject me. Stick me. Do whatever you got to do. Maybe it helps me. If not, maybe it'll help my family. I don't think anything's going to cure me, but if I could find something that will help someone else, why not?"

Such altruistic participation in research can also strengthen a sense of meaning and purpose in one's life. These links to future beneficiaries may thus also increase rates of research participation.

Many of these patients also appeared more willing than IRBs to allow researchers to conduct future as-yet-undetermined genetic tests on biological specimens. IRBs tend to hesitate to allow participants to donate samples without knowing what exactly will be done with them. But the individuals here tend to value potential benefits to their relatives and descendants, which IRBs might not consider. As Albert, the policeman with the HD mutation, explained,

> My mother died, and her body is in the Midwest somewhere, just sitting there. Does that bother me? No. If they think it can help research down the road, I don't mind. My blood was taken because they need research, and it goes off somewhere.

He is not sure where or why, but this ignorance does not perturb him.

Many interviewees acknowledge potential risks, including possible violation of confidentiality, but feel that the benefits to other individuals outweigh these concerns. Benjamin, for example, the engineer with Alpha, gave his blood to a DNA databank.

> A lot of people said, "Why are you doing this?" and need more protection so their names don't get out. They want to remain anonymous. That's just not me. This DNA bank might help. I don't think it can hurt. I suppose the information could be compromised, but it wouldn't bother me. I suppose somebody could make a lot of money on it, and steal it. But I trust them.

He considered, weighed, and ultimately dismissed these objections. If a company might profit financially from such research, he would still participate, but would wish that any therapeutic benefits would then be inexpensively distributed. "If they said, 'We're going to make a lot of money out of it,' I'd want a commitment that they're going to try to make it readily available."

Simone, the bookkeeper with the HD mutation who learned of the disease only after getting engaged, saw research participation as an ethical mandate of community members and was angry at individuals, including even those in her own family, who declined.

> I was annoyed at my father for not wanting to get involved. That was very selfish. If you have HD, and there's nothing you can do, at least get involved in research and do your own little bit.

Nonetheless, not everyone wants to participate in studies. Patty, for instance, who pushes her risk "under a rug," "would not volunteer, because I don't want to be a guinea pig. And I react differently than a lot of people." She cites two reasons—not wanting to be experimented on, and being biologically atypical.

Gauging herself in her body sculpting class, the possibility of having HD also still terrifies her. For her, these fears and potential risks outweigh potential community benefits, loyalties, or needs.

Political Action

Given the relative newness, the miscomprehension, and the potential discrimination of genetics, many organizations also develop and propose public policy. But here, too, challenges arise. Such policies usually concern Medicare, Medicaid, insurance, and treatment.

Genetic communities can exert pressure on professional and governmental leaders, pushing for a variety of interventions to help patients, and motivating members to become more politically active. But these organizations may have only limited or uncertain power and effectiveness. Nonetheless, such activities can feel very gratifying and empowering. "I picked up the political stuff as a challenge," Jennifer, with Alpha, said. "It really felt good to contribute in that way. It strengthens me." Mounting economic pressures can further the political activities and needs of these organizations and individuals. As Dorothy, the former TV producer, added, "We had our first advocacy day in Washington. Medicare was going to cut medication payments. We got an exemption on Prolastin. Only three drugs got it. That was exciting!" Such activities aimed at shaping legislation can serve to help both oneself, psychologically, and the organization.

These communities can also push to change public images about diseases. Dorothy added,

> We can't use the term "A1AD." No one knows it, so no one cares. We came up with the name "Alpha," and use it in public information. And we've got to get rid of self-destructive terminology. We can't use the words emphysema or cirrhosis. People think: smoking and alcohol—you've done it to yourself.

Thus, organizations can help reverse negative images of a diagnosis helping patients and the broader public. Groups can also alter stereotypes of who gets a disease. As Bonnie, the 24-year-old without testing or symptoms whose sister had breast cancer, said,

> A lot of breast cancer organizations give an image that it's only an older woman's disease. One organization doesn't, and says it can happen at *any* age: 17 and 18. It's important to get rid of that other image.

Yet despite these needs, individuals vary dramatically in *how* involved in these ways they want to be, or feel comfortable being. Patients may agree with the legislative goals, but not feel at ease "going public" or being politically engaged. Such overt activities may be especially difficult for HD, given its psychiatric symptoms and potentially higher stigma.

Patients must also balance a sense of obligation to the group against competing demands and preferences (e.g., desires for solitude). "I'm more quiet, not so active," said Rhonda, the nurse with breast cancer and a mutation. "Except if I'm asked to call a newly diagnosed person."

These men and women must decide, too, how much time to devote to the disease as opposed to other aspects of their lives. "I try not to make it my be-all and end-all," Rhonda added. These limits may be based on these individuals' own needs or those of their family versus those of non-kin. Some people strive to aid their own immediate family rather than the broader community. Smaller, tangible efforts may be more rewarding. In addition, certain people simply dislike meetings and groups. As Karl concluded, "The biggest help I can now be is personal: just helping my brother."

FACTORS INVOLVED

Given these complex and competing issues, individuals vary in their community engagements, related to several factors, such as disease state. Serious or debilitating symptoms can thwart some or all of these endeavors, forcing hard choices.

Genetic communities can differ, too, based on aspects of each specific disorder. Psychiatric symptoms, for instance, can impair social interactions. Hence, individuals with HD may be less politically active, given cognitive and psychiatric problems and higher stigma. Wilma, with both breast cancer and bipolar disorder, compared the value and nature of the support groups for each of these diagnoses.

> I get the mood disorder newsletter, and have gone to some lunches, but don't care for their support groups. You sit around and get dragged down. But the breast cancer support group is very uplifting. We are just buddies: you want to see what my breast surgery looks like, I'll show you. So we close the door, and I show you. With the mood disorder, a lot of the people have self-esteem problems, which I don't.

Community involvements can reflect and shape identities to differing extents. Many want a community, but not an identity, or vice versa. Some people become integral parts of a disease community, which powerfully shapes their sense of self. Yet the boundaries between individuals and communities can be fluid, porous, or ambivalent. People face quandaries about how and where to erect boundaries. Karen, the lawyer with breast cancer, said,

> Do I feel part of the breast cancer community or cancer community? Yes and no. I've done Race for the Cure, where survivors wear pink t-shirts and everyone else wears white. I always feel weird wearing a pink one. In some ways, it's very nice: I can "out" myself. But I walked into a restaurant, and saw someone I knew.

She then had to explain why she was wearing that shirt.

As we saw earlier, illness can represent a whole or only a part of one's life—giving meaning to as opposed to consuming one's life. Even online, individuals make choices of how engaged to be. Denise, with breast cancer, bases her involvement on how helpful she thinks she can be. "I read message boards a lot, but don't post anything unless somebody has a question that I know a lot about," she said. Since she works for a bank that may read employees' emails, she is extra-cautious.

Seeing Sicker Patients: Acceptance versus Denial

These communities can generate deep ambivalence when individuals observe sicker patients with the same illness. Sufferers are thrown together, fostering both bonds and tensions. Individuals range in the degrees to which they accept or minimize or deny their illness, affecting how much they want to participate. At times, anxieties and discomfort expressed themselves through humor. "You're in an exclusive club," Charles, the accountant, said, "that nobody wants to belong to, if they had a choice."

Seeing more advanced cases of one's own disease can be terrifying. Some people may even avoid going to clinics, because patients there may be sicker. Mary, with early symptoms of HD, said, "I don't even like sitting in the waiting room, because I don't want to see my future."

Evidence of others' treatment side effects can be disturbing, too. Jennifer, who described her first Alpha meeting as "a high," nevertheless said, "People I met are not in very good shape now. I can only have so many death announcements around me."

Observing others who are more or less sick can make one feel either better or worse about oneself. Healthier patients can stimulate depression and jealousy. Patients compare their relative degrees of illness, at times making themselves feel better, even if it represents schadenfreude—that is, based on the suffering of others. Awkwardness can result, as individuals may not be able to disguise their distress or glee. Sherry, the waitress with breast cancer but no family history or mutation, explained,

> One woman in the group is not going to make it. She's had three ovarian cancer surgeries, and got cancer again. I said, "I've had four breast surgeries." She said, "You beat me. I'll never feel sorry for myself again!" I thought, "But *I'm* going to make it." Still, she got a lift from knowing she hadn't had as many surgeries as me.

Individuals struggle with deciding when they have witnessed "too much" disease in others, and modulate their involvement, balancing benefits against psychological burdens. Relatively healthy, asymptomatic individuals at risk may shirk support groups because of fears of seeing worse symptoms. Such exposures may in fact feel psychologically harmful, forcing tradeoffs between support and fear. Patty, who sweeps her HD risk "under the rug," said, "The support group is depressing, so I ignore it. The people there are really ill. It's almost *worse* for me. I'd rather live in my own little world, than with these shattered lives."

For patients with Alpha, immunocompromised from treatment, exposure to others can in fact exacerbate disease. Such patients may thus eschew these interactions even more. Betty, the designer with Alpha, does not go to "big meetings." She is afraid of "getting a germ, traveling, being around strangers."

Individuals may also be wary of fellow patients' anger, fear, or depression. Others' psychiatric symptoms can generate stress, with which patients might not cope well or directly. Frustrated patients may displace their rage onto others. As Sherry reported,

> The first time I went to the yoga class through this breast cancer organization, two of the women started arguing over which way to place the mats. Then, I went to the clay class, and one woman made a one-and-a-half breasted woman, and started to cry.

Sherry stopped attending.

An Internet community, too, can force participants to confront stresses more than they want. Even a listserv can be upsetting. "On the e-list they do a lot of griping," Jennifer said. "So I took my name off."

Desires for Anonymity

Varying wishes for privacy and anonymity also shape subsequent decisions about community involvements. To join an organization can necessitate divulgence of personal information, mutations, disease, and other stigmatizing aspects of one's life. People differ in how they weigh concerns about these risks to privacy against the possible benefits of engagement. On the one hand, concerns about privacy may be relatively low. Benjamin, the engineer who lost his job when his employer realized he could go on disability due to Alpha, acknowledged but accepted the costs of openness. "Everybody has things they want to keep private, but I've always been open," he said. "I have a big mouth, shoot from the hip, and tell you what I think. Politically, it's not too savvy."

Instead, as indicated earlier, many others seek anonymity. Even Denise, the banker who discussed on the web anal fissures she received from chemotherapy, draws a line, remaining unidentified in these interchanges. Discomfort and embarrassment about anal lesions may also contribute to physician silence on the topic. She weighs altruistic sharing against desires to maintain privacy and avoid shame: "When anybody wanted detailed information about anal fissures, I never gave out my phone number or screen name."

Such online anonymity provides both benefits and limitations. Non-identifiability has advantages in facilitating discussions of taboo topics. Denise continued, "Discussion boards are great because you're anonymous, and can tell people the real down and dirty side of it: *You make up a name.*"

Outside the web, one may not know these other persons, thereby preserving confidentiality. Other individuals make finer-grained choices of where and when exactly to draw the line, identifying themselves in some, but not all, types of communication.

Yet even with promises of anonymity, online interactions about genetic risk may feel too personal. Isabelle, the social worker with breast cancer and a mutation, said,

> Being anonymous was good about the Internet—you can go to a message board and have tons of people in your same situation. Yet how much are you going to expose yourself? I go there once in a while. I look at research studies, but don't converse with anyone. I'm not in touch with any people specifically. I don't go to chats. I subscribe to a breast cancer network listserv. It sends you news. I once went to a chat to see what it was like. A few people seemed very nice, but it's just not my thing. It's too personal.

Over time, maintaining anonymity while communicating about deeply personal experiences can also become increasingly hard. Threats to confidentiality can occur from not only fellow website visitors, but others. As we saw earlier, men and women face challenges at the workplace, sending or receiving emails about medical issues, and even visiting disease websites. As Denise, the banker, reported, "Everything you write can go through the company's Compliance Division."

Responsibilities to Communities

Patients also have to balance obligations to the community versus to themselves and other aspects of their lives. "I do the support group, but it's not my life," explained Rhonda, the nurse with breast cancer and a mutation. "They did help me when I was going through it, so it's the least I could do."

However, this sense of obligation can clash with other personal needs, and individuals may wish at a certain point to reduce their voluntarism, which can consume substantial amounts of time. Patients must then decide how to weigh time with these communities against other priorities. But clear limits can be difficult to erect and maintain. Rhonda continued, "Sometimes I feel: why do I put myself out like this? If I get busy, I think, 'I have too much going on!'"

Individuals confront dilemmas of *how long* to remain involved after initial diagnosis. They can feel threatened, seeing sicker patients, yet feel badly deserting them. Karen, the lawyer, said,

> *How much cancer is too much cancer?* I'm debating whether to stop. I didn't have a real desire to continue with those people. But I still go once a week. Some of the most interesting things that have happened to me have been seeing the different ways in which people die.

Internal Politics

Both within and between groups, organizational missions can conflict, creating stress. Members may view differently the nature or function of any one organization, leading to clashes. Generally, the majority of members, or the antecedent mission of the group, prevail. But given individual and organizational shifts, members of an association may also self-select to stay or not. Jennifer, who felt the Alpha meeting was "a high," later took her name off the e-list and became more aware of the nuanced pros and cons of such organizations.

> The support group has become important to some people, and not to others. Some come once or twice, are very angry, and attack people who don't agree with them. That's not how I see this group.

For these organizations, multiple foci and agenda can produce inter-group synergy, complementarity, and linkages or tension. One organization may promote research, while another may establish support groups. They can collaborate, mutually assisting each other, or fight for resources. "Two organizations used to bicker," Dorothy elaborated. "Now, they are joined at the hip."

Even groups addressing the same disease can end up battling. Benjamin said about such conflicts regarding Alpha,

A couple of organizations seem to be butting heads. One was more focused on supporting the individual, the other on finding a cure. Now, one is severely in debt. If one didn't help, it was killing the other. If it did help, it was taking over.

Other sociodemographic issues can produce strains as well. For instance, questions emerge as to whether some support groups may too exclusively represent certain patient characteristics—age, ethnicity, or social class. Hilda, the African American home health aide with breast cancer, questioned the diversity, outreach, and perceived openness of some organizations, including medical institutions. "At *other* hospitals, people come in and talk to you," she reported. "When I was in the last hospital, nobody did that. They don't give support, or books. Nobody comes, or tries to help."

Genetic Communities versus the Outside World

Genetic communities can have complex, complementary, or conflictual relationships with outsiders as well. Patients may observe tensions between these communities and unaffected individuals, including mutation-free family members. Outsiders can either encourage or discourage community engagements, and pressure patients to increase or decrease these activities. External observers may not appreciate the benefits of these communities and may be wary or antagonistic. Jan's sister told her to focus less on breast cancer groups.

My sister cannot comprehend anything I have gone through. She says, "You're so boring, all you do is go to breast cancer seminars. Everything is: cancer. *Get a life!*" I tried to explain. She said I've just given up. She can't understand that this *is* my life. When I was diagnosed, she couldn't help me. She said, "Oh my God, it's going to happen to me next!"

This sister's reaction may thus result from her own anxieties, but nonetheless creates stress.

Changes Over Time

Over months or years, interactions with a disease community can evolve. Many people become involved initially and then less so over time. Yet these temporal alterations are not always wholly planned or controllable; relationships can take on a life of their own. Ori said about a telephone buddy with whom a patient organization had paired her:

> At the beginning, we would call each other every week, sometimes twice a week. Then I felt less need to call, and she'd leave me alone. In the beginning, we talked at least 50 or 60 times. Now, it's monthly, or every two months. She stays on the phone until I want to get off. That's taxing, because I don't know when it's polite to get off . . . "Oh, how are the kids?"

Roles can change from assigned patient "buddies" to "friends," yet questions then emerge as to responsibilities in these new relationships. Beyond a certain point, individuals may in fact continue difficult involvements, and must then balance these against other needs. Betty said, regarding Alpha,

> I liked going to support groups, but then had enough. It's probably more detrimental to me to be surrounded by this, than not. Recently, a woman in the group had a lung transplant. She seemed good, but then did badly and died. She was forty-something.

Individuals may change not only what activities they engage in but how they do so. For instance, individuals may initially enter online groups anonymously, but subsequently choose to reveal their identities. Dilemmas then surface of whether and how to transition from unnamed to named, and what to do if these decisions are not wholly mutual. Individuals can wrestle with the pros and cons, feeling uncertain. Denise, the banker, said,

> I go to Internet support sites, but not support groups. I was very active on the boards, and we had a get-together at a restaurant. People were talking about who's coming. I would watch that thread, but not put anything down. I wasn't going to commit. That morning, it was raining. I really wanted to go, but was afraid people would look really sick. I looked pretty healthy. A friend said, "You can always leave." So, I went. We had so much fun. I never laughed so hard. I didn't have my wig anymore at that point, but the women still in wigs all exchanged them. People who had brown hair were putting on the blonde wigs; the long wig for short wigs. A couple

of women had their husbands there, who put on the wigs. Then, every-body took their wigs off at once.

Yet even here, tensions between identity and anonymity quickly arose. These individuals each suddenly had to decide how to proceed.

> In the restaurant, we decided to have name tags. Initially, it was just going to be pseudonyms, but everybody ended up writing their real name. A lot of the pseudonyms were nicknames they had as children, or their cats' or children's name: like, "David's mom" or "Sunshine." It's part of people's identity—just not their given name.

Over time, groups may evolve and develop new functions or structures. Specialized organizations can form for particular niches—for example, for young breast cancer survivors. As Bonnie, the 24-year-old, reported: "On other organizations' websites, I didn't see pictures of 22-year-olds. I couldn't relate to that, or say, 'Wow, that's me.'" Such organizations can sprout spontaneously from the ground up. She continued,

> A group of friends found a support system. We're professionals. One's a lawyer. They're not just housewives with nothing better to do. It became *a network system*. "You know who else has cancer? My coworker."

This subgroup was based in part on socioeconomic status, and expanded over time as each new member knew other potential members, creating a network.

IMPLICATIONS

As suggested, genetic communities can help patients cope and make health decisions regarding testing, treatment, disclosure, and research participation. These groups affect these decisions both directly and indirectly. For instance, genetic communities can help one accept and disclose one's disease more widely. Jennifer explained, "Since I have become comfortable in the Alpha community, I now tell everyone. The first Alpha-1 conference I went to, everyone wore a little button. 'Alpha-What?'"

Communities can provide language and vocabulary for disclosing and understanding the disease—even specifics of how to talk about it. Further disclosure can assist in coping and strengthening the degrees to which patients incorporate their genetic risk into their sense of identity. Jennifer added,

I learned how to talk about it in a way that people can handle. I say I have "genetic emphysema." That's better than "Alpha-1 Antitrypsin Deficiency." I don't want to get into a whole big conversation with somebody who isn't going to understand.

CONCLUSIONS

These men and women reveal how genetic communities range widely in structures and functions, with groupings varying from formal to informal, online to in-person, large to small, anonymous to public, and rigid to fluid. Prior research has suggested several advantages and disadvantages to patient groups,[9] but the individuals here highlight areas that have received less attention, concerning how patients actually make decisions about these possible involvements, what tensions they face, and how they often struggle in weighing these and vary in doing so over time. Patients confront choices between in-person support groups, one-on-one phone interactions, online chat rooms, and message boards—each with pros and cons, and complex relationships to each other. People differ in when and how they enter these communities, how involved they become, and for how long they remain. These individuals and communities grapple with how to weigh anonymity versus the need for information, and how to assess whom to trust. Anonymity can make the quality of available online information hard to judge. As a result, over time, these communities evolve, with both individuals and organizations shifting to meet changing needs, modulating their activities. Groups form anew or refocus.

Involvement in these communities requires a certain degree of acceptance—as opposed to denial or minimization—that these engagements can in turn further enhance. Similarly, participation can beget added involvement, creating a positive feedback loop. These patients suggest a process of *socialization* as they enter and become part of these groups, altering both their inner and outer worlds—their identities and social networks.

Yet individuals may enter too late, or leave too early, reducing the benefit they may otherwise accrue. Individuals may also reach a point at which they perceive that the harms (seeing sicker patients) outweigh the benefits (support). They may weigh, too, perceived moral responsibilities to aid others against individual psychological costs.

Given at-risk relatives, patients may view the risks and benefits of research participation differently when confronting diseases that are strongly associated with genetic markers as opposed to other disorders. Providers, patients, family members, and others need to know about these community sources of potential support. Broad education is vital, since individuals may be unaware that they are at risk and may be able to benefit from these organizations. Clinicians should also be aware of these complex issues, in order to assist patients and family members in making decisions about these groups, which can potentially affect testing, treatment, and quality of life.

Further efforts are needed to better understand how communities might most assist individuals, and individuals might make most use of these groups. Past studies have tended to focus on just one type of organization rather than the wide assortment from which people choose. Thus while some investigators have compared participants and nonparticipants of a particular type of group, future research can also examine participants of different kinds of groups (e.g., online versus in-person). Differences may emerge due to logistics and other issues.

Moreover, communities and clinicians can potentially work better together, yet it is unclear how physicians view and interface with these associations—whether, when, and how often providers refer patients to such organizations. Dissatisfied patients, more than others, may promulgate their opinions in such groups.

On-line, given rapidly evolving scientific understandings, websites face challenges in optimizing both the quality and anonymity of postings. Needs exist for quality control—for mechanisms to correct any errors. Consumer, provider, and governmental groups or standards can potentially help. As the amount of genetic information expands, physicians, either individually or through professional bodies or governmental agencies, could monitor websites and help them provide the most accurate, user-friendly information.

These men and women thus illuminate the complex tensions within genetic and other communities that many of us may one day encounter.

CHAPTER 12

"Testing Everyone?":

Gene Politics

The individuals in this book reflected on their experiences to try to help others facing similar predicaments, and suggested many implications for broader social and political institutions. They spontaneously discussed these ramifications, pondering how not only they and their families but society as a whole should confront genetic risks. In so doing, they considered several types of policies that could affect genetics.

As we saw, many mistrust confidentiality protections or do not grasp the full details. Assessing privacy regulations is difficult. This confusion, perhaps deliberately created by insurance companies, leads many people to view privacy laws warily. Generally, these individuals sensed they had few, if any, options.

Ultimately, many perceived only one solution: universal health care. Given their genetic risks, they saw broad benefits to such universal coverage, extending to many aspects of their lives. Barbara, the part-time professor with Alpha, argued, "You should be able to have insurance, lead your life, find out your purpose, and have a chance at whatever your life path is." President Barack Obama's health care reform legislation of 2010 will surely help address many concerns about pre-existing conditions. But as of this writing, many details concerning the implementation and enforcement of this legislation remain unclear. The men and women here highlight the need for ongoing attention to these issues.

SCREENING

These individuals also voiced strong views concerning policy debates about whether to widen genetic testing or screening. Some here are aware of the possible broad public health benefits, and feel that more testing should be done since it could potentially help save lives. As Carmen, the Latina, said, "Doctors should check genetic testing for everybody, not just for cancer, but for all medical problems, to see what defects you have in your genes, so they could correct them." The fact that she had breast and thyroid cancer and a mutation shaped her views.

Yet these attitudes may at times be ill-informed, and not always fully reflect the possible complexities involved. Carmen suggests an ability to "correct" these mutations, which is generally not yet the case. Barbara, a former smoker, added—more realistically—about Alpha,

> All kids should be tested for Alpha, because you can make lifestyle choices early. I made the wrong ones. There probably are dangerous insurance implications. And if you're a kid, and your parents find out you have something incurable, it's tough.

But she still feels that the pros of wider screening outweigh the cons.

Benjamin, the engineer, thinks that smokers should all be screened for Alpha, though he recognizes the potential controversies involved.

> I don't know if smokers would agree to it. I probably would not have agreed to it, when I smoked. But people are now identified when they've already lost a lot of lung function, not when they're *starting* to lose it.

He feels that the advantages to patients who would be identified override the potential political problems involved.

He appreciates the importance of individual rights, but remains unswayed. "We've got to be very careful with screening, but people can then make the right smoking decisions," he said.

A few argued that more assays should be performed for HD as well. Roger, who tested mutation-positive, said,

> More people should be tested for Huntington's, but a lot of people just aren't ready. When I first saw my genetic counselor, he told me I *shouldn't* get tested. But if you're having early signs, you should at least get in touch with a Huntington's group.

Questions arise about screening for other diseases as well—for example, hemochromatosis, which affects 10% of the population.

Yet others are far more cautious about widespread probing. Several feel that genetic testing is appropriate only if patients could then act on the information in some way. Rachel, with breast cancer and a mutation, said that she "wanted to find out, because maybe there's something I can do . . . I have two young children. If my future was only about me, I might not have tested." She wanted to help her family—even if she was not clear how.

Others support increased screening to eliminate a mutation from the population. But they, too, had generally not thought through the full implications. "If you can remove the HD mutation," said Kate, the former nurse with Alpha, "it's much better." She does not see the possible problems of eugenics here—the potential slippery slope.

Others more readily acknowledged these complicated tradeoffs. Peter, the retired businessman now leading an Alpha support group, cited other potentials for exploitation of the information—not eugenics—though still favoring wider Alpha testing. "The earlier you learn about it, the better," he said. "But you have to protect against corruption and misuse of the information."

Another potential problem with screening concerns false positives and negatives, and determinations of what rates of these are acceptable. As Simone, the bookkeeper with the HD mutation, pointed out, a "false positive rate of three in 1,000 is still not great, if you're going to tell someone: life or death." But what error rate would legitimize broader evaluation is not clear. Complex tradeoffs and political decisions are involved here.

Some recommend wider testing that would not be mandated by policy makers, but encouraged and adopted by patients and communities more informally. In various social worlds, individuals frequently seek to persuade others to test. Gilbert, the factory worker, for example, advises smokers to be checked. "If I encounter a smoker, even casually, I will encourage them to get an Alpha test," he said. "Maybe it will give somebody that last little bit of incentive to stop smoking."

GENETIC DATABASES

Many law enforcement and elected officials continue to seek the establishment of large genetic databanks for apprehending and convicting criminals, posing additional social and ethical quandaries. Such proposals spark anxieties about potential violations of confidentiality. Interviewees expressed concern that existing DNA research banks could be subpoenaed, and searched to discover identities of perpetrators or others. Simone, familiar with private industry, added,

> You could track down criminals, but now schools want test results, too. They would look and say, "This person is going to have HD. I'd better send a little note to my buddy at the insurance company." And then they don't

give the person insurance. *If you open a door, you never know what's going to come out.* You introduce legislation for a certain reason, and 20 years down the road, it's twisted. It sounds great to have the DNA for finding criminals, but they can't take care of people in prisons now, anyway.

Still, if the predictive accuracy of assays increases, views of some of these issues might change. She continued, "It should be more up to the person, if they want to get tested. In 20 years, if they can tell you that in two years you're going to get sick, it would make more sense to find out."

HOPES FOR RESEARCH

Genetic communities actively encourage research and hope, galvanizing resources. But how fast genetic research will proceed, and how soon a cure will be developed for HD or other disorders, is unclear. The timetable, whether years or decades, is unknown. Many people see great promise from science, but also hazards. Barbara, the part-time professor and former smoker who was "relieved" to learn she had Alpha, remained optimistic: "They're working on stem cell research . . . a baby could be helped in the future—maybe not in my generation, but in several generations." She readily accepts the long-term frame of scientific progress. More individuals will have more information about their fate. But even she recognizes the double-edged sword. What people will do with that information—whether it will be good or bad—remains unknown. She continued,

Everybody should live with the knowledge of their own death. But it's going to cause problems for the haves and have-nots. Rich people could get three livers. Our society is going to need more equal access.

Further skepticism arises, too, about these potential gains. Given her neuroscience training and familiarity with the slow pace of research, Antonia thinks that a cure for HD is far off. She is struck by how much scientists still do not know.

For 10 years, we have known that the disease results from just one gene. But we still don't know what the gene *does*. Without it, mice die, so it's needed. But we still don't know its normal function.

Still, overall, even nonscientists here remain sanguine about research. Karl perceived impressive advances in scientists' abilities to pinpoint disease causes.

"It's a *miracle*," he said, "that you can glimpse into the human genome. Ultimately, that is going to be incredibly valuable to all people."

As mentioned earlier, many feel, altruistically, that participating in research is therefore important. They recognize that genetics is still experimental, but they are undeterred.

Nonetheless, several remain wary about too much genetic tampering. Some feel cautious, for instance, about cloning and stem cell research. Bill, the salesman who cares closely for his HD-affected brother, said, "You're screwing with Mother Nature. Understanding genetics is great. But once you mix genes, and clone sheep, you don't know the repercussions."

Others are cautious about specific details involved in conducting research. For instance, long informed consent forms may end up not being user-friendly or well-understood. Still, other interviewees, such as Charles, the accountant with Alpha who had worked for a major corporation, understood the needs of researchers in industry and elsewhere.

> The forms are too long, but that's the way they are. I don't have a problem with everybody protecting themselves, as long as it's not at my expense. And if there are potential downsides to a study, I want to know.

Individuals thus view these issues in widely diverging ways based on a range of personal, professional, and medical factors.

Researchers Testing Samples in the Future

Increasingly, new tests will be conducted in the future on DNA collected in the past. Yet such assays pose additional conundra—who should own these samples, how useful will these tests be, and who should receive the results? Many of the men and women here would want to know the findings of such future tests conducted on their DNA—an integral part of themselves. Interviewees felt, too, that researchers should disclose future test results to past research participants, since these data may be important to know. Jan, with breast cancer but no mutation, said, "Researchers should tell me. If they're doing a genetic test, and are not going to tell me, I should know why."

Carol, who chose prophylactic surgery despite her boyfriend's opposition, would also want to be notified about future tests, because she thinks these might aid her. "If they found something that would benefit me, and didn't tell me, I would be really *mad*." She recognizes the possible logistical impediments to contacting research participants from years earlier, but feels that these barriers would not necessarily exist ("I haven't moved in 15 years").

Yet such tests may yield only very slight, if any, direct benefit, and may be experimental. The results may not be replicable, and the tests may not be run in standardized government-certified labs. The results may be only minimally significant, and very difficult to interpret.

Though some are wary of such future tests without notification of patients, others support it, accepting the limitations of alternatives. Charles, with Alpha, downplayed potential problems:

> I just gave blood to a study, and allowed them to keep it as long as they want, and use it for whatever they want. I don't have any problem with that. I can't imagine why anybody would.

He cannot even conceive of reasons for caution.

Individuals may support such future testing since they have already been diagnosed with a major disorder. Yvonne doesn't care about future tests on her genetic samples—in part because she already has Alpha: "I'm already sick, so it doesn't matter with me."

Other people may be uninterested in the results in part because these can be threatening. Vera said that her siblings gave blood for breast cancer research, but did not want to learn the results.

> One sister said, "Why do you need to know? The test wasn't available 20 years ago, and people still lived and died. Why put myself through the anguish of trying to decide what to do if I have the gene?"

In part, Vera feels her siblings simply would not be able to "handle the news well."

Altruism—stemming from the fact that such future testing might aid subsequent patients—could legitimize researchers not disclosing these results. Some people would prefer to know, but would forego that right if other patients were being helped. Bonnie, having seen breast cancer in her mother and sister, said, "If 50 years down the line they could find a cure because I gave blood—fine. I *should* know. But if they just want to keep testing the blood, that's fine." She valued altruism over her own rights.

Others support future testing, but would want to know the outcome, because they are interested in science.

Still others expressed caveats, seeing a clear tradeoff: they would let their DNA be used for future studies because it may help others, as long as confidentiality is protected. Gilbert said, regarding Alpha,

> I give carte blanche permission for researchers to look at my blood any time in the future. If I'm contributing to the solution of a problem, go

ahead. But confidentiality is the key. I would not give that up. As long as you don't reveal my name, rank, and serial number, I don't have a problem.

Until now, many researchers and IRBs have concurred that DNA donors will simply *not* be told the results. But patients may nevertheless *want* to know. It remains unclear what exactly the threshold for notification should be, given the diversity of preferences and beliefs. Further public discussion is essential.

IMPLICATIONS FOR EDUCATION

These men and women also highlight ways of enhancing education about genetics. Providers need to increase their knowledge and sensitivity concerning these issues. Beatrice, the math teacher who had breast cancer along with her sister, but no mutation, described an inadvertently callous physician her sister had encountered.

> The resident was just not very nice or comforting. When my sister came back to the hospital having to go through surgery again, he said, "What are you doing here?" My sister said, "I have to come back for another mastectomy." He said, "Shit happens!" My sister was very upset by that. It was very insensitive.

Clinicians may also need to become more attentive to the diverse psychological and ethical issues that patients and their family members face in testing, disclosure, and reproductive decisions. In many regards, these issues differ from those posed by other diseases. Here, providers need to assist and communicate with not just one "index" patient, but broader families who may require help as well. Chloe added,

> Doctors should talk to caretakers, along with the actual patient. It's really hard for the caretaker. I help my nephew do his homework, because my sister can't, due to HD. Doctors should talk to the whole family.

These interviewees reveal needs for increased public education about genetics as well, but dilemmas emerge of what and how much to say at what level. The public needs more information, but may not be interested—unless they feel it directly impacts them. As Albert, the policeman with the HD mutation, said, "If it doesn't affect you, people just aren't interested. If they're not aware of genetic problems in their family, most don't care about it." For breast and ovarian cancer, given the relatively high prevalences, more public education is especially critical since many at-risk individuals do not know that genetic testing exists. Public understanding of cancer as a whole is improving, but could be further enhanced.

Yet tensions arise, since heightened information about genetics could fuel unrealistic expectations—which have already begun to surface—about the "power" of the field. Sarah, the computer programmer with a family history of breast cancer, but no symptoms or mutation, said,

> A lot of people assume that there's one single magic cure coming—like with smallpox vaccination. But for breast cancer, the treatments are horrible—being unable to walk, bathe yourself, or control your bowels.

CONCLUSIONS

Confronting their genetic risk shapes how these men and women view not only their own lives, but how they view broader social policy and educational issues as well. Their experiences affect their perspectives on public debates about health care reform, broad population screening, genetic databases sought by law enforcement officials and schools, and future research on DNA samples. These individuals underscore the pressing need for more education of patients, providers, and the public at large. The newness of the field, the rise of the Internet, and other social phenomena all make genetics both personal and far more broadly social, affecting one's immediate as well as larger worlds. These men and women do not always agree on what specific policies are needed—but they all see wide social repercussions of their struggles.

PART VI

Conclusions

CHAPTER 13

Genes in Everyday Life

We have come to the end of our odyssey, but in many ways, it is, of course, just a beginning. I have charted these individuals' journeys to illustrate how genetics shapes multiple issues in their lives. I have raised more questions than I have wholly answered, but that has been part of my intent: to illuminate the wide range of complexities and challenges that genetics can pose, to help ready us—as individuals and as a broader society—for the onslaught of genetic information that is fast approaching, whether we want it or not.

Many of us—whether as patients, family members, friends, coworkers, employers, neighbors, providers, policy makers, or citizens—will increasingly confront genetic information, however ambiguous and incomplete, about ourselves and others. This information will have various degrees of predictiveness, as well as social, psychological, and ethical implications. Unfortunately, the growth of this information is far outpacing our abilities to fathom its meaning and impact. This knowledge should be used to maximize benefits and minimize harms. But how exactly to do that is unclear.

In the meantime, each year innumerable people consider and proceed to obtain genetic tests. They interpret these in highly subjective ways based on their personal and cultural beliefs, values, and agendas. Both public health priorities and commercial enterprises are propelling much research and practice. Gene patenting has unleashed industrial interests that seek profit from tests, and thus "oversell" the predictiveness and potential clinical value of certain assays, further confusing patients.

Importantly, these interviewees each struggle to make sense of the genetic risks they confront in individual ways, drawing on their own personal, medical, and familial histories. Initially, I had assumed that patients would see genetic information more similarly to the way physicians do—primarily as objective. Yet in fact, these men and women view it far more subjectively than I had anticipated—in many ways that have not been described before.

The number of domains that genetics impacts surprised me—from birth to death, personal to social identity, and work to love, fate, luck, and religion. Genetics shape these men and women in multiple and at times conflicting ways, affecting virtually all aspects of their lives. These individuals each embark on different—but related—voyages. They face quandaries concerning testing, disclosing to families and others, understanding genetics, integrating this information into their identity, and deciding about treatment, reproduction, and involvements in patient communities. In each of these domains, multiple gray areas loom. These men and women were themselves astonished at the breadth of the implications they had to confront. Providers, too—even genetic counselors—often appeared ill prepared to handle this wide array of issues. Yet increasing numbers of people confront genetic testing decisions each day, highlighting the importance of beginning to address these concerns more fully.

Across these broad realms, several key underlying characteristics of genetics interact. The field is new and filled with uncertainties about future probabilities that can be interpreted in myriad ways. This knowledge affects not just single patients, but multiple family members—past, present, and future—and can lead to discrimination, at times subtle and unprovable. These and other characteristics shape a series of decisions that in turn mold each other.

Beliefs about the degree to which a disease has a genetic component can frame decisions about testing and treatment. Within a family, disclosure of genetic risk by one person can beget further divulgences. Conversely, silence and ignorance perpetuate each other. A patient's community engagements can prompt and result from testing, understandings of genetics, and disclosures to families and others. Disease organizations can impact testing, treatment, and reproductive decisions. Whether and when people test affects when and how they tell their family, have children, and participate in patient organizations. Whether they tell family members can shape whether these members then test or screen embryos.

People confront and address these dilemmas in intricate social contexts that can profoundly influence these decisions. Clinicians, families, and communities play crucial roles in identifying additional patients. Particularly for rare diseases, these social inputs can be vital. Individuals respond to both broad social and political phenomena (for example, media coverage of genetics), as well as specific local contexts of families, friends, and work. These diverse worlds are closely interlinked, and hence need to be seen and addressed in integrated ways by clinicians, patients, families, and others.

Some critics have been very wary of the advent of genetic information. As indicated by the titles of recent books such as DNA: Promise and Peril[1] and The Troubled Helix[2] many scholars view genetics with great caution, while countless scientists seem to embrace it, and companies invest hundreds of millions of dollars into it.

The interviewees here echo both sides of this debate, often in unique ways. These men and women tend to grasp that complexities exist, even if, like scholars, they are unable to fully resolve all of these intricacies. They are not wholly swayed by genetic determinism, but tend to have innate faith in their ability to shape their fate in some way.

Many of these people feel that genetic testing has in fact helped them. Those with Alpha are relieved to learn they have a mutation, because they can now be treated. Their relief may be akin to that which future patients may experience through pharmacogenetics—though it is too early to know how predictive and effective such future tests will be. At the same time, in confronting these paradoxes, the individuals here receive input from a variety of people who often fail to appreciate these stresses.

In their daily lives, genetics presents these men and women with additional quandaries, embodying broader, long-standing issues and conflicts about determinism versus free will, nature versus nurture, and science versus the soul.

Since antiquity, questions of how we confront key aspects of our biological nature—the fact of death, and the raw power of potentially destructive emotions within us—have troubled writers and philosophers. From Plato to Freud, authors have probed conflicting parts of our selves. Like these thinkers, patients here struggle to grasp the degrees to which they can control the biological forces inside them. Clearly, in many ways, we are products of our genes. Yet these individuals illuminate the difficulties of grappling with what that means—to be molded by genes and other phenomena. Resistance to genetic determinism reflects not only the roles of possible environmental factors, but deep yearnings for freedom, hope, and control. To conceptualize these tensions between our innate biology and our beliefs in our own agency is daunting.

Few of these individuals adopt wholly deterministic views. Rather, almost all opt for combinations, based in large part on their other needs. To think of oneself as the product of genes is both counterintuitive and disturbing. Generally, these men and women feel that their lives are not exclusively determined by biology. Granted, environmental factors play important roles for most diseases and traits, but people also don't want to believe that their genes control them. These interviewees manifest persistent and inextinguishable desires to avoid despair, fatalism, and anxiety, and find narrative coherence, meaning, and hope.

Yet at the same time, people tend to draw a line in the sand, believing that in the end, the disease they confront is mostly genetic or not—that is, that they can or cannot control it, and do or do not need to worry about it. But these decisions are not easy—is a 15% chance of disease a lot or a little? Does it warrant undergoing PGD to select embryos without the genetic marker? Black or white, all-or-none scenarios seem easier and more comfortable than coping with shades of gray. Yet our own genetics may make it difficult for us to understand our genes. The ways our brains have evolved—our desires for control and lucid answers, and our fears of disease—can impede our open-mindedness. Cognitively, people tend to want one cause—a culprit. To figure out how to parse blame is far more onerous. Thus, these individuals frequently try to find a unified view in some way, to integrate these competing perspectives. They attempt to mediate conflicts (e.g., between desires for control versus realities of mutation-positive tests) by trying to draw lines between genetic determinism and other causes. They seek to make distinctions—for example, that genes determine whether but not when or how severely they will get sick, or whether anything can be done about it, and if so, what. People seek "wiggle room"—even for HD. They then wrestle with what aspects of each disease result from each cause, to what degree, and with what implications.

But genetics is presenting us as individuals and as a society with far more information than we know how to process. In many ways it is asking too much of patients—to comprehend complex data that scientists and physicians cannot yet fathom. In part, the field is a moving target. Each month, research uncovers new facets of how our genes operate, interact with each other and the environment, and mold key parts of our bodies. Similarly, for millennia scientists have sought to chart the universe, countless details of which remain mysterious. When Columbus first landed, he thought he had reached India. Subsequent voyages over decades slowly revealed the contours of two continents, and the full landscape took hundreds of years to map. The complete explanation of genetic mechanisms and their effects will also surely take decades, if not centuries. Hence, newly identified genetic markers that contribute to our makeup, but have less predictiveness—say 10% or 20%, rather than 50% or 100%—may pose more rather than fewer challenges, and be more rather than less difficult to grasp.

The interviewees here strive to understand the cause of these diseases, elucidating a fundamental human drive: to understand the roots of events that befall us. Yet the bases of disease can be multiple, complex, and elusive. Nonetheless, given severe shortages of genetic counselors, physicians and other providers will need to aid patients and families in grappling with these questions. Families and friends can benefit by learning how to approach these issues as well.

In some regards, these questions resemble the conclusions of the philosopher Daniel Dennet—that we should consider what particular aspects of free will we care about and want to uphold. But the real-life situations here underscore the emotional—as opposed to philosophical—underpinnings of these tensions. Over the past century, philosophical questions about free will may have received more attention than those about causation, but that imbalance may now need to shift. The psychological needs chronicled here mold many crucial decisions. While some scholars abhor genetic determinism in the media, as if these depictions wholly decide and reflect prevailing social views, the men and women here are fortunately wary of such determinism—in part due to these competing needs and beliefs.

These individuals offer insights, too, on issues extending beyond genetics alone to broader underlying aspects of the human condition—how we view and make sense of ourselves, and seek meaning. While certain theorists highlight culturally constructed concepts of disease and identity, the men and women here draw on not only broad cultural and social categories but also unique personal and familial experiences, and biological phenomena. These factors will no doubt continue to influence how people perceive genetics—that is, based on not just cultural or political structures, but individual needs. These individuals also illuminate how certain aspects of biology are more open to subjective interpretations. These interviewees develop senses of personal epidemiology, taking into account *who* gets sick—how many family members, who they are, and what specific factors (genetic or biological) may be involved. They confront and try to make sense of several biological phenomena, and choose *which* medical events to focus on, frequently based on prior beliefs. Yet as these medical events evolve, so, too, do these views. People here tend to see themselves in ways that are not wholly socially constructed, essentialist, or biological, but rather simultaneously draw on various social, personal, and biological aspects of themselves, creating intricate collages on their own. Interpretations of tests, symptoms, and diagnoses in oneself and one's family are subjective, but choices of biological phenomena on which to focus are not unlimited—test results almost always reveal that a mutation, whatever its predictiveness, is or is not present.

Genetics also raises profound existential issues that have received relatively little attention in this context. Discovery that one possesses a mutation can challenge one spiritually and religiously. Around the globe, as science advances, many individuals turn to metaphysics for meaning. Religion and spirituality emerge here as integral to notions of fate, attempts to understand genetics and answers to questions of "why me" and whether to meddle with perceived destiny through assisted reproductive technologies—creating life, and therefore "playing God." Many of these interviewees try to fit genetics into their prior spiritual and religious beliefs—for example, that God must have wanted them to have a mutation. These men and women suggest free-floating sets of metaphysical beliefs about destiny—"what is meant to be." These beliefs often involve superstitions, not necessarily connected to any specific religion. Rather, these beliefs seem in some ways similar to pagan and ancient Greek conceptions of fate, antedating the major organized religions. These notions also appear to reflect a will to wholeness, and a desire for temporal coherence in one's life.

Similarly, while psychologists such as Daniel Kahneman and Amos Tversky have examined through experiments issues of risk aversion, here, in the rich fabric of people's lives, these issues appear fully intertwined with other phenomena. These interviewees often compare not risk of loss versus possibility of gain (as in many experiments), but two or more relative risks (e.g., the chance of disease recurrence versus the likelihood of harmful side effects from prophylactic surgery). These individuals balance and make utilitarian choices—for example, accepting threats to themselves over those to their offspring. Altruism—testing for the benefit of one's children—can trump risk aversion.

Moreover, these interviewees suggest how rational choice theories more broadly tend to downplay the roles of factors such as fear, hope, horror, superstition, and magical thinking that emerge here as important. While the philosopher Søren Kierkegaard described the vast existential terror of jumping into the void concerning the existence of God, the individuals here make difficult, frightening existential leaps concerning fate and the ultimate causes of their disease. They suddenly find themselves surrounded by vagaries and doubts about the sources of key aspects of their very lives.

Whereas many historians and philosophers of science describe scientists as "constructing" interpretations of phenomena in various ways, the nonscientists here act both similarly and differently. These patients do not primarily seek truth (as do scientists), but instead pursue health. Hence, as goals in making sense of genetics, these men and women seek—far more than do scientists—to avoid stress, depression, and anxiety; to resolve dilemmas about testing, disclosure, treatment, and reproduction; and to obtain social support. While Michel Foucault and others have illustrated how historical epochs shape perspectives on disease, individual patients here frame their views based on a wide range of personal factors and needs as well.

While health belief models and theories of reasoned action seek to explain objective health behaviors, these interviewees often draw on highly subjective notions—for example, about luck and God. These beliefs in turn affect their decisions and senses of self. Research has been conducted on the roles of religion in medicine, often using numeric scales to assess religiosity,[1] but the men and women here highlight the knotty ambiguities of these realms, defying easy statistical analyses. Many concepts here are exceedingly elusive, if not impossible, to measure quantitatively. But analyses of patients' narratives, as suggested in these pages, can reveal crucial portions of their lives.

As such, these men and women illustrate the importance of perspectives from the humanities and social sciences. These interviewees' own words best convey their experiences. Hence, they highlight needs to pay more attention to language and narratives in medicine, and to draw on the social sciences and the humanities in other ways as well. With science burgeoning, and more colleges and universities underfunding and deemphasizing the liberal arts, it is vital not to lose sight of the inherent subjectivity involved in how we incorporate scientific knowledge into our daily lives. Genetic researchers are giving us more data than we may want or know how to use, creating confusion. How we should employ this information is highly individual. Yet unfortunately, the vast majority of research on coping and other psychological aspects of responses to illness are quantitative. Hence, key phenomena may be missed.

These men and women underscore, too, limitations in language concerning a variety of terms. They confront abstract genetic concepts that they often do not understand, but that nonetheless profoundly shape their lives. Established vocabulary fails to capture the full meanings, implications, and boundaries of genes. Existent terms do not wholly fit experiences: these men and women do not feel wholly "sick," "diseased," "disabled," or completely "healthy." Rather, they strive to redefine themselves, often in unique, amalgamated ways. They struggle to assess if mutations in fact cause their disease, what that means, and whom or what to blame. Deep ambiguities emerge regarding terms such as "fate," "luck," "predisposition," "self," "disclosure," "closeness," "privacy," "secrecy," "trust," "family," "kin," "friend," "altruism," and "community."

A critic may argue that the experiences here refer only to risks for particular conditions, and consequently have little, if any, pertinence to the choices other individuals will face in the future concerning less predictive genetic tests. Arguably, questions about causality, blame, and sharing test results may make sense only with highly predictive tests.

Clearly, these issues vary somewhat with the specific type of disease—for example, chronic versus acute, rare versus common, treatable versus fatal, and those involving psychiatric or visible symptoms as opposed to those that do not. "Genetic disease" is not monolithic. Rather, the diversity of disorders displayed here sheds light on a wide range of both similarities and differences. For instance, since Alpha is less prevalent, it is often missed as a diagnosis. Doctors do not always know to test for it, yet treatment is available. For breast cancer, especially for those who have a mutation but no symptoms, these issues can be more abstract: decisions surface about whether to undergo prophylactic surgery based on possible future symptoms that in fact may never occur. HD produces severe psychiatric problems and lacks treatment, posing additional challenges. These diseases generate many common concerns, but also some differences, as shown.

Indeed, in many ways, HD—the first human disease for which a genetic marker was identified—has not been a very generalizable model. HD is very predictable, following straightforward patterns of Mendelian genetics, and affects patients at the same age as their parents. For most people confronting a disease for which a genetic marker has been identified, HD is in many ways an anomaly. But the experiences here are still valuable in and of themselves, revealing how people respond to the quandaries and stresses posed by at least certain kinds of genetic information. Moreover, we do not yet know whether combinations of mutations (perhaps in conjunction with certain environmental factors) may be found in the future that will be somewhat predictive of additional diseases for which single markers have not yet been identified. As further genetic research in conducted and applied, it behooves us to be prepared for such diverse scenarios.

The term "genetic disease" is also in itself problematic, often used to cover a wide range of disorders that result, to highly ranging degrees, from genetics as opposed to environmental or other factors. In the case of breast cancer, one of two mutations have been found in about 10% of cases and, if present, contribute to the disease approximately 50% of the time. Mutations have been found to be associated with Alzheimer's and other diseases even more rarely. Each such disease may thus be genetic for some patients, but not others. Eventually, with ongoing research, scientists may come to identify subtypes of these diseases that result from different sets of factors. Breast cancer in which *BRCA* mutations are present may turn out to differ from cases where the mutations are absent. Until then, using the term "genetic disease" can be problematic, given such complex diseases of mixed cause.

Diseases with an identified genetic marker differ from other disorders in several ways—for example, having more explicit implications for future generations, and affecting more directly not only one individual, but his or her family as well. With other disorders, a person's illness may upset one's family, and thus impact their health indirectly. But genetics can implicate these kin far more, highlighting biological links that in turn shift social bonds and moral responsibilities. The individuals here, more directly than those confronting other kinds of disease, appear to value benefits to future generations over potential harms to themselves. But they also confront quandaries concerning how much exactly to help their kin, and whether to push family members to engage in testing, treatment, or preventive health measures.

Surely, individuals who test for other genetic markers, especially in other cultures, will differ in various ways from the men and women here, but the experiences here are noteworthy even by themselves. These experiences may also have critical relevance in the future, even if in as yet unclear ways. Among future patients confronting genetic data about themselves, similar challenges may well emerge. In upcoming years and decades, patients will no doubt continue to encounter difficulty in making sense of this information, and view it in highly subjective ways that may differ from how physicians perceive it. Future tests that predict disease less fully may indeed be harder, not easier, to grasp. Many people will inevitably use or misconstrue or misuse this information in a variety of ways. People will no doubt continue to, struggle to grasp, interpret, and integrate this knowledge into their stories and notions about themselves and their past experiences, reconstructing or maintaining their identities, deciding whether to test, and to divulge the information to others. Individuals with less education will most likely encounter additional obstacles as well.

Increasingly, healthy people without known genetic risks may confront whole genome sequencing by their physicians and direct-to-consumer marketing of tests. When these individuals develop symptoms, testing, as it improves and advances from sampling only tiny bits of chromosomes to assaying the whole genome itself, may begin to provide results that are more informative than at present concerning various disorders and treatments, even if only partly so. Moreover, as suggested earlier, combinations of three or four genetic markers, at times in conjunction with various environmental factors, may prove more predictive than many current tests, increasing even more the importance of issues presented here. Even if some of the biggest challenges here shift as science advances, these narratives will, I anticipate, remain vital, in the very least, as presenting a valuable and unique snapshot in time. The tales here shed crucial light on how people are responding at a transformative juncture in the history of science and society, revealing, for instance, how searches for personal meaning trump scientific understandings alone.

Importantly, these men and women suggest the need to expand discussions from whether genetics is hyped or not to how we should best prepare for increasing amounts of genetic data that we will no doubt confront in upcoming years—in whatever muddled and incomplete forms it takes.

We need to prepare for these challenges now—to avoid pitfalls and misunderstandings as much as we can.

These interviews have implications for public policy as well. Testing needs to be optimized—to be made available to those whom it might help. But how exactly to do that is unclear. Presently, doctors under-test for relatively rare diseases (such as Alpha and hemochromatosis, which can be treated), while direct-to-consumer marketing appears to seek to over-test for common diseases for which genetic tests provide little if any useful information. Given the complexities here, education of policy makers, providers, and the public at large about these issues is crucial.

The need to make testing more widely available and affordable poses issues of justice, too. Insurance companies should expand their coverage of testing without discrimination. Life and disability insurance should become more flexible and available. Justice may also dictate that governmental regulations require health care insurers to cover a certain amount of reproductive technologies for some patients. Insurance companies may argue that they have other priorities, but unfortunately, profit-making is one of these. Still, to decide how much coverage, and for whom and when, will be hard. For instance, PGD may make sense for HD, but not for many other diseases. These issues will require careful ongoing attention.

These phenomena have additional implications for clinicians as well. For instance, it is not clear how providers do or should assess what exactly patients have disclosed to at-risk family members. More cases may directly pose questions of whether providers ever have a responsibility to notify third parties (i.e., family members) of genetic risks, and if so, when.

We should fully neither embrace the hype around genetics nor dismiss the field—but rather, as individuals and a society, carefully judge how best to proceed. Given the inherent ambiguity of genetics, we will continue to struggle to make sense of this knowledge and construct, frame, and negotiate meanings. As the men and women here suggest, the ways in which people respond will reflect and affect many aspects of their lives. We will draw on our understandings, misunderstandings, and uncertainties about science, personal experiences, cultural myths, desires for hope and control, and wishes to avoid anxiety and despair.

Rapidly advancing genetic research will confront us with ever-new complexities, dilemmas, ambiguities, and tensions. The experiences of the individuals here can help us prepare.

CHAPTER 1

1. Steenhuysen J. "Consumer gene test results misleading: U.S. probe." *Reuters*. July 22, 2010. http://www.reuters.com/article/idUSTRE66L5QF20100722. Accessed June 28, 2011.
2. Gibson DG, Glass JI, Lartigue C, et al. "Creation of a bacterial cell controlled by a chemically synthesized genome." *Science* 329(5987) (2010): 52–56.
3. Rothman, BK. *The Book of Life: A Personal and Ethical Guide to Race, Normality and the Human Gene Study*. Boston, MA: Beacon Press, 2001.
4. Geertz C. *Interpretation of Cultures: Selected Essays*. New York: Basic Books, 1973.
5. Harper B. "Huntington disease." *Journal of the Royal Society of Medicine* 98(12) (2005): 550.
6. Harper PS. "The epidemiology of Huntington's disease." *Human Genetics* 89(4) (1992): 365–376.
7. Oveson L, Yarborough M. "Aspen report: 'ethical issues in occupational genetics.'" The Ramazzini Institute for Occupational and Environmental Health Research 2(2) (2001). http://www.ramazziniusa.org/apr01/geneticp. Accessed May 21, 2008.
8. Jones NL, Smith AM. *Genetic Information: Legal Issues Relating to Discrimination and Privacy*. CRS Report for Congress. Washington, D.C.: Congressional Research Service: Library of Congress, 2005.
9. Laurell CB, Erikson S. "The electrophoretic alpha1 globulin pattern of serum in alpha antitrypsin deficiency." *Scandinavian Journal of Clinical and Laboratory Investigation* 15(2) (1963): 132.
10. Rachelefsky G, Hogarth DK. "Issues in the diagnosis of alpha 1-antitrypsin deficiency." *Journal of Allergy and Clinical Immunology* 121(4) (2008): 833–838.
11. Browne BS, Rozalinde J, Mannino DM III, et al. "Alpha 1-antitrypsin deficiency deaths in the United States from 1979–1991: an analysis using multiple-cause mortality data." *Chest* 110(1) (1996): 78–83.
12. Campos MA, Wanner A, Zhang G, et al. "Trends in the diagnosis of symptomatic patients with alpha-1-antitrypsin deficiency between 1968 and 2003." *Chest* 128(3) (2005): 1179–1186.

13. Stolk J, Seersholm N, Kalsheker N. "Alpha-1 antitrypsin deficiency: current perspective on research, diagnosis, and management." *International Journal of Chronic Obstructive Pulmonary* Disease 1(2) (2006): 151–160.

14. Stolk J. "Case detection of alpha-1 antitrypsin deficiency: does it help the patient or the doctor?" *European Respiratory Journal* 26(4) (2005): 561–652.

15. Sveger T, Thelin T, McNeil TF. "Neonatal Alpha-1 antitrypsin screening: parents' views and reactions 20 years after the identification of the deficiency state." *Acta Paediatrica* 88(3) (1999): 315–318.

16. World Health Organization. "Global strategy for the diagnosis, management, and prevention of chronic obstructive pulmonary disease." *Global Initiative for Chronic Obstructive Lung Disease* (2006). http://www.who.int/respiratory/copd/GOLD_ WR_06.pdf. Accessed June 16, 2008.

17. American Thoracic Society. "American Thoracic Society/European Respiratory Society statement: standards for the diagnosis and management of individuals with Alpha-1 Anti-trypsin deficiency." *American Journal of Respiratory and Critical Care Medicine* 168 (2003): 818–900.

18 "Cancer facts and figures." *American Cancer Society* (2009): 9–11. http:// www.cancer.org/docroot/STT/content/STT_1x_Cancer_Facts__Figures_2009.asp. Accessed May 27, 2010.

19. Hall JM, Lee MK, Newman B, et al. "Linkage of early-onset familial breast cancer to chromosome 17q21." *Science* 250(4988) (1990): 1684–1689.

20. Wooster R, Neuhausen SL, Mangion J, et al. "Localization of a breast cancer suscep- tibility gene, BRCA2, to chromosome 13q12–13." *Science* 265(5181) (1994): 2088– 2090.

21. "BRCA1 and BRCA2: Cancer Risk and Genetic Testing." National Cancer Institute (2009). http://www.cancer.gov/cancertopics/factsheet/Risk/BRCA. Accessed May 27, 2010.

22. Saslow D, Boetes C, Burke W, et al. "American Cancer Society guidelines for breast screening with MRI as an adjunct to mammography." *CA: A Cancer Journal for Clinicians* 57(2) (2007): 75–89.

CHAPTER 2

1. Kessler S, Field T, Worth L, Mosbarger H. "Attitudes of persons at risk for Huntington disease toward predictive testing." *American Journal of Medical Genetics* 26(2) (1987): 259–270.

2. Markel DS, Young AB, Penney JB. "At-risk persons' attitudes toward presymptom- atic and prenatal testing of Huntington disease in Michigan." *American Journal of Medical Genetics* 26(2) (1987): 295–305.

3. Mastromauro C, Myers RH, Berkman B. "Attitudes toward presymptomatic testing in Huntington disease." *American Journal of Medical Genetics* 26(2) (1987): 271– 282.

4. Meissen GJ, Berchek RL. "Intended use of predictive testing by those at risk for Huntington disease." *American Journal of Medical Genetics* 26(2) (1987): 283–293.

5. Creighton S, Almqvist EW, MacGregor D, et al. "Predictive, pre-natal and diagnos- tic genetic testing for Huntington's disease: the experience in Canada from 1987 to 2000." *Clinical Genetics* 63(6) (2003): 462–475.

6. Hayden M. "Predictive testing for Huntington's disease: the calm after the storm." *The Lancet* 356(9246) (2000): 1944–1945.

7. Cox SM. "Stories in decisions: how at-risk individuals decide to request predictive testing for Huntington disease." *Qualitative Sociology* 26(2) (2003): 257–280.

8. Wexler NS. "Presymptomatic testing for Huntington's disease: Harbinger for the new genetics." In Bankowski Z, Caprons AM, eds. *Genetics, Ethics and Human Values: Human Genome Mapping, Genetic Screening and Gene Therapy.* Geneva, Switzerland: CIOMS, 1991.

9. Quaid K, Brandt J, Faden R, Folstein, S. "Knowledge, attitude, and the decision to be tested for Huntington's disease." *Clinical Genetics* 36(6) (1989): 431–438.

10. Evers-Kiebooms G, Decruyenaere M. "Predictive testing for Huntington's disease: a challenge for persons at risk and for professionals." *Patient Education and Counseling* 35(1) (1998): 15–26.

11. Meissen G, Mastromauro CA, Kiely DK, McNamara DS, Myers RH. "Understanding the decision to take the predictive test for Huntington disease." *American Journal of Medical Genetics* 39(4) (1991): 404–410.

12. Robins-Wahlin TB, Backman L, Lundin A, Haegermark A, Winblad B, Anvert M. "High suicidal ideation in persons testing for Huntington's disease." *Acta Neurologica Scandinavica.* 102(3) (2000): 150–161.

13. Quaid K, Morris M. "Reluctance to undergo predictive testing: the case of Huntington disease." *American Journal of Medical Genetics* 45(1) (1993): 41–45.

14. Baum A, Friedman AL, Zakowski SG. "Stress and genetic testing for disease risk." *Health Psychology* 16(1) (1997): 8–19.

15. Struewing JP, Lerman C, Kase RG, Giambarresi TR, Tucker MA. "Anticipated uptake and impact of genetic testing in hereditary breast and ovarian cancer families." *Cancer Epidemiology, Biomarkers & Prevention* 4(2) (1995): 169–173.

16. Brunger JW, Murray GS, O'Riordan M, Matthews AL, Smith RJH, Robin NH. "Parental attitudes toward genetic testing for pediatric deafness." *American Journal of Human Genetics* 67(6) (2000): 1621–1625.

17. Lerman C, Hughes C, Trock BJ, et al. "Genetic testing in families with hereditary nonpolyposis colon cancer." *The Journal of the American Medical Association* 281(17) (1999): 1618–1622.

18. Jacobsen PB, Valdimarsdottir HB, Brown KL, Offit K. "Decision-making about genetic testing among women at familial risk for breast cancer." *Psychosomatic Medicine* 59(5) (1997): 459–466.

19. Lerman C, Narod S, Schulman K, et al. "*BRCA1* testing in families with hereditary breast-ovarian cancer." *The Journal of the American Medical Association* 275(24) (1996): 1885–1892.

20. Prochaska JO, DiClemente CC, Norcross JC. "In search of how people change: applications to addictive behavior." *American Psychologist* 47(9) (1992): 1102–1114.

21. Houlihan GD. "The evaluation of the 'stages of change' model for use in counselling client's undergoing predictive testing for Huntington's disease." *Journal of Advanced Nursing* 29(5) (1999): 1137–1143.

22. Taylor SD. "Predictive genetic test decisions for Huntington's disease: elucidating the test/no-test dichotomy." *Journal of Health Psychology* 10(4) (2005): 597–612.

23. Littell JH, Girvin H. "Stages of change: a critique." *Behavior Modification* 26(2) (2002): 223–273.

24. Rosenstock IM, Strecher VJ, Becker MH. "Social learning theory and the health belief model." *Health Education Quarterly* 15(2) (1988): 175–183.

25. Fang CY, Dunkel-Schetter C, Tatsugawa ZH, et al. "Attitudes toward genetic carrier screening for cystic fibrosis among pregnant women: the role of health beliefs and avoidant coping style." *Women's Health* 3(1) (1997): 31–51.

26. Folkman S, Lazarus RS. "An analysis of coping in a middle-aged community sample." *Journal of Health and Social Behavior* 21(3) (1980): 219–239.

27. Gooding H, Organista K, Burack J, Bowles Biesecker B. "Genetic susceptibility testing from a stress and coping perspective." *Social Science & Medicine* 62(8) (2006): 1880–1890.

28. Wilson TD. "On user studies and information needs." *Journal of Documentation* 37(1) (1981): 3–15.

29. Miller SM. "Monitoring and blunting: validation of a questionnaire to assess styles of information seeking under threat." *Journal of Personal Social Psychology* 52(2) (1987): 345–353.

30. Case DO, Andrews JE, Johnson JD, Allard S. "Avoiding versus seeking: the relationship of information seeking to avoidance, blunting, coping, dissonance and related concepts." *Journal of the Medical Library Association* 93(3) (2005): 48–57.

31. Shiloh S, Ben-Sinai R, Keinan G. "Effects of controllability, predictability, and information-seeking style on interest in predictive genetic testing." *Personality and Social Psychology Bulletin* 25(10) (1999): 1187–1195.

32. Van Zuuren FJ, Wolfs HM. "Styles of information seeking under threat: personal and situational aspects of monitoring and blunting." *Personality and Individual Differences* 12(2) (1991): 141–149.

33. Tversky A, Kahneman D. "The framing of decisions and the psychology of choice." *Science* 211(4481) (1981): 453–458.

34. Kahneman D, Tversky A. "Judgment under uncertainty: heruristics and biases." *Science* 185(4157) (1974): 1124–1131.

35. Gifford SM. "The meanings of lumps: a case study of the ambiguities of risk." In Janes, C, Stall, R, Gifford, SM, eds. *Anthropology and Epidemiology: Interdisciplinary Approach to the Study of Health and Disease (Culture, Illness and Healing)*. Boston: Reidel., 1986.

36. Goffman E. *Stigma: Notes on the Management of Spoiled Identity*. Englewood Cliffs, NJ: Prentice-Hall, 1963.

37. Downing C. "Negotiating responsibility: case studies of reproductive decision-making and prenatal genetic testing in families facing Huntington's disease." *Journal of Genetic Counseling* 14(3) (2005): 219–234.

38. Sher C, Romano-Zelekha O, Green MS, Shohat T. "Factors affecting performance of prenatal genetic testing by Israeli Jewish women." *American Journal of Medical Genetics* 120A(3) (2003): 418–422.

39. Freedman AN, Wideroff L, Olson L, Davis W, et al. "US physicians' attitudes toward genetic testing for cancer susceptibility." *American Journal of Medical Genetics* 120A(1) (2003): 63–71.

40. Cho MK, Sankar P, Wolpe PR, Godmilow L. "Commercialization of BRCA1/2 testing: Practitioner awareness and use of a new genetic test." *American Journal of Medical Genetics* 83(3) (1999): 157–163.

41. Parsons T. "On the concept of influence." In Parsons, T. *Sociological Theory and Modern society*. New York: Free Press, 1967.

42. Meiser B, Dunn S. "Psychological impact of genetic testing for Huntington's disease: an update of the literature." *Journal of Neurology, Neurosurgery & Psychiatry* 69(5) (2000): 574–578.

43. Beck AT, Brown G, Berchick RJ, Stewart BL, Steer RA. "Relationship between hopelessness and ultimate suicide: a replication with psychiatric outpatients." *The American Journal of Psychiatry* 147(2) (1990): 190–195.

44. Broadstock M, Michie S, Marteau T. "Psychological consequences of predictive genetic testing: a systematic review." *European Journal of Human Genetics* 8(10) (2000): 731–738.

45. Tibben A, Duivenvoorden HJ, Vegter-van der Vlis M, et al. "Presymptomatic DNA testing for Huntington disease: identifying the need for psychological intervention." *American Journal of Medical Genetics* 48(3) (1993): 137–144.

46. Decruyenaere M, Evers-Kiebooms G, Cloostermans T, et al. "Predictive testing for Huntington's disease: relationship with partners after testing." *Clinical Genetics* 65(1) (2004): 24–31.

47. Brain K, Soldan J, Sampson J, Gray J. "Genetic counselling protocols for hereditary non-polyposis colorectal cancer: a survey of UK regional genetics centres." *Clinical Genetics* 63(3) (2003): 198–204.

48. Chase GA, Geller G, Havstad SL, Holtzman NA, Bassett SS. "Physicians' propensity to offer genetic testing for Alzheimer's disease: results from a survey." *Genetics in Medicine* 4(4) (2002): 297–303.

49. Menasha JD, Schechter C, Willner J. "Genetic testing: a physician's perspective." *The Mount Sinai Journal of Medicine* 67(2) (2000): 144–151.

50. Sifri R, Myers R, Hyslop T, et al. "Use of cancer susceptibility testing among primary care physicians." *Clinical Genetics* 64(4) (2003): 355–360.

51. Wideroff L, Freedman AN, Olson L, et al. "Physician use of genetic testing for cancer susceptibility: results of a national survey." *Cancer Epidemiology, Biomarkers & Prevention* 12(4) (2003): 295–303.

52. Graham J, Maugh TH. "Mammogram guidelines spark heated debate." *Los Angeles Times*. November 17, 2009. http://www.latimes.com/news/nationworld/nation/la-na-mammogram17-2009nov17,0,3942708.story. Accessed January 20, 2011.

53. Appelbaum PS, Roth LH, Lidz C. (1982). "The therapeutic misconception: informed consent in psychiatric research." *International Journal of Law & Psychiatry* 5(3-4), 319–329.

54. Aktan-Collan K, Mecklin JP, de la Chapelle A, Peltomäki P, Uutela A, Kääriäinen H. "Evaluation of a counselling protocol for predictive genetic testing for hereditary non-polyposis colorectal cancer." *Journal of Medical Genetics* 37(2) (2000): 108–113.

55. Harper PS, Lim C, Craufurd D. "Ten years of presymptomatic testing for Huntington's disease: the experiences of the UK Huntington's Disease Prediction Consortium." *Journal of Medical Genetics* 37(8) (2000): 567–571.

56. Sermon K, De Rijcke M, Lissens W, et al. "Preimplantation genetic diagnosis for Huntington's disease with exclusion testing." *European Journal of Human Genetics* 10(10) (2002): 591–8.

57a. Simpson SA, Harper PS, United Kingdom Huntington's Disease Prediction Consortium. "Prenatal testing for Huntington's disease: experience within the UK 1994–1998." *Journal of Medical Genetics* 38(5) (2001): 333–335.

57b. Stern HJ, Harton GL, Sisson ME, et al. "Non-disclosing preimplantation genetic diagnosis for Huntington disease." *Prenatal Diagnosis* 22(6) (2002): 503–507.

58. Forrest K, Simpson SA, Wilson BJ, et al. "To tell or not to tell: Barriers and facilitators in family communication about genetic risk." *Clinical Genetics* 64(4) (2003): 317–326.

59. Evers-Kiebooms G, Welkenhuysen M, Claes E, Decruyenaere L. "The psychological complexity of predictive testing for late onset neurogenetic diseases and hereditary cancers: implications for multidisciplinary counseling and for genetic education." *Social Science & Medicine* 51(6) (2000): 831–841.

60 Keats J. "To George and Thomas Keats, December 21, 27 (?), 1817." In *Selected Poems and Letters*. Boston, MA: Houghton Mifflin, 1959.

61. Hundert EM. "A model for ethical problem solving in medicine, with practical applications." *American Journal of Psychiatry* 144(7) (1987): 839–846.

62. Fins JJ, Miller FG, Bachetta MD. "Clinical pragmatism: Bridging theory and practice." *Kennedy Institute of Ethics Journal* 8(1) (1998): 37–42.

CHAPTER 3

1. Sobel S, Cowan D. "Impact of genetic testing for Huntington disease on the family system." *American Journal of Medical Genetics* 90(1) (2000): 49–59.

2. Sorenson JR, Jennings-Grant T, Newman J. "Communication about carrier testing within hemophilia A families." *American Journal of Medical Genetics* 119C(1) (2003): 3–10.

3. Green J, Richards M, Murton F, Statham H, Hallowell N. "Family communication and genetic counseling: the case of hereditary breast and ovarian cancer." *Journal of Genetic Counseling* 6(1) (1997): 45–60.

4. Forrest Keenan K, Simpson SA, Wilson BJ, et al. "'It's their blood not mine': who's responsible for (not) telling relatives about genetic risk." *Health Risk and Society* 7(3) (2005): 209–226.

5. Lerman C, Peshkin BN, Hughes C, Isaacs C. "Family disclosure in genetic testing for cancer susceptibility: determinants and consequences." *Journal of Health Care Law & Policy* 1 (1998): 353–372.

6. Wilson BJ, Forrest Keenan K, van Teijingen ER, et al. "Family communication about genetic risk: the little that is known." *Community Genetics* 7(1) (2004): 15–24.

7. Ayme S, Macquart-Moulin G, Julian-Reynier C, Chabal F, Giraud F. "Diffusion of information about genetic risk within families." *Neuromuscular Disorders* 3(5-6) (1993): 511–514.

8. Suslak L, Price DM, Desposito F. "Transmitting balanced translocation information within families: a follow-up study." *American Journal of Medical Genetics* 20(2) (1985): 227–232.

9. Julian-Reynier C, Eisinger F, Chabal F, et al. "Disclosure to the family of breast/ovarian cancer genetic test results: patient's willingness and associated factors." *American Journal of Medical Genetics* 94(1) (2000): 13–18.

10. Fanos JH, Johnson JP. "Barriers to carrier testing for adult cystic fibrosis sibs: the importance of not knowing." *American Journal of Medical Genetics* 59(1) (1995): 85–91.

11. Tercyak KP, Hughes C, Main D, Snyder C, Lynch JF, Lynch HT, et al. "Parental communication of *BRCA 1/2* genetic test results to children." *Patient Education and Counseling* 42(3) (2001): 213–224.

12. Tercyak KP, Peshkin BN, Tiffani A, et al. "Parent-child factors and their effect on communicating *BRCA 1/2* test results to children." *Patient Education and Counseling* 47(2) (2002): 145–153.

13. Hughes C, Lerman C, Schwartz M, et al. "All in the family: evaluation process and content of sisters' communication about *BRCA 1/2* genetic test results." *American Journal of Medical Genetics* 107(2) (2002): 143–150.

14. Peterson SK. "The role of the family in genetic testing: Theoretical perspectives, current knowledge, and future directions." *Health Education & Behavior* 32(5) (2005): 627–639.

15. Plantinga L, Natowicz M, Kass N, Chandros S, Gostin L, Faden R. "Disclosures, confidentiality, and families: experiences and attitudes of those with genetic versus nongenetic medical conditions." *American Journal of Medical Genetics* 119C(1) (2003): 51–59.

16. Klitzman R. *Being Positive: The Lives of Men and Women With HIV.* Chicago: Ivan R. Dee, 1997.

17. Klitzman R, Bayer R. *Mortal Secrets: Truth and Lies in the Age of AIDS.* Baltimore, MD: Johns Hopkins University Press, 2003.

18. Dudok deWit AC, Meijers-Heijboer EJ, Tibben A, et al. "Effect on a Dutch family of predictive DNA-testing for hereditary breast and ovarian cancer." *The Lancet* 344(8916) (1994): 197.

19. Rosenstock IM, Strecher VJ, Becker MH. "Social learning theory and the health belief model." *Health Education Quarterly* 15(2) (1988): 175–183.

20. Goffman E. *Stigma: Notes on the Management of Spoiled Identity.* Englewood Cliffs, NJ: Prentice-Hall, 1963.

21. Parsons T. *The Social System.* London: Routledge and Kegan Paul, 1951.

22. Buckner F, Firestone M. "'Where the public peril begins': 25 years after Tarasoff." *The Journal of Legal Medicine* 21(2) (2000): 187–222.

23. Offit K, Groeger E, Turner S, Wadsworth E, Weiser M. "The 'duty to warn' a patient's family members about hereditary disease risks." *The Journal of the American Medical Association* 292(12) (2004): 1469–1473.

24. Palner J, Mittelmark MB. "Differences between married and unmarried men and women in the relationship between perceived physical health and perceived mental health." *Norwegian Journal of Epidemiology* 12(1) (2002): 55–61.

25. Pienta AM, Hayward MD, Jenkins KR. "Health consequences of marriage for the retirement years." *Journal of Family Issues* 21(5) (2000): 559–586.

26. Osborne C, Ostir GV, Du X, Peek MK, Goodwin JS. "The influence of marital status on the stage at diagnosis, treatment, and survival of older women with breast cancer." *Breast Cancer Research and Treatment* 93(1) (2005): 41–47.

27. Sherbourne CD, Hays RD. "Marital status, social support and health transitions in chronic disease patients." *Journal of Health and Social Behavior* 31(4) (1990): 328–343.

28. Sherbourne CD, Meredith LS, Rogers W, Ware JE. "Social support and stressful life events: age differences in their effects on health-related quality of life among the chronically ill." *Quality of Life Research* 1(4) (1992): 235–246.

29. Booth A, Johnson D. "Declining health and marital quality." *Journal of Marriage and the Family* 56(1) (1994): 218–223.

30. Wikrama KAS, Lorenz FO, Conger RD, Elder Jr. GH. "Marital quality and physical illness: a latent growth curve analysis." *Journal of Marriage and the Family* 59(1) (1997): 143–155.

31. Hollingshead AB. "Cultural factors in the selection of marriage mates." *American Sociological Review* 15(15) (1950): 619–627.

32. South SJ. "Sociodemographic differentials in mate selection preferences." *Journal of Marriage and the Family* 53(4) (1991): 928–940.

33. Belot M, Francesconi M. "Can anyone be 'the' one? Evidence on mate selection from speed dating." Institute for the Study of Labor, University of Bonn (2006).

34. Li NP, Bailey JM, Douglas TK, Linsenmeier JAW. "The necessities and luxuries of mate preferences: testing the tradeoffs." *Journal of Personality and Social Psychology* 82(6) (2002): 947–955.

35. Surra CA. "Research and theory on mate selection and premarital relationships in the 1980s." *Journal of Marriage and the Family* 52(4) (1990): 844–865.

36. D'agincourt-Canning L. "Experiences of genetic risk: disclosure and the gendering of responsibility." *Bioethics* 15(3) (2001): 231–247.

37. Bok S. *Lying: Moral Choice in Public and Private Life.* New York: Vintage, 1999.

38. Nyberg D. *The Varnished Truth.* Chicago, IL: University of Chicago Press, 1995.

Chapter 4

1. Klitzman R, Daya S. "Challenges and changes in spirituality among doctors who become patients." *Social Science & Medicine* 61(11) (2005): 2396–2406.

2. Klitzman R. *When Doctors Become Patients.* New York: Oxford University Press, 2008.

3. Kleinman A. *The Illness Narratives: Suffering, Healing, & the Human Condition.* New York: Basic Books, 1988.

4. Kuhn T. *The Structure of Scientific Revolutions.* Chicago, IL: University of Chicago Press, 1996.

5. Shiloh S, Rashuk-Rosenthal D, Benyamini Y. "Illness causal attributions: an exploratory study of their structure and associations with other illness cognitions and perceptions of control." *Journal of Behavioural Medicine* 25(4) (2002): 373–394.

6. Henderson BJ, Maguire BT. "Three lay mental models of disease inheritance." *Social Science & Medicine* 5(2) (2000): 293–301.

7. Wulff H. "Comments on Hesslow's 'What is genetic disease?'" In L Nordenfelt, BIB Lindahl, eds., *Health, Disease and Causal Explanations in Medicine.* Dordrecht: D. Reidel, 1984: 195–197.

8. Weil J. "Mothers' postcounseling beliefs about the causes of their children's genetic disorders." *The American Journal of Human Genetics* 48(1) (1991): 145–153.

9. Shiloh S. "Illness representations, self-regulation, and genetic counseling: a theoretical review." *Journal of Genetic Counseling* 15(5) (2006): 325–337.

10. Bottorff JL, Ratner PA, Johnson JL, Lovato CY, Joab SA. "Communicating cancer risk information: the challenges of uncertainty." *Patient Education and Counseling* 33(1) (1998): 67–81.

11. Dekkers W, Rikkert MO. "What is a genetic cause? The example of Alzheimer's disease." *Medicine, Health Care and Philosophy* 9(3) (2006): 273–284.

12. Smith KC. "A disease by any other name: musings on the concept of a genetic disease." *Medicine, Health Care and Philosophy* 4(1) 2001: 19–30.

13. Popper KR. *The Logic of Scientific Discovery.* London: Routledge, 2002.

14. Evans-Pritchard EE. *Witchcraft, Oracles and Magic Among the Azande.* New York, NY: Oxford University Press, 1976.

15. Farmer P. *AIDS and Accusation: Haiti and the Geography of Blame (Comparative Studies of Health Systems and Medical Care).* Berkeley, CA: University of California Press, 1993.

16. Phelan JC, Bromet EJ, Link BG. "Psychiatric illness and family stigma." *Schizophrenia Bulletin* 24(1) (1998): 115–126.

17. Brown L, ed. *The New Shorter Oxford English Dictionary on Historical Principles (Vol. 1, A–M).* New York, NY: Oxford University Press, 1973.

18. Pritchard D, Smith M. "The psychology and philosophy of luck." *New Ideas in Psychology* 22(1) (2004): 1–28.

19. Nagel T, 1979. *Mortal Questions.* Cambridge: Cambridge University Press, 1979.

20. Weiner B. *An Attribution Theory of Achievement, Motivation and Emotion.* New York: Springer, 1986.

21. Langer EJ. "The illusion of control." *Journal of Personality and Social Psychology* 32(2) (1975): 311–328.

22. Strenski I. (Ed.) *Malinowski and the Work of Myth.* Princeton, NJ: Princeton University Press, 1992.

23. Lawson KL. "Perceptions of deservedness of social aid as a function of prenatal diagnostic testing." *Journal of Applied Social Psychology* 33(1) (2003): 76–90.

24. Dennett DC. *Elbow Room: The Varieties of Free Will Worth Wanting.* Cambridge, MA: The MIT Press, 1984.

25. Sivell S, Elwyn G, Gaff CL, et al. "How risk is perceived, constructed and interpreted by clients in clinical genetics, and the effects on decision-making: systematic review." *Journal of Genetic Counseling* 17(1) (2008): 30–63.

26. Senior V, Marteau TM, Peters TJ. "Will genetic testing for predisposition for disease result in fatalism? A qualitative study of parents responses to neonatal screening for familial hypercholesterolaemia." *Society Science & Medicine* 48(12) (1999): 1857–1860.

27. Santos S. "The diversity of everyday ideas about inherited disorders." *Public Understanding of Science* 15(3) (2006): 259–275.

28. Gifford SM. "The meanings of lumps: a case study of the ambiguities of risk." In Janes C, Stall R, Gifford SM, eds. *Anthropology and Epidemiology: Interdisciplinary Approach to the Study of Health and Disease (Culture, Illness and Healing).* Boston: Reidel, 1986.

29. Floyd DL, Prentice-Dunn S, Rogers RW. "A meta-analysis of research on protection motivation theory." *Journal of Applied Social Psychology* 30(2) (2000): 407–429.

30. Parsons T. *The Social System.* London: Routledge and Kegan Paul, 1951.

CHAPTER 5

1. Klitzman R. *Being Positive: The Lives of Men and Women With HIV*. Chicago, IL: Ivan R. Dee, 1997.
2. Kleinman A. *The Illness Narratives: Suffering, Healing, & the Human Condition*. New York: Basic Books, 1988.
3. Shiloh S. "Illness representations, self-regulation, and genetic counseling: A theoretical review." *Journal of Genetic Counseling* 15(5) (2006): 325–337.
4. Walter FM, Emery J. "'Coming down the line'–patients' understanding of their family history of common chronic disease." *Annals of Family Medicine* 3(5) (2005): 405–414.
5. Riessman CK. "Performing identities in illness narrative: masculinity and multiple sclerosis." *Qualitative Research* 3(1) (1988): 5–33.
6. Mathieson C, Stam H. "Renegotiating identity: cancer narratives." *Sociology of Health and Illness* 17(3) (1995): 283–306.
7. Adams S, Pill R, Jone A. "Medication, chronic illness and identity: the perspective of people with asthma." *Social Science & Medicine* 45(2) (1997): 198–201.
8. Scharloo M, Kaptein AA, Weinman J, et al. "Illness perceptions, coping and functioning in patients with rheumatoid arthritis, chronic obstructive pulmonary disease and psoriasis." *Journal of Psychosomatic Research* 44(5) (1998): 573–585.
9. Bradley EJ, Calvert E, Pitts MK, Redman CWE. "Illness identity and the self-regulatory model in recovery from early stage gynaecological cancer." *Journal of Health Psychology* 6(5) (2001): 511–521.
10. Petrie KJ, Weinman J, Sharpe N, Buckley J. "Role of patients' view of their illness in predicting return to work and functioning after myocardial infarction: longitudinal study." *British Medical Journal* 312(7040) (1996): 1191–1194.
11. Kelly M. "Self, identity and radical surgery." *Sociology of Health and Illness* 14(3) (1992): 390–415.
12. McConkie-Rosell A, Spiridgliozzi G, Melvin E, Dawson DV, Lachiewicz AM. "Living with genetic risk: effect on adolescent self-concept." *American Journal of Medical Genetics Part C* 148C(1) (2008): 56–69.
13. Zeiler K. "Who am I? When do 'I' become another? An analytic exploration of identities, sameness and difference, genes and genomes." *Health Care Analysis* 15(1) (2007): 25–32.
14. Armstrong D, Michie S, Marteau T. "Revealed identity: a study of the process of genetic counseling." *Social Science & Medicine* 47(11) (1998): 1653–1658.
15. Juengst ET. "FACE facts: why human genetics will always provoke bioethics." *Journal of Law, Medicine & Ethics* 32(2) (2004): 267–275.
16. Elliott C, Brodwin P. "Identity and genetic ancestry tracing." *British Medical Journal* 325(7378) (2002): 1469–1471.
17. Parsons T. *The Social System*. London: Routledge and Kegan Paul, 1951.

CHAPTER 6

1. Emery J, Watson E, Rose P, Andermann A. "A systematic review of the literature exploring the role of primary care in genetic services." *Family Practice* 16(4) (1999): 426–445.

2. Walter FM, Emery J, Braithwaite D, Marteau TM. "Lay understanding of familial risk of common chronic diseases: a systematic review and synthesis of qualitative research." *Annals of Family Medicine* 2(6) (2004): 583–593.

3. Kessler L, Collier A, Hughes Halbert C. "Knowledge about genetics among African-Americans." *Journal of Genetic Counseling* 16(2) (2007): 191–200.

4. DeVries H, Mesters I, van de Steeg H, Honing C. "The general public's information needs and perceptions regarding hereditary cancer: an application of the integrated change model." *Patient Education and Counseling* 56(2) (2005): 154–165.

5. Lanie AD, Jayaratne TE, Sheldon JP, et al. "Exploring the public understanding of basic genetic concepts." *Journal of Genetic Counseling* 13(4) (2004): 305–320.

6. Shaw A, Hurst JA. "'What is this genetics, anyway?' Understandings of genetics, illness causality and inheritance among British Pakistani users of genetic services." *Journal of Genetic Counseling* 17(4) (2008): 373–383.

7. Condit CM, Dubriwny T, Lynch J, Parrott R. "Lay people's understanding of and preference against the word 'mutation.'" *American Journal of Medical Genetics* 130A(3) (2004): 245–250.

8. Shaw A, Hurst JA. "'What is this genetics, anyway?' Understandings of genetics, illness causality and inheritance among British Pakistani users of genetic services." *Journal of Genetic Counseling* 17(4) (2008): 373–383.

9. Emslie C, Hunt K, Watt G. "A chip off the old block? Lay understandings of inheritance among men and women in mid-life." *Public Understanding of Science* 12(1) (2003): 47–65.

10. Sivell S, Elwyn G, Gaff CL, et al. "How risk is perceived, constructed and interpreted by clients in clinical genetics, and the effects on decision-making: systematic review." *Journal of Genetic Counseling* 17(1) (2008): 30–63.

11. D'Agincourt-Canning L. "The effect of experiential knowledge on construction of risk perception in hereditary breast/ovarian cancer." *Journal of Genetic Counseling* 14(1) (2005): 55–69.

12. Appelbaum PS, Roth LH, Lidz C. "The therapeutic misconception: informed consent in psychiatric research." *International Journal of Law & Psychiatry* 5(3-4) (1982): 319–329.

13. "BRCA1 and BRCA2: Cancer risk and genetic testing." National Cancer Institute (2009) http://www.cancer.gov/cancertopics/factsheet/Risk/BRCA. Accessed May 27, 2010.

14. Whittemore AS, Gong G, John EM, et al. "Prevalence of *BRCA1* mutation carriers among U.S. Non-Hispanic Whites." *Cancer Epidemiology, Biomarkers & Prevention* 13(12) (2004): 2078–2083.

15. Walter FM, Emery J. "'Coming down the line'—Patients' understanding of their family history of common chronic disease." *Annals of Family Medicine* 3(5) (2005): 405–414.

16. Shiloh S. "Illness representations, self-regulation, and genetic counseling: a theoretical review." *Journal of Genetitc Counseling* 15(5) (2006): 325–337.

17. Etchegary H, Perrier C. "Information processing in the context of genetic risk: implications for genetic-risk communication." *Journal of Genetic Counseling* 16(4) (2007): 419–432.

18. Berkenstadt M, Shiloh S, Barkai G, Katznelson M, Goldman B. "Perceived personal control (PPC): A new concept in measuring outcome of genetic counseling." *American Journal of Medical Genetics* 82(1) (1999): 53–59.
19. Tversky A, Kahneman D. "The framing of decisions and the psychology of choice." *Science* 211(4481) (1981): 453–458.
20. Tversky A, Kahneman D. "Judgment under uncertainty: Heuristics and biases." *Science* 185(4157) (1974): 1124–1131.
21. Almqvist EW, Brinkman RR, Wiggins S, Hayden MR. "Canadian collaborative study of predictive testing. Psychological consequences and predictors of adverse events in the first 5 years after predictive testing for Huntington's disease." *Clinical Genetics* 64(4) (2003): 300–309.

CHAPTER 7

1. Fox R, Swazey J. *Spare Parts: Organ Replacement in American Society*. New York: Oxford University Press, 1992.
2. "Genetic/familial high-risk assessment: breast and ovarian." NCCN Guidelines. National Comprehensive Cancer Network. 2010. http://www.nccn.org. Accessed May 27, 2010.
3. Bermajo-Perez MJ, Marquez-Calderon S, Llanos-Mendez A. "Effectiveness of preventive interventions in *BRCA1/2* gene mutation carriers: a systematic review." *International Journal of Cancer* 121(2) (2007): 225–231.
4. Anderson K, Jacobson JS, Heitjan DF, et al. "Cost-effectiveness of preventive strategies for women with *BRCA1* or *BRCA 2* mutation." *Annals of Internal Medicine* 144(6) (2006): 397–406.
5. Lerman C, Hughes C, Croyle RT, et al. "Prophylactic surgery decisions and surveillance practices one year following *BRCA 1/2* testing." *Preventive Medicine* 31(1) (2000): 75–80.
6. Schwartz MD, Kaufman E, Peshkin, BN, et al. 2003. "Bilateral prophylactic oophorectomy and ovarian cancer screening following *BRCA1/BRCA2* mutation testing." *Journal of Clinical Oncology* 21(21) (2003): 4034–4041.
7. Meijers-Heijboer EJ, Verhoog LC, Brekelmans CTM, et al. "Presymptomatic DNA testing and prophylactic surgery in families with a *BRCA 1* or *BRCA 2* mutation." *The Lancet* 355(9220) (2000): 2015–2020.
8. Metcalfe KA, Lubinkski J, Ghadirian P, et al. "Predictors of contralateral prophylactic mastectomy in women with *BRCA 1* or *BRCA 2* mutation: the hereditary breast cancer clinical study group." *Journal of Clinical Oncology* 26(7) (2008): 1093–1097.
9. Metcalfe KA, Ghadirian P, Rosen B, et al. "Variation in rates of uptake of preventive options by Canadian women carrying the *BRCA 1* or *BRCA 2* genetic mutation." *Open Medicine* 1(2) (2007): 92–98.
10. Metcalfe KA, Birenbaum-Carmeli D, Lubinski J, et al. and the Hereditary Breast Cancer Clinical Study Group. "International variation in rates of uptake of preventive options in *BRCA 1* and *BRCA 2* mutation carriers." *International Journal of Cancer* 122(9) (2008): 2017–2022.
11. Bradbury AR, Ibe CN, Dignam JJ, et al. "Uptake and timing of bilateral prophylactic salpingo-oophorectomy among *BRCA 1* and *BRCA 2* mutation carriers." *Genetics in Medicine* 10(3) (2008): 161–166.

12. Kram V, Peretz T, Sagi M. 2006. "Acceptance of preventive surgeries by Israeli women who had undergone BRCA testing." *Familial Cancer* 5(4) (2006): 327–335.

13. Miller SM, Roussi P, Daly MB, et al. "Enhanced counseling for women undergoing BRCA 1/2 testing: impact on subsequent decision making about risk reduction behaviors." *Health Education and Behavior* 32(5) (2005): 654–667.

14. Van Dijk S, Otten W, Zoeteweij MW, et al. "Genetic counseling and the intention to undergo prophylactic mastectomy: effects of a breast cancer risk assessment." *British Journal of Cancer* 88(11) (2003): 1675–1681.

15. Madalinska JB, van Beurden M, Bleiker EMA, et al. "Predictors of prophylactic bilateral salpingo-oophorectomy compared with gynecologic screening use in BRCA 1/2 mutation carriers." *Journal of Clinical Oncology* 25(3) (2007): 301–307.

16. Antill Y, Reynolds J, Young M, et al. "Risk-reducing surgery in women with familial susceptibility for breast and/or ovarian cancer." *European Journal of Cancer* 42(5) (2006): 621–628.

17. Hallowell N, Jacobs I, Richards M, Mackay J, Gore M. "Surveillance or surgery? A description of the factors that influence high risk premenopausal women's decisions about prophylactic oophorectomy." *Journal of Medical Genetics* 38(10) (2001): 683–726.

18. Tiller K, Meiser B, Butow P, et al. "Psychological impact of prophylactic oophorectomy in women at increased risk of developing ovarian cancer: a prospective study." *Gynecologic Oncology* 86(2) (2002): 212–219.

CHAPTER 8

1. Sermon K, De Rijcke M, Lissens W, et al. "Preimplantation genetic diagnosis for Huntington's disease with exclusion testing." *European Journal of Human Genetics* 10(10) (2002): 591–598.

2. Simpson SA, Harper PS, United Kingdom Huntington's Disease Prediction Consortium. "Prenatal testing for Huntington's disease: experience within the UK 1994–1998." *Journal of Medical Genetics* 38(5) (2001): 333–335.

3. Stern HJ, Harton GL, Sisson ME, et al. "Non-disclosing preimplantation genetic diagnosis for Huntington disease." *Prenatal Diagnosis* 22(6) (2002): 503–507.

4. Lavery SA, Aurell R, Turner C, et al. "Preimplantation genetic diagnosis: patients' experiences and attitudes." *Human Reproduction* 17(9) (2002): 2464–2467.

5. Elger B, Harding T. "Huntington's disease: do future physicians and lawyers think eugenically?" *Clinical Genetics* 64(4) (2003): 327–338.

6. Alonso Vilatela ME, Ochoa Morales A, Garcia de la Cadena C, Ruiz Lopez I, Martinez Aranda C, Villa A. "Predictive and prenatal diagnosis of Huntington's disease: attitudes of Mexican neurologists, psychiatrists, and psychologists. *Archives of Medical Research* 30(4) (1999): 320–324.

7. Drake H, Reid M, Marteau T. "Attitudes towards termination for fetal abnormality: comparisons in three European countries." *Clinical Genetics* 49(3) (1996): 134–140.

8. Hayden M. "Predictive testing for Huntington's disease: the calm after the storm." *The Lancet* 356(9246) (2000): 1944–1945.

9. Richards FH, Rea G. "Reproductive decision making before and after predictive testing for Huntington's disease: an Australian perspective." *Clinical Genetics* 67(5) (2005): 404–411.

10. Creighton S, Almqvist EW, MacGregor D, et al. "Predictive, pre-natal and diagnostic genetic testing for Huntington's disease: the experience in Canada from 1987 to 2000." *Clinical Genetics* 63(6) (2003): 462–475.

11. Lesca G, Goizet C, Dürr A. "Predictive testing in the context of pregnancy: experience in Huntington's disease and autosomal dominant cerebellar ataxia." *Journal of Medical Genetics* 39(7) (2002): 522–525.

12. Maat-Kievit A, Vegter-van der Vlis M, Zoeteweij M, et al. "Experience in prenatal testing for Huntington's disease in The Netherlands: procedures, results and guidelines (1987–1997)." *Prenatal Diagnosis* 19(5) (1999): 450–457.

13. Taylor CA, Myers RH. "Long-term impact of Huntington disease linkage testing." *American Journal of Medical Genetics* 70(4) (1997): 365–370.

14. Goizet C, Lesca G, Durr A. "Presymptomatic testing in Huntington's disease and autosomal dominant cerebellar ataxias." *Neurology* 59(9) (2002): 1330–1336.

15. Evers-Kiebooms G, Nys K, Harper P, et al. "Predictive DNA-testing for Huntington's disease and reproductive decision making: a European collaborative study." *European Journal of Human Genetics* 10(3) (2002): 167–176.

16. Adam S, Wiggins S, Whyte P, et al. "Five year study of prenatal testing for Huntington's disease: demand, attitudes, and psychological assessment." *Journal of Medical Genetics* 30(7) (1993): 549–556.

17. Henn W. "Consumerism in prenatal diagnosis: A challenge for ethical guidelines." *Journal of Medical Ethics* 26(6) (2000): 444–446.

18. Robertson JA. "Extending preimplantation genetic diagnosis: the ethical debate: Ethical issues in the new uses of preimplantation genetic diagnosis." *Human Reproduction* 18(3) (2003): 465–471.

19. Braude PR, De Wert GM, Evers-Kiebooms G, Pettigrew RA, Geraedts JP. "Non-disclosure preimplantation genetic diagnosis for Huntington's disease: practical and ethical dilemmas." *Prenatal Diagnosis* 18(13) (1998): 1422–1426.

20. Downing, C. "Negotiating responsibility: Case studies of reproductive decision-making and prenatal genetic testing in families facing Huntington disease." *Journal of Genetic Counseling* 14(3) (2005): 219–234.

21. Houlihan GD. "The evaluation of the 'stages of change' model for use in counselling client's undergoing predictive testing for Huntington's disease." *Journal of Advanced Nursing* 29(5) (1999): 1137–1143.

22. Taylor SD. "Predictive genetic test decisions for Huntington's disease: elucidating the test/no-test dichotomy." *Journal of Health Psychology* 10(4) (2005): 597–612.

23. Coleman PK, Reardon DC, Strahan T, and Cougle JR. "The psychology of abortion: a review and suggestions for future research." *Psychology and Health* 20(2) (2005): 237–271.

24. Hundert, EM. "A model for ethical problem solving in medicine, with practical applications." *American Journal of Psychiatry* 144(7) (1987): 839–846.

25. Robertson JA. "Ethics and the future of preimplantation genetic diagnosis." Reproductive BioMedicine Online., 2005. 10, Supp 1: 97–101.

26. Healy M. "Embryo diagnosis stirs controversy." *Los Angeles Times*, July 29, 2003.

27. Bankole A, Sing S, Haas T. "Reasons why women have induced abortions: Evidence from 27 countries." *International Family Planning Perspectives* 24(3) (1998): 117–152.

28. Sihvo S, Bajos N, Ducot B, Kaminski M, the Cocon Group. "Women's life cycle and abortion decision in unintended pregnancies." *Journal of Epidemiology & Community Health* 57(8) (2003): 601–605.

29. Thomassen R, Tibben A, Niermeijer MF, vand der Does E, van de Kamp JJP, Verhage F. "Attitudes of Dutch general practitioners towards presymptomatic DNA-testing for Huntington disease." *Clinical Genetics* 43(2) (1993): 63–68.

30. Richards F, Williams K. "Impact on couple relationships of predictive testing for Huntington Disease: a longitudinal study." *American Journal of Medical Genetics* 126A (2004): 161–169.

31. Uniform Adoption Act. 1994. http://www.law.upenn.edu/bll/ulc/fnact99/1990s/uaa94.htm. Accessed March 27, 2006.

CHAPTER 9

1. Greenhouse S. "Ex-Worker says her firing was based on genetic test." *New York Times*, April 30, 2010.

2. Nowlan W. "A rational view of insurance and genetic discrimination." *Science* 297(5579) (2002): 195–196.

3. Nowlan W. "A scarlet letter or a red herring?" *Nature* 241(6921) (2003): 313.

4. Wertz D. "Genetic discrimination—an overblown fear?" *Nature Reviews Genetics* 3(7) (2002): 496.

5. Otlowski M. "Exploring the concept of genetic discrimination." *Journal of Bioethical Inquiry* 2(3) (2005): 165–176.

6. Otlowski MF, Taylor SD, Barlow-Stewart KK. "Genetic discrimination: too few data." *European Journal of Human Genetics* 11(1) (2003): 1–2.

7. Treloar S, Taylor S, Otlowski M, Barlow-Stewart K, Stranger M, Chenoweth K. "Methodological considerations in the study of genetic discrimination: a review." *Community Genetics* 7(4) (2004): 161–168.

8. Taylor S, Treloar S, Barlow-Stewart K, Otlowski M, Stranger M. "Investigating genetic discrimination in Australia: perceptions and experiences of clinical genetics service clients regarding coercion to test, insurance and employment." *Australian Journal of Emerging Technologies and Society* 5(2) (2007): 63–83.

9. Taylor S, Treloar S, Barlow-Stewart K, Stranger M, Otlowski M. "Investigating genetic discrimination in Australia: a large-scale survey of clinical genetics clients." *Clinical Genetics* 74(1) (2008): 20–30.

10. Rawls J. *A Theory of Justice.* Cambridge, MA: Harvard University Press, 1971.

CHAPTER 10

1. Klitzman R. *When Doctors Become Patients.* New York: Oxford University Press, 2008.

CHAPTER 11

1. Plass A, Koch U. "Participation of oncological outpatients in psychosocial support." *Psycho-Oncology* 10(6) (2001): 511–520.

2. Ussher J, Kirsten L, Butow P, Sandoval M. "What do cancer support groups provide which other supportive relationships do not? The experience of peer support groups for people with cancer." *Social Science & Medicine* 62(10) (2006): 2565–2576.

3. Docherty A. "Experience, functions and benefits of a cancer support group." *Patient Education and Counseling* 55(1) (2004): 87–93.

4. Taylor SE, Falke RL, Shoptaw SJ, Lichtman RR. "Social support, support groups, and the cancer patient." *Journal of Consulting and Clinical Psychology* 54(5) (1986): 608–615.

5. Grande GE, Myers LB, Sutton SR. "How do patients who participate in cancer support groups differ from those who do not?" *Psycho-Oncology* 15(4) (2006): 321–334.

6. Shaw BR, Hawkins R, Arora N, McTavish F, Pingree S, Gustafson DH. "An exploratory study of predictors of participation in a computer support group for women with breast cancer." *CIN: Computers, Informatics, Nursing* 24(1) (2006): 18–27.

7. Winzelberg AJ, Classen C, Alpers GW, et al. "Evaluation of an internet support group for women with primary breast cancer." *Cancer* 97(5) (2003): 1164–1173.

8. Classen C, Butler LD, Koopman C, et al. "Support-expressive group therapy and distress in patients with metastatic breast cancer." *Archives of General Psychiatry* 58(5) (2001): 494–501.

9. Finfgeld DL. "Therapeutic groups online: the good, the bad, and the unknown." *Issues in Mental Health Nursing* 21(3) (2000): 241–255.

10. Coulson NS, Buchanan H, Aubeeluck A. "Social support in cyberspace: a content analysis of communication within a Huntington's disease online support group." *Patient Education and Counseling* 68(2) (2007): 173–178.

11. Van Uden-Kraan CF, Drossaert CH, Taal E, Shaw BR, Seydel ER, van de Laar MAFJ. "Empowering processes and outcomes of participation in online support groups for patients with breast cancer, arthritis, or fibromyalgia." *Qualitative Health Research* 18(3) (2008): 405–417.

12. Radin P. "'To me, it's my life': medical communication, trust, and activism in cyberspace." *Social Science & Medicine* 62(3) (2006): 591–601.

13. Barker KK. "Electronic support groups, patient-consumers, and medicalization: the case of contested illness." *Journal of Health and Social Behavior* 49(1) (2008): 20–36.

14. Appelbaum PS, Roth LH, Lidz C. "The therapeutic misconception: informed consent in psychiatric research." *International Journal of Law & Psychiatry* 5(3–4) (1982): 319–329.

CHAPTER 13

1. McCabe LL, McCabe ERB. *DNA: Promise and Peril.* Berkeley, CA: University of California Press, 2008.

2. Marteau T, Richards M. (eds.) *The Troubled Helix: Social and Psychological Implications of the New Human Genetics.* Cambridge, England: Cambridge University Press, 1999.

3. Klitzman R, Daya S. "Challenges and changes in spirituality among doctors who become patients." *Social Science & Medicine* 61(11) (2005): 2396–2406.

Genetic Testing 101

Based on his experiments with pea plants, Gregor Mendel, a monk living in the Austro-Hungarian Empire, formulated basic tenets of genetics in 1865. He found that when he crossed a white-flowered and a purpled-flowered plant, the offspring were not all purplish white, or 50% purple and 50% white. Rather, 75% of the offspring were purple, and only 25% were white. Yet when he cross-pollinated the purple plants, 25% of their progeny were white. Thus, he hypothesized that certain traits were controlled by "factors" (later termed "genes"), of which offspring inherited one each from each parent. In addition, genes for traits such as flower color could be dominant or recessive.

Since then, scientists have discovered that in humans and other species, this so-called "classical" Mendelian pattern applies to certain diseases and traits, but not most. Common diseases such as high blood pressure and diabetes may be influenced by multiple genes, as well as by the environment.

We now know that each person has 46 chromosomes—23 from each parent—that consist of deoxyribonucleic acid (DNA). DNA is a double stranded molecule, each strand of which contains a sequence of four different amino acids—adenine, cytosine, thymine, and guanine (abbreviated A, C, T, G). Sequences of these "letters" A C T G form "genes," each of which constitutes the cellular instructions for a particular function (e.g., making a particular protein). Our chromosomes contain two copies of each of the three billion letters that make us. These letters form approximately 25,000 genes.

Each cell in our body contains these 46 chromosomes. The DNA sequences on the chromosomes in each of us differ from the sequences in anyone else's body by 0.1%. The only exception is if one is an identical twin (or if one were to have a clone).

Occasionally, as a single fertilized egg or embryo keeps dividing to become a multi-billion cellular mass, a mistake—or mutation—gets made. If the mutation occurs in a cell that becomes an egg or sperm, this mutation could get passed on to our children. Usually, a single such error has no consequences. But sometimes, such an error can cause major problems. A single broken link in the DNA chain can make a protein misfold and dysfunction. Similarly, in retyping text, an occasional error does not ordinarily change the overall meaning. But at times, a single error could lead to problems. King Louis XIV's diction *L'etat c'est moi* ("*I* am the state") could accidentally become *L'etat c'est toi* ("*You* are the state"), completely altering the implications. *War and Peace* could end up being titled *Car and Peace*, or *Bar and Peace*. Similarly, the play *Wit* concerned ambiguity over whether the poet John Donne meant to use a comma or a semicolon in the last line of one of his Holy Sonnets—the meaning of his poem is different in each instance. (A typo could also change the title of this play to *Bit*, *Hit*, or *Win*).

In the case of HD, *BRCA*, and Alpha, these mutations can be deadly. Yet these three diseases differ in certain regards. HD follows a so-called Mendelian pattern—one gene is dominant, and is solely responsible for the disease. The mutation actually consists of a few accidental added repeats of the sequence CAG on the gene that makes the Huntington protein. A person who has this error on this gene from either parent will develop this deadly disease. Each child then has a 50% chance of inheriting this defective chromosome (with the mutation), rather than the other, normal chromosome that the ill parent has (and received from his or her healthy parent).

In contrast, breast cancer appears not to follow a classic Mendelian pattern. Rather, multiple factors may be involved. Two mutations have been identified—named *BRCA 1* and *BRCA 2*—that predispose to the disease. The presence of one of these two mutations gives a person a 40%–60% chance of developing the disorder. Yet only approximately 10% of breast cancer is due to one of these two mutations.

In the case of Alpha, a person can inherit the mutation from only one parent (in which case one is a carrier, and may develop some mild symptoms), or from both parents (in which case, one develops a more severe form of the illness).

Sample Questions from Semi-Structured Interviews

When did you first find out you were at risk for a genetic disorder, and how did you respond? What are your understandings of what it means to be at risk for a genetic disorder?

Do you feel genetic information is different than other kinds of health information, and if so, how and why?

Do you feel you are "disabled," or "sick," or not?

Do you see genetic information as part of your identity, and if so, how?

Has your genetic risk affected you in any way, and if so, how?

PRIVACY AND DISCLOSURE DECISIONS

What do you feel comfortable or uncomfortable having others know about you, and why, concerning genetic or other medical information?

How concerned are you about threats to privacy of genetic information? Of other information?

Who have you decided to tell or not to tell about your genetic risk?

Have you told family members (spouse/significant other, sisters, brothers, parents, children, other extended family members, in-laws), friends, coworkers, employers, neighbors, healthcare professionals (primary physician, other physicians in different contexts), researchers, insurers (health insurers, life insurers, disability insurers), and others? How do you make these decisions?

What have you disclosed, and when and why?

Have you told your offspring, and if so, when?

Have you told healthcare professionals or institutions? Why or why not?

Have you ever had to hide the fact that you are at risk of, or have a genetic or other disorder?

Have other family members ever told *you* that you may be at risk of a genetic disorder? If so, what was said and when?

Have your views about whom to tell changed over time, and if so, how?

What is it like to face these decisions?

DISCRIMINATION

Have you ever experienced limitations on privacy?

Have you ever encountered stigma or discrimination as a result of a diagnosis? How do you view these?

Have you ever not disclosed potentially relevant information to physicians, and if so, what kind of information, when, and why?

Have physicians ever discussed with you limitations on confidentiality or risks of genetic discrimination, and if so, what was said?

How do you feel about healthcare professionals and institutions having access to private aspects of yourself?

Are there differences in doctors having access to personal information, medical history, or laboratory tests (including DNA), and if so, how?

Have you ever requested or considered requesting that certain information not be included in your record, or ever delayed or avoided treatment because of privacy concerns? How have you made these decisions?

Have privacy concerns affected your use of the Internet in any way, and if so, how?

Have concerns about privacy of genetic information affected you in other ways, and if so, how?

Has your health information ever "leaked out" or led to discrimination, and if so, how?

Do you feel employers have access to health information, or would under new laws?

Do you feel your employer has ever used health information in work decisions (e.g., hiring or promotions) with employees?

Do you know of others who have faced discrimination or stigma as a result of genetic or other health information? What experiences have these others had?

Have you ever disclosed that you are at risk of or have a genetic or other disorder to individuals who then in turn communicated that information to others?

HEALTH BEHAVIORS, TESTING, AND TREATMENT

Have any family members considered or sought testing? How did they make their decisions? What factors were involved? Have these experiences affected your views in any way?

How have you made decisions concerning testing?

Have you made any decisions about treatment of a genetic condition? If so, what?

VIEWS OF TRADEOFFS AND POLICY ISSUES

How do you weigh privacy against other concerns or benefits in choosing to have tests or treatment?

How do you balance individual rights to privacy with other concerns?

Do you feel you would be more likely to take tests if better treatment were available? How effective would the treatment have to be?

Do you feel third parties have a right to some types of information, and if so, what or when? What if you would risk losing health insurance coverage or other benefits if you did not grant permission?

What do you feel should be done when it may not be possible to request such consent (e.g., on records collected in the past)?

Do you feel it should ever be permissible to share such information when authorization cannot be obtained?

Would you be willing to pay additional costs to protect privacy? Why or why not?

What factors would you take into account in deciding whether to consent or not to your genetic information being shared?

What do you think doctors should do if patients with a genetic disorder do not inform family members who may be at risk? Do you think the physician has a "duty to warn" family members?

Do you feel loss of privacy is inevitable? Have you felt coerced to accept such limitations?

How do you feel such decisions concerning privacy safeguards should be made?

Do you have any other thoughts about these issues?

Additional Details Concerning Methods

Chapter 1 presents a brief overview of the methods. More fully, I had the interviews transcribed, and analyzed them during the period I was conducting them. I conducted interviews until I reached "saturation"—that is, until the major and minor themes became clear.

I tried to recruit additional African Americans and Latinos, but to do so proved difficult in part because Caucasians undergo genetic testing far more than these other groups do. These different rates of testing result from various reasons including finances and wariness, given the history of eugenics in the United States. Nonetheless, several African Americans and Latinos agreed to participate.

I analyzed the interviews, informed by grounded theory.[1] Once the full set of interviews was conducted, subsequent analyses were conducted in two additional phases, by myself and research assistants who had social science training. We independently examined a subset of interviews to assess factors that shaped participants' experiences, identifying categories of recurrent themes and issues to which we subsequently gave codes. We assessed similarities and differences between participants, examining categories that emerged, ranges of variation within categories, and variables that may be involved. We thus developed a coding manual and examined areas of disagreement until reaching consensus. We discussed new themes that did not fit into the original coding framework, and then modified the manual when appropriate. In phase two of the analysis, we refined and merged subdivided categories into secondary or sub-codes, when suggested by associations, or overlap in the data. We then used these codes and sub-codes in analyzing of all of the interviews. To ensure reliability, two coders analyzed all interviews. We triangulated methods, referring to anecdotal reports and prior literature.

The Columbia University Department of Psychiatry Institutional Review Board approved the study.

---

1. Strauss, A, and Corbin, J. *Basics of Qualitative Research—Techniques and Procedures for Developing Grounded Theory.* Thousand Oaks, CA: Sage Publications, 1990.

_____ DATE